Artificial Intelligence for Innovative Healthcare Informatics

Shabir Ahmad Parah • Mamoon Rashid
Vijayakumar Varadarajan
Editors

Artificial Intelligence for Innovative Healthcare Informatics

Springer

Editors
Shabir Ahmad Parah
PG Department of Electronics and
Instrumentation Technology
University of Kashmir
Srinagar, India

Mamoon Rashid
Department of Computer Engineering
Faculty of Science and Technology
Vishwakarma University
Pune, India

Vijayakumar Varadarajan
University of New South Wales
Sydney, NSW, Australia

ISBN 978-3-030-96568-6 ISBN 978-3-030-96569-3 (eBook)
https://doi.org/10.1007/978-3-030-96569-3

This Springer imprint is published by the registered company Springer Nature Switzerland AG
The registered company address is: Gewerbestrasse 11, 6330 Cham, Switzerland

Contents

Part I
Medical Image Analysis Using Artificial Intelligence

Chapter 1
Use of Deep Learning in Biomedical Imaging

N. Shanu and R. S. Ganesh

Contents

1 Introduction

There is an ever-increasing demand for automated algorithms in biomedical image analysis. These algorithms are crucial for medical diagnosis, treatment initiation, and analysis of disease progression. Electronic transmission of medical images for automated diagnosis or expert opinion is becoming popular. This suggests the need for encryption of images applied in health care to improve the security and authentication of data [1–8]. There is a wide variety of imaging modalities that aid radiologists in visualizing a disease condition—X-rays, computed tomography (CT), ultrasound, and magnetic resonance imaging (MRI). X-rays are used in

N. Shanu (✉)
College of Engineering, Karunagapally, Kerala, India
e-mail: shanu@ceconline.edu

R. S. Ganesh
Noorul Islam Centre for Higher Education, Kumaracoil, Tamilnadu, India
e-mail: ganesh@niuniv.com

S. A. Parah et al. (eds.), *Artificial Intelligence for Innovative Healthcare Informatics*,
https://doi.org/10.1007/978-3-030-96569-3_1

radiography—contrast and normal, mammography, fluoroscopy, and arthrography. CT is an important modality for the abdomen, bladder, brain, chest, kidney, and cervix. Owing to the absence of ionizing radiation, ultrasounds are preferred for analysis of the gallbladder, spleen, breast, cranial, transrectal, abdominal, and transabdominal. Radiologists rely on MRI for neuroimaging, cardiovascular, liver, and brain. Functional MRI is used to study brain activities assessing changes in blood flow [9, 10]. In phase-contrast, an MRI signal is used to analyze blood flow velocity [11]. The challenging nature of medical image analysis is due to the similarity of tissues, intensity variations, shadowing, and noise. For example, in B-mode ultrasound, the appearance of jugular veins and common carotid artery are similar which makes delineation of carotid artery challenging. These challenges are common across different modalities [12].

Classification, segmentation, and registration are the fundamental operations in biomedical image analysis. Segmentation refers to algorithms for the delineation of an interesting area (tissue or lesion) from its background. Classification represents methods to detect abnormality in a scan and tagging it diseased or normal. Image registration is a process of aligning images to a single coordinate system having multiple applications. The original images are multi-modal (different modalities), multi-temporal (2D or 3D), or captured at different instances [13]. Traditional image analysis methods rely on handcrafted techniques to derive features to solve challenging problems. As the dimension of data increased, attempts were made for a data-driven approach. This led to the application of deep learning algorithms to solve such challenges. At first, the scientific community enjoyed the application of CNN for lung nodule detection [14]. However, parameter training was challenging and [15] developed the backpropagation algorithm for handwritten character recognition. Later, deeper architectures like AlexNet appeared in competitions and have now become the trend in computer vision challenges [16].

Prior information on modality and classification criterion—intensity, edge, color, or shape, often favours segmentation. These pixel-based approaches later gave way to supervised methods. Depending on the prior information applied the supervised methods are classified as model-based—warping, elasticity function, and atlas-based—deformable functions. These methods applied handcrafted feature engineering and are a rule-based approach. Programs (a set of rules) and images are applied to the system, and based on the underlying rule an output (segmented tissue) is produced. However, machine learning (ML) algorithms are data-driven. The input image and target are applied to a system—tracking down the underlying relation between them (learning). *Learning* refers to a transformation from the input data to the target with minimum error. Supervised, unsupervised, self-supervised, and reinforcement learning are four classes of machine learning. Supervised involves learning methods to map input data to the target. Classification, segmentation, and regression are examples of supervised learning. Methods such as dimensionality reduction and clustering, that avoid a target for learning implies unsupervised learning. Autoencoders implement self-supervised learning, where the output generated utilizes the input data as targets for training. In reinforcement learning, an agent accumulates observations and takes actions to maximize the reward for correct learning. Based on the number of layers networks are either *shallow* or *deep*. A shallow network refers to models with comparatively fewer layers, whereas deep networks have more layers between the input layer and output layer.

Deep Learning (DL) is a subset of ML where each layer hierarchically learns the relation between input data and the targeted output. Every layer is composed of neural networks that are characterized by the weights of the layers—weights are parameters of the layer. These weights are found by showing instances of data and desired target to the network. In this context, learning is redefined as finding suitable layer weights that transform input data to the target. To assess the performance of the model a loss function is computed; loss function is the variation of model output from the target output. An optimizer, often based on a backpropagation algorithm, is then executed to update weights and reduce the loss function. It is a common viewpoint that two or more layers of neural networks combined with non-linear activation functions are capable of approximating any function (relation) between input data and target. Further, while reducing the number of network parameters, even training with small dataset yields good results. This is implemented in Convolutional Neural Networks (CNNs), which is the most useful model in computer vision and biomedical image analysis. CNN-based models are applied for tissue characterization [17], lung pattern classification [18], thyroid nodule detection [19], breast cancer diagnosis/detection [20, 21] and Alzheimer classification [22]. Several clinical applications applying CNN are summarized in [23].

Researchers have offered varieties of DL algorithms that are successful in challenging biomedical analysis. There are several layers in a DL architecture and training requires large labeled datasets—a scarce resource in medical imaging. Also, DL algorithms are computationally intense and are affected by underfitting—model is not able to obtain sufficiently low training error; overfitting—the gap between testing error and training error is large; and convergence issues [24]. To reduce the computational complexity, often a few initial pre-trained layers are applied. Further, layers are added on top of the pre-trained layers and fine-tuning of the entire network is performed. Prevalent pre-trained networks applied are Xception [25, 26], ResNet, VGG, and Inception [27]. One way to reduce overfitting is to provide additional training data to the model. Another practical method is to diminish the model size. Such a model has reduced the number of parameters to be learned; *dropout* is one such method. Yet another method to fight to overfit is *weight regularization*—forcing weights to take smaller values. *L1 regularization* and *L2 regularization* are two popular weight regularization methods. In this method, randomly selected output features are set to zero during training.

There is hardly any single algorithm that is suited for vessel segmentation in all modalities. Conventional methods for vessel segmentation depend on variations in intensity, morphology, curvature, centerline, and smoothness [28]. Vessels regularly inhibit nodule detection and the performance of automatic nodule detection algorithms significantly improves after vessel segmentation [29]. Further, vessel segmentation is crucial in the design of automated interstitial lung disease [30]. Guo et al. compared the performance of traditional and deep learning-based methods for vessel segmentation on lung CT [31]. They implemented a cascade of two networks for vessel segmentation. At first, a binary classifier was used to segregate vessels and nodules together from lung CT. Then, applying a multiclass classifier vessels are segmented from nodules. They studied that the mean Dice score (0.943 ± 0.013) improved and missed scans diminished in applying DL-based methods. Vessel parameters in retinal fundus images are an indicator of diabetic retinopathy [32], cardiovascular and renal disease [33]. Traditional vessel segmentation methods are challenging due to low image resolution [34], equipment variability, thin vasculature [35], and small dataset. CNN-based approaches [36], U-Net [37] and stacked autoencoders [38] presented accurate segmentation results.

Researchers have sounded the importance of automatic lesion detection in multiple sclerosis amidst challenges due to variation in shape, location, and texture of the lesion. Scientists applied CNN on a fusion of multiple modalities and obtained human-like performance [39]. Aslani et al. proposed architecture with three parts: ResNet, multi-modal feature fusion (MMFF), and multiscale feature up-sampling (MSFU) [40]. The information from different MRI modalities is down-sampled with ResNet50 architecture pre-trained on ImageNet. Representations from different modalities and resolutions are combined and up-sampled. Further, the team proposed a modified slice-based approach with two pathways, developed on the encoder/decoder CNN architecture, and achieved better results on the ISBI challenge dataset [41].

This chapter analyses important biomedical imaging modalities in Sect. 2. Stacked Auto-Encoder, Deep Belief Network, Deep Boltzmann Machine, CNN, Recurrent Neural Network, LSTM, and U-Net are studied in Sect. 3. Application of DL algorithms on biomedical images and its performance analysis are described in Sects. 4 and 5. Moreover, significant challenges in the application of DL algorithms are portrayed before the conclusion.

2 Imaging Modalities

2.1 X-Rays

As early as 1895, Wilhelm Röntgen created X-rays. In an X-ray tube, a current heat up the filament of the cathode and releases electrons which are accelerated towards the anode. Hitting the target material, these electrons interact with either the nucleus or the shell of the target. The electrons interacting with the nucleus are slowed down by the Coulomb effect of the proton and a photon equivalent of the loss in kinetic energy is released (Bremsstrahlung). Further, the electrons interacting with the shell releases characteristic radiations. Thus, when X-rays pass through matter when applied for imaging either absorption or scattering occurs. Scattering can be either coherent (Thomson effect) or non-coherent (Compton effect). The absorption coefficient of the material μ is unique and is mapped to grayscale to display the image. The absorption equation is represented in Eq. (1.1).

$$I = \int I_0(E) e^{\int \mu(z,E)dz} dE \quad (1.1)$$

The radiation intensity I is dependent on photon energy E and μ. Five basic densities are identified in an X-ray: air (pass-through), fat, fluid/soft tissue, bone, and metal (attenuated). Often, multiple views—orthogonal, are required for analysis. X-rays are applied for detecting fractures, abdominal emergencies, and chest imaging.

2.2 Computed Tomography (CT)

In an X-ray image, the ordering information of the objects is lost because of attenuation coefficients along the path overlap. Also, there is limited differentiation of different densities: water and soft tissue are identical. However, CT applies multiple slices to determine the volumetric information, and algorithms are employed for image reconstruction. Popular reconstruction algorithms are Filtered backpropagation (FBP), Algebraic reconstruction techniques (ART), Simultaneous Iterative Reconstruction (SIRT), or Simultaneous Algebraic Reconstruction Technique (SART). Hounsfield unit (HU) is a value used to measure density on CT scans. Water has 0 HU and air has −1000 HU are applied as reference values; tissues with higher HU appear brighter in the CT. Different gray levels that can be differentiated in a CT depend on the *window width*. *Window level* is the central number at a particular window width.

2.3 Magnetic Resonance Imaging (MRI)

MRI is based on electromagnetic effects of the nucleus; more significantly that of hydrogen because of the presence of water molecules in our body. The nucleus is always in continuous motion and has an associated magnetic moment and precision frequency. In tissue, there are several atoms and there is a superimposed magnetic moment. With the application of an external magnetic field, the superimposed magnetic moment aligns itself either parallel or anti-parallel to the field. Further, to excite the spinning electrons an external impulse in the form of radiofrequency is applied. Varying amplitude and time of excitation the direction of magnetic moment can be altered. As the system is restoring its equilibrium state a relaxation signal is released. This signal is detected and used for image reconstruction.

There are two effects with distinct relaxation times that superimpose in the relaxation signal. A spin-spin effect with relaxation time T_2 and a spin-lattice effect with relaxation time T_1. To obtain a high-quality relaxation signal spin-echo sequences with different radio frequency impulses are applied and if necessary, T_1 and T_2 relaxation signals are processed in between. Further, gradient fields are superimposed to the external magnetic field to obtain spatial alignment with the signal. Contrary to the methods in CT, mechanical rotation is not required in MRI as these gradient fields are generated using gradient coils and altered using current. MRI images are composed of multiple sequences of several 3D volumes and these are combined to a single volume before image processing is applied. Pre-processing techniques applied for transforming MRI slices in different planes into a composite image are referred to as image registration. Functional MRI (fMRI) is a method for analyzing brain activity by monitoring blood oxygen level-dependent signals. A summary of recent observations on the analysis of fMRI applying deep learning algorithms is presented in another study [42].

2.4 *Ultrasound*

Ultrasound is an imaging modality based on sound waves (2–20 MHz) and hence free from ionizing radiations. A transducer composed of a piezoelectric crystal that changes shape with electric impulse is used for analysis. At any interface, the sound wave is transmitted by fluids (anechoic, black), reflected by bone and air (hyperechoic, white), or partly reflected/transmitted by soft tissues (iso/hypo/hyperechoic, shades of gray). These sound waves deform the crystal resulting in an electrical impulse that gets recorded in a computer.

3 Popular Deep Learning Architectures

3.1 *Unsupervised Feature Learning*

3.1.1 Stacked Auto-Encoder (SAE), Deep Belief Network (DBN), and Deep Boltzmann Machine (DBM)

An autoencoder is a simple model that learns an optimal representation of the input by minimizing reconstruction error between input and output—learned representation of the input. This simple model learns very few features and for better representation, several autoencoders are stacked leading to a stacked autoencoder [43]. DBNs are stacked Restricted Boltzmann Machines (RBMs), a two-layered network with no connections between neurons of the same layer. DBN has one visible layer, several hidden layers, and is trained “greedily” [44]. A DBM [45] is an undirected model with multiple layers of hidden random variables. It is composed of several visible and hidden layers with no interconnection between nodes in the same layer. They are constructed by stacking multiple DBNs hierarchically. Each layer is fine-tuned using parameters from adjacent layers. The unsupervised learning techniques discussed here are not trained with a target vector and classification results are not guaranteed. Generally, an output layer is added to the highest hidden layer and a pre-trained network is used to initialize the model. To prevent the model from tracking local minima the output layer is first randomly initialized and then the entire network is trained with the target using a gradient descent algorithm [46]. SAEs are applied for mammographic risk scoring, breast lesion, and pulmonary nodule detection [47]. Some applications of DBNs are vertebrae segmentation [48], liver segmentation [49], and tracking of Parkinson's disease progression [50].

3.2 *Convolutional Neural Network (CNN)*

CNN is a DL-based algorithm with a stack of alternate convolutional and pooling layers followed finally by one or two dense layers. Convolution is a filter-based operation that aids in parameter sharing and sparsity of connections. A feature learned from one image section is re-usable (parameter sharing) and each time only a subset of the image is processed—leading to sparse connections. They learn local patterns in the input image and the learning is hierarchical. They learn lower-level features such as edges and textures in earlier layers and higher-level abstractions constructed from these features in later layers. Pooling is a down-sampling operation that helps in reducing the number of feature map coefficients; enabling subsequent layers to have a broader perspective. In a dense layer, each neuron is connected to every neuron in the previous layer and they learn global patterns in the input image. Figure 1.1 shows the layer-wise representation of a basic CNN architecture.

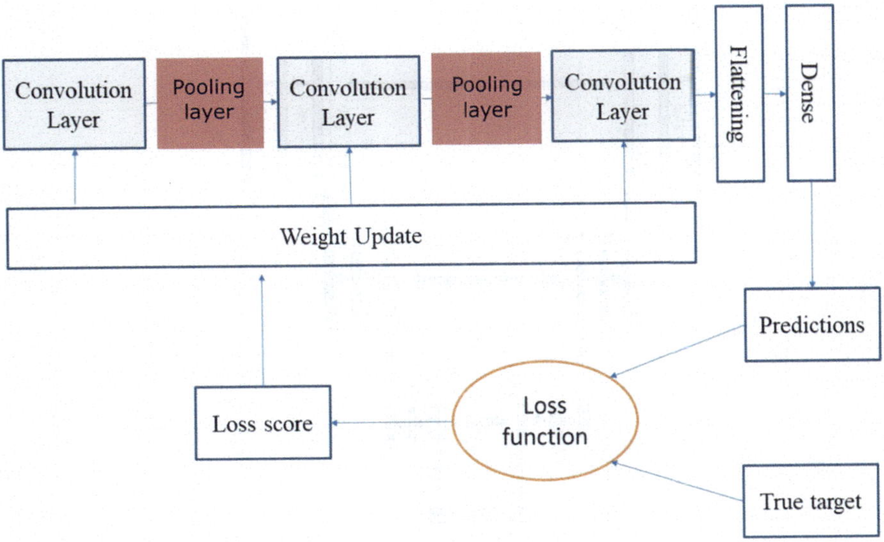

Fig. 1.1 Layer-wise representation of basic CNN

3.3 U-Net Architecture

The U-Net architecture [51] has two parts: contraction path and expansion path. Figure 1.2 illustrates the U-Net architecture. It consists of convolutional layers followed by: pooling layers (down-sampling) in the contraction path and up-sampling in the expansion path. In the contraction path, down-convolutions and down-sampling are applied. The feature maps decrease in size after each step. The expansion path takes the smaller feature map, applies a series of up-sampling and up-convolutions; and gets back to the original image size. It also concatenates the up-sampled versions with corresponding high-resolution features from the contraction path. Finally, the last layer provides a segmentation map corresponding to the input image.

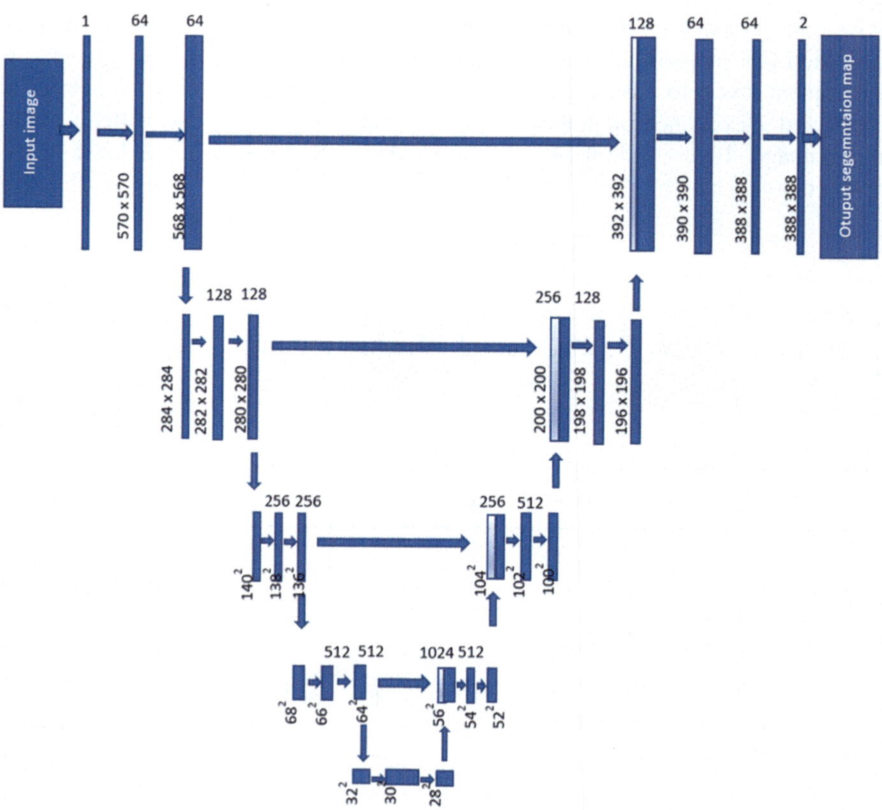

Fig. 1.2 Basic U-Net architecture. (Courtesy: Ronneberger et al. [51])

3.4 *Recurrent Neural Network (RNN) and Long Short-Term Memory (LSTM)*

Dense networks are ineffective in storing sequential information; they are feedforward networks. This is crucial in some applications such as slice-level examination, a radiologist may investigate adjacent slides for haemorrhage confirmation. Current solutions are implemented with RNN, LSTM, and Gated Recurrent Unit (GRU). In a slice-level examination of a subject, RNN stores information in the form of *loops* and *states*—the information between two slices of the same subject. Each time the network is refreshed before the application of images from the next subject. The RNN suffers *from the vanishing gradient problem*—the network becomes un-trainable after many iterations. To overcome this LSTM and GRUs are proposed. They store additional *carry* information that can be processed when required even after many timesteps.

3.5 *Workflow Optimization in DL Algorithms*

DL algorithms have a crucial role in medical diagnosis. Figure 1.3 illustrates the workflow of a DL algorithm. Previous works have focused on the application of DL to segmentation and classification tasks. Dataset preparation in supervised DL involves a pairwise arrangement of input data and target (labels or segmentation mask) and pre-processing. The pre-processing tasks are subjective and include cropping, scaling, intensity thresholding, rotating, normalization, and data augmentation. This is followed by model preparation—selection of network type and its hyper-parameters (learning rate, epochs, batch size). A brief discussion on the performance parameters is provided in the upcoming section.

4 Deep Learning in Medical Image Diagnosis

A disease diagnosis model based on biomedical images involves several processes depicted in Fig. 1.4.

Each time the model is invoked, it yields a (disease) probability associated with the image, and based on a threshold the image is classified as normal or abnormal. The probability computation is crucial for accurate classification and depends on the samples shown to the model during training. Prominent challenges that lead to miscomputations are class imbalance, multi-label association, and the size of the dataset. Frequently in datasets with low variability, the number of normal cases outnumbered the diseased case (class imbalance) and models trained on such a dataset are biased to the normal class. To discuss the class imbalance problem and methods to overcome it let us discuss the binary classification problem. Here, a

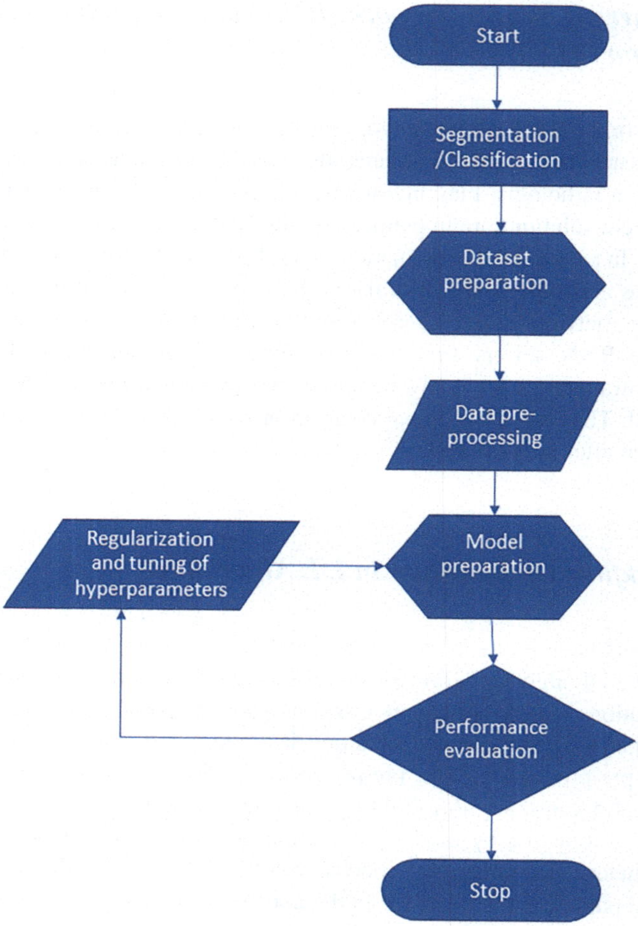

Fig. 1.3 Workflow of a DL algorithm

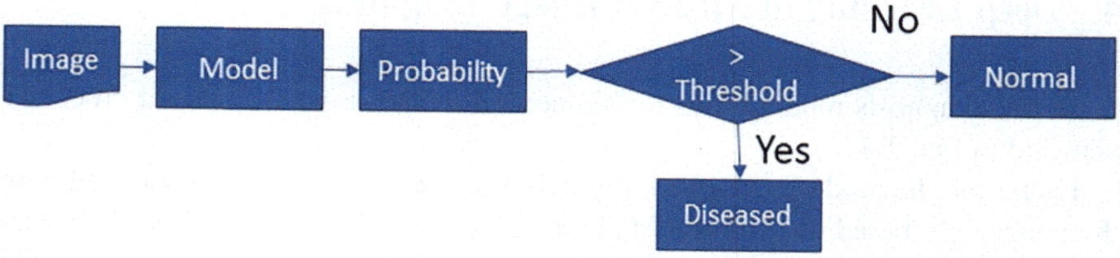

Fig. 1.4 Medical image diagnosis model

binary cross-entropy function, $L(X, y)$, is computed to measure the performance of the model with y as label and X as the input feature vector as shown in Eq. (1.2).

$$L(X,y) = \begin{Bmatrix} -\log P(Y=1|X)\ \mathit{if}\ y=1 \\ -\log P(Y=0|X)\ \mathit{if}\ y=0 \end{Bmatrix} \tag{1.2}$$

$P(Y = 1| X)$ and $P(Y = 0| X)$ are the model outputs for each input and total loss is defined as

$$H(q) = -\frac{1}{N}\sum\nolimits_{i=1}^{N} y_i.\log\left(p(y_i)\right) + (1-y_i).\log\left(1-p(y_i)\right) \tag{1.3}$$

The loss in Eq. (1.3) favors the more probable class and the performance of the model tuned with a biased loss function leads to class imbalance. One solution is to apply a weighted cross-entropy function as defined in Eq. (1.4).

$$L(X,y) = \begin{Bmatrix} W_p \times -\log P(Y=1|X)\ \mathit{if}\ y=1 \\ W_n \times -\log P(Y=0|X)\ \mathit{if}\ y=0 \end{Bmatrix} \tag{1.4}$$

where, $w_p = \frac{N_{-ve}}{N}$ and $w_n = \frac{N_{+ve}}{N}$, N_{-ve} is the number of normal samples, N_{+ve} is the number of diseased samples and N is the total number of samples. This provides a balanced approach to reducing the class imbalance effect. Another solution is to perform re-sampling—to have equal representations from a diseased and normal class. Further, the binary cross-entropy function is applied to evaluate the performance.In some applications, there are multiple classification tasks associated with the same problem. For example, the model needs to assess the presence/absence of a lesion, and classify a scan as diseased or normal at the same time. In such situations, each input scan has multiple labels associated with it. The models are trained for multiple labels with required samples from each class. Superposition of different loss functions is computed to obtain the total loss. Moreover, weighted cross-entropy functions are applied to avoid any class imbalance. Another challenge is the unavailability of a large dataset. A solution is to apply a pre-trained network and fine-tune it on the available dataset. This technique is referred to as *transfer learning*. Data augmentation that includes translation, rotation, zoom, flip, crop, and intensity transformations are applied to generalize to the variability in the image. However, care should be taken to preserve the image label even after data augmentation.

4.1 Evaluation of Model Performance

To evaluate a model often the dataset is split into three sets: train, test, and validation. Model is trained on the training set, evaluated on the validation set, and if necessary, fine-tuned. Finally, the model is tested on the unseen test data. Multiple ways to split data are hold-out validation, K-fold cross-validation, and iterative K-fold validation. In hold-out validation, a portion of the dataset is assigned as a validation set and the rest as the training set. In K-fold cross-validation, the dataset is split into K-partitions and for each partition *i*, the model is trained on K − 1 and evaluated on i^{th} partition. The final performance measure is the average of the K-measures obtained. When limited data is available, K-fold validations are repeated multiple times shuffling the data on each iteration—iterative K-fold validation.

Challenges in evaluating a model include sample overlap, unequal sampling, and ground truth preparation. Sometimes, a scan of the same subject appears in both the training and test set. This is referred to as *sample overlap* and the model tries to memorize (biased to) some features of the scan. Care should be taken in data preparation and all scans of the same subject should appear in the same set. Another challenge is the number of minority class samples in the test set and validation set. Often a minimum percentage of minority class samples are chosen for the test set and validation set. The remaining samples are allocated to the training set. Another problem in the ground truth preparation is the interobserver variability. Consensus voting and additional confirmation tests are performed to overcome this challenge. In consensus voting, weightage is given to opinions from a majority of experts.

4.2 Accuracy, Sensitivity, Specificity, and Prevalence

Accuracy is defined as the ratio of the number of samples correctly classified to the total number of samples and is applied to assess the quality of a model. Consider a dataset with diseased and normal samples. Here, the model accuracy is defined in Eq. (1.5).

$$ACC = P(correct|disease) + P(correct|normal) \tag{1.5}$$

where, $P(correct|disease)$ is the probability that the model is correctly classifying when the subject is diseased and $P(correct|normal)$ is the probability that the model is correctly classifying when the subject is normal. Importantly, $P(correct|disease)$ in Eq. (1.5) is the true positives (TP) and $P(correct|normal)$ is the true negatives (TN). Moreover, $P(correct|disease) = P(positive|disease)$ and $P(correct|normal) = P(negative|normal)$. Importantly, sensitivity (Eq. 1.6) is the fraction of diseased that are also positive and specificity (Eq. 1.7) is the fraction of normal subjects that are also negative.

$$Sensitivity = \frac{TP}{TP + FN} \tag{1.6}$$

Fig. 1.5 Confusion matrix

		Model response	
		Positive	Negative
GT	Disease	TP	FN
	Normal	FP	TN

$$Specificity = \frac{TN}{TN + FP} \tag{1.7}$$

Prevalence is defined as the probability of having disease and is denoted by *P*-(*disease*), so the probability of having no disease is *P*(*normal*). This leads to an alternate definition for accuracy as shown in Eqs. (1.8 and 1.9).

$$ACC = Sensitivity \times P(disease) + Specificity \times P(normal) \tag{1.8}$$

Or

$$ACC = Sensitivity \times Prevalance + Specificity \times (1 - Prevalance) \tag{1.9}$$

In clinical evaluation physicians are interested in the reverse probabilities: Positive Predictive Value (PPV = *P*(*positive*|*disease*)) and Negative Predictive Value (*NPV* = *P*(*negative*|*normal*)). A confusion matrix (Fig. 1.5) is a basic table applied to describe the performance of a classification model. Rows of the confusion matrix represent the ground truth and columns represent the model response. The confusion matrix portraits the relationship between specificity, sensitivity, PPV, and NPV.

4.3 ROC Curve and Threshold

In a binary classifier, the model's response is a probability value associated with the input image. Based on a threshold the response is classified as positive or normal—response above the threshold is positive and below the threshold is normal. ROC curve is the plot of sensitivity vs. specificity for different threshold values.

Significant performance parameters are calculated using the following Eqs. (1.10–1.12):

$$Precision = \frac{TP}{TP + FP} \tag{1.10}$$

$$Re\,call = \frac{TP}{TP + TN} \tag{1.11}$$

$$F1_{score} = 2 \times \frac{precision \times recall}{precision + recall} \tag{1.12}$$

$$Dice\,score = \frac{2 \times |P \cap G|}{|P| + |G|} \tag{1.13}$$

Where P is the prediction and G is the ground truth in Eq. (1.13). $F1_{score}$ is a measure of a test accuracy; a value near unity indicates high accuracy.

5 Application of DL Algorithms in Biomedical Images

5.1 Vessel Segmentation in Retinal Fundus Images

Vessel segmentation is crucial in retinal fundus images. Changes in vessel diameter are a biomarker and early indicator of several diseases. It is strongly associated with mortality in both cardiovascular [52] and end-stage renal disease [33]. Segmentation includes the application of *priori* on color, thickness, central reflex, and branching details around optic discs. Typically, veins are darker red, thicker, and less recognizable than arteries. The inherent variability in these characteristics along with the different image resolutions used in fundus cameras makes automatic classification a computationally challenging task [34]. Manual and semiautomatic segmentation methods are time-consuming and operator-dependent. For years, reliable automatic algorithms have been the focus of several research groups. Recently, deep learning algorithms provided accurate segmentation results and this section provides a brief review of recent literature in this area.

Traditionally, vessel segmentation in fundus images involves the extraction of a vessel from the background. Liu et al. studied that a densely connected CNN applied on the DRIVE dataset achieved accuracy >95% [53]. The dense connections tackled the vanishing gradient problem effectively. Segmentation is studied as a boundary detection task and Fu et al. utilized CNN with RNN-based Conditional Random Field (CRF)—*Deep Vessel*, for delineation [54]. The method includes deep supervision with probability maps generated by CNN for classification and the final classifier extracts pixels with high correlation. They achieved ~95% accuracy on the DRIVE, CHASE_DB1, and STARE datasets. Lahiri et al. analyzed the DRIVE dataset with an ensemble of two stacked autoencoders—one for training with patch-based images and the other for architectural revision [38]. The method finetuned with SoftMax achieved an average accuracy of 95.3%. Lepetit-Aimon et al. proposed a modified approach for segmentation that diminishes the computational and memory requirements [55]. They applied a CNN—trained on low-resolution images for feature extraction, and an autoencoder FCCN—trained on the CNN output.

Before testing, they retrained the entire network on high-resolution patches and observed an accuracy of 96.1% on the DRIVE database.

In semantic segmentation, the primary goal is the identification of a structure of interest. Girard et al. suggested a CNN-based algorithm followed by a graph-based approach for segmentation and classification on the DRIVE and MESSIDOR datasets [36]. The team investigated five training methods: three with original and enhanced images, one with bypass connections similar to U-Net, and another with a likelihood score. The score-based method improved classification accuracy by 2% and performed well even in challenging small vessels. Hemelings et al. applied U-Net architecture for semantic segmentation of artery and vein in fundus images on two public datasets DRIVE and HRF [37]. The system validated by an ophthalmologist achieved >94% accuracy and the study reported a 25% error reduction compared to traditional pixel-based methods [56]. Li et al. proposed a modified U-Net architecture [57] replacing the convolution layers with Selective Kernel units [58] and Attention models [59]. This improved the quality of segmentation and the architecture achieved high sensitivity, specificity, accuracy, and AUC on multiple datasets. Generally, segmentation algorithms apply pixel-wise loss for training unintentionally introducing class imbalance for thick and thin vessels. Yan et al. attributed this as the reason for the inadequate performance of thin vessel segmentation [35]. To overcome this, the team proposed a three-stage DL approach: thick vessel segmentation, thin vessel segmentation, and vessel fusion. The first two stages are trained separately on respective data and the final stage removes uninterested pixels. The algorithm excelled on the DRIVE, STARE, and CHASE_DB1 datasets. Table 1.1 shows recent benchmarking studies in this area.

5.2 *Multiple Sclerosis Lesion Segmentation in Brain MRI*

Multiple sclerosis (MS) is a neurological disease where the protective covering of nerves degenerates leading to lesion formation. Detection and visualization of the lesion are crucial for diagnosis and treatment. Several automatic and semiautomatic methods trivial to other delineation applications are available for MS, especially in MR images. However, clinical routine follows manual segmentation and these are often time-consuming, operator dependent, and challenging. Recently, successful deep learning-based algorithms have been proposed. They are fast, robust, avoid operator bias, and capable of providing clinical diagnosis support.

Automatic MS lesion segmentation is challenging due to the variety in morphology, position, and texture. Birenbaum et al. observed that a lesion appears brighter in FLAIR images and darker in T1-weighted images [39]. They applied a mask-based approach with this priori for classifying voxels and compared the performance of four DL-architectures: a CNN, longitudinal CNN, multi-view CNN, and multi-view longitudinal CNN. Longitudinal CNN applies patches at different time instants; multi-view CNN applies data from orthogonal planes and longitudinal multi-view applies longitudinal data from orthogonal planes. To avoid overfitting

Table 1.1 Benchmarking studies for vessel segmentation in retinal fundus images

Study	Dataset size	Dataset	Pre-processing and method	Result
Hemelings et al. (2019)	40 45	DRIVE HRF	Contrast enhancement, Gaussian filter, Normalization, Data augmentation, **U-net, FCN**, Dropout 20%	**Vessel segmentation:** Accuracy 96.75% **Artery-vein discrimination**: Accuracy 94.25% Benchmarking: 25% reduction in mistakes
K. Li et al. (2020)	40 20 28	DRIVE STARE CHASE_DB1	Gray transformations, Green channel extraction, CLAHE, Clipping, **FANet**	Sensitivity 80% Specificity 0.97 Accuracy 0.97 AUC 0.98
Girard et al. (2019)	40 1200	DRIVE MESSI-DOR	Median filtering, Normalization, **CNN**, Likelihood score propagation, Graph-based approach, tenfold cross-validation	**DRIVE** Sensitivity 93.7 ± 4%, Specificity 92.9 ± 5%, Time 0.5 s **Vessel segmentation** AUC 0.972 Specificity 78.4% Sensitivity 98.1% Accuracy 95.7%
Lepetit-Aimon et al. (2018)	40	DRIVE	Patch-based FCNN Encoder-decoder	Accuracy 96.1%, +5% improvement over U-Net
Z.-F. Liu et al. (2018)	40	DRIVE	17-layer Dense CNN	Accuracy >95%
Fu et al. (2016)	40 20 28	DRIVE STARE CHASE_DB1	Deep Vessel Multi-scale and multi-level CNN (4 stages), Conditional Random Field, Side-output fusion	**DRIVE** Accuracy 0.95 Sensitivity 0.76 **STARE** Accuracy 0.95 Sensitivity 0.74 **CHASE_DB1** Accuracy 0.94 Sensitivity 0.71
Lahiri et al. (2016)	40	DRIVE	Green-channel extraction, CLAHE, Image skeletonization, Dilation, Stacked Denoised Autoencoder, Ensemble of two Stacked Denoising Autoencoder	Accuracy 0.953 Kappa agreement 0.709

FANet Fully Attention-based Network, *CLAHE* Contrast Limited Adaptive Histogram Equalization

Table 1.2 Benchmarking studies in multiple sclerosis lesion segmentation

Study	Dataset size Subjects	Dataset	Pre-processing and method	Result
Birenbaum and Greenspan (2016)	19	Longitudinal images Multiple Sclerosis Segmentation Challenge 2015	Image registration, Brain extraction, Bias-field correction, Intensity normalization **Longitudinal Multi-view CNN**	Dice 0.627 Human-like Segmentation accuracy
Vaidya et al. (2015)	19	Longitudinal Multiple Sclerosis Segmentation Challenge 2015	Histogram matching, Normalization, 3D CNN classifier, Data sampling to reduce the class imbalance	Dice 81.63 Jaccard 68.97 Sensitivity 76.26
Roy et al. (2018)	5 (21 scans) 14 (61 scans) 128	(ISBI 2015): ISBI-21 ISBI-61 MS-100	Image registration, Skull-stripping, Intensity normalization, Convolutional filter banks, FC layer, **FLEXCONN**	**ISBI-61** Dice 0.5243 LFPR 0.1103 PPV 0.8660 VD 0.5207 **MS-100** Dice 0.5639 LFPR 0.3077 PPV 0.6040 VD 0.1978
Valverde et al. (2017)	27,000 patches	MICCAI 2008	Cascaded 3D CNN	Dice 0.5639, LFPR 0.3077, PPV 0.6040, VD 0.1978

CNN Convolutional Neural Network, *FC* Fully Connected, *FLEXCONN* Fast Lesion Extraction using CNN Neural Networks

weight-sharing, dropout, and data augmentation are applied. The authors achieved human-like performance by training on a small dataset of only five subjects. Roy et al. proposed a method with two convolutional pathways for lesion segmentation [60]. In the first pathway, patches from T1-w and FLAIR images are passed separately through the five layers of convolutional filter banks. Its output is concatenated and applied to the second pathway, a fully convolutional network that predicts a membership value for each voxel. They achieved a lesion false positive rate (LFPR) of 0.1102 and a positive predictive value (PPV) of 0.866. However, the algorithm achieved a weaker score than Birenbaum et al. on the ISBI 2015 challenge. In a different approach, Vaidya et al. applied sparse convolutions with SoftMax activation function on multichannel 3D patches and achieved high accuracy and DICE score for lesion segmentation [61]. Valverde et al. used T1-w, T2-w, and FLAIR images from the MICCAI2008 challenge dataset [62]. They observed that cascaded architectures performed well on small datasets and the application of two 3D CNNs achieved better ranking scores. The algorithm validated on clinical MS data observed a high correlation ($\geq$0.97) between predicted lesion volume and expected lesion volume. Recent research works in this area applying cascaded CNNs are displayed in Table 1.2.

Table 1.3 Benchmarking studies in lymph node biopsy segmentation

Study	Number of images	Dataset	Pre-processing and method	Result
Jin et al. (2020)	327,680	PatchCamelyon	Stain normalisation Morphological transformations, **ConcatNet**	AUC 0.924 Sensitivity 82% Specificity 87.8% Accuracy 84.1%
Vesal et al. (2018)	400	BACH 2018 grand challenge	Stain normalization, Data augmentation **Inception-V3, ResNet50** **Transfer learning**	**Inception-V3** Accuracy 97.08% **ResNet50** Accuracy 96.66%
Y. Liu et al. (2019)	399 108	Camelyon16	Colour normalization, **Deep learning**	Tumor-level sensitivity 91% **Camelyon16** AUC 99% **DS2** AUC 99.6%

5.3 Segmentation in Lymph Node Biopsy

Early detection of metastatic tissue in sentinel lymph nodes is crucial in the prognosis of breast cancer. Traditionally, analysis is performed by a trained histopathologist and often is time-sensitive—a decision on surgery or follow-up treatment depends on the outcome of the analysis. Deep learning architectures improved the diagnostic potential of clinicians. Jin et al. proposed a concatenated U-Net architecture to detect lymph node metastases [63]. They added four channels trained with annotated datasets for segmentation mask generation of nucleus, mitosis, tubule, and epithelium. This introduced a focussed approach to training and model performance improved significantly. DL-based computer-aided approaches elevated histopathologic interpretation and treatment procedures. Studies reported an 8% improvement in micrometastases detection while reducing average review time [64]. Vesal et al. applied transfer learning on the image patch after stain normalization [65]. Their method illustrated the capability of transfer learning approaches in the accurate classification of breast cancer histology images. Another team [66] proposed a DL-based algorithm Lymph Node Assistant (LYNA) for detection and workflow integration. They achieved an AUC of 99.6% and found that the algorithm detected metastases even in the presence of histopathologic artifacts. These are summarized in Table 1.3.

5.4 Intracranial Haemorrhage Detection in Head CT

Intracranial haemorrhage is a critical condition with death or severe disability as the primary outcome [67]. A community-based study reported that in first-ever stroke patients, ICH accounted for 10% of stroke [68]. Further in ICH, the mortality rate in the first month or first 3 years is very high [69]. Even though initial clinical evaluation is crucial, misdiagnosis and misinterpretations lead to a blackout, aneurysm, hydrocephalus, and vasospasm [70, 71]. To overcome this accurate detection and early treatment is the need of the hour. When physicians applied computer-aided diagnosis, the mean accuracy improved 6% and the figure-of-merit moved from 0.78 to 0.82 [72]. The diagnosis time improved by 96% with workflow integration of DL-based algorithms [73] and faster processing of scans [74]. The following section reviews the latest state-of-the-art studies in ICH detection, classification of subtypes, and segmentation.

Majumdar et al. applied postprocessing with CNN to detect ICH on a dataset of 134 subjects and achieved a sensitivity of 0.81 and specificity of 0.98 [75]. They applied a frame-by-frame approach and on detecting an ICH, the postprocessing block analyzed consecutive frames at the same location for confirmation. Chilamkurthy et al. analyzed the performance of a deep learning algorithm for the detection of calvarial fracture, midline shift, and mass effect in addition to the five subtypes of ICH on two datasets of 21,095 scans and 491 scans [76]. Further, they validated the outcomes on a separate dataset and evaluated the accuracy of the algorithm with ground truth from three radiologists. Further, studies observed that automated ICH detection improved triage and diagnostic accuracy [77].

Several researchers reported improved performance applying a fusion of architectures. Cho et al. proposed two separate algorithms: a CNN-based binary classifier and an FCN-based multi-class classifier [78]. The method reported sensitivity improvement (1%) and overall segmentation enhancement (3.44%) compared to single FCN methods. The classifiers were trained separately with varying window levels. Ye et al. proposed a fusion of CNN and RNN to detect ICH and classify its subtypes on 3D scans [79]. On a dataset of 2836 Asians, they reported an AUC $\geq$ 0.98 for binary classifiers and an AUC > 0.8 for the subtype classifier. Moreover, the algorithm processed a 3D scan in <30 s elevating its application as a tool for diagnostic assistance [80]. However, the layer weights were updated using backpropagation algorithms that lead to the vanishing gradient problem. To deal with the vanishing gradient problem Arab et al. applied CNN with deep supervision (CNN-DS) for the evaluation of haemorrhage (segmentation) and its volume computation [74]. Each hidden layer had a separate objective function in addition to the overall objective function. The study improved both the Dice score and recall compared to U-Net and had a faster processing time. The varying morphology of haemorrhage forced Kuo et al. to apply semantic segmentation to detect acute ICH [81]. They applied a single patch-based FCN for classification and abnormality localization and trained on a small dataset. They combined three consecutive images as a multi-channel input to mimic common radiologist practice. The patch-based

FCN technique achieved an AUC of 0.991, sensitivity and specificity of 100%, and the algorithm outperformed radiologists.

The mean accuracy (+6%), figure-of-merit, and reading time improved significantly when clinicians applied DL-based computer-aided diagnosis for ICH detection [72]. However, the false-positive rate is crucial in clinical diagnosis. Watanabe et al. applied the Random Forest algorithm on probability heat maps generated by a U-Net classifier for false-positive removal and observed improved sensitivity, specificity, and accuracy [72]. This favored the application of a DL-based computer-aided approach for workflow optimization in emergency rooms. Up to a 96% reduction in the time to diagnosis for new outpatient was observed in the case of ICH [73]. They successfully re-prioritized cases overlooked by radiologists, particularly subtle ICH, and achieved an AUC of 0.846. Chang et al. developed a mask ROI-based network for haemorrhage detection and quantification [82]. They trained the network on 10,159 subjects and tested it on 862 subjects with multiple scans per subject. The obtained varying Dice scores for SAH (0.772), IPH (0.931), and epidural/subdural (0.863). However, the study reported the performance from only a single institution.

Further, Danilov et al. demonstrated a classification accuracy >0.81 using a ResNext-based deep learning architecture trained on a dataset of 674,258 scans provided by Kaggle competition on haemorrhage classification [83]. The method displayed AUC ranging from 0.71 to 0.8 for various subtypes on another dataset of 752,807 scans. Ker et al. analyzed 3D-CNN on brain volumetric images after thresholding adapted for haemorrhage detection [84].They achieved an $F1_{score}$ of 0.684 for multiclass classification and the detection worked perfectly for all classes except SAH. Ko et al. proposed a deep CNN-LSTM model for classification [85]. They trained the Xception based CNN model on 4,516,842 scans and tested on 727,392 scans and achieved an accuracy of 93% on balanced data and 89% on unbalanced data. Lee et al. proposed an integrated approach imitating the workflow of the radiologist for ICH detection on a dataset of 904 scans [86]. At first, they constructed a multi-channel composite image from multiple versions of the input image (multiwindow approach). Then, interpolated images from adjacent slices are applied to the model (slice-level interpolation). The model generates attention maps and using a distance measure with class-specific activation maps a predictive basis is computed. The features generated by the model for prediction matched with the features selected by a radiologist for classification. Table 1.4 summarizes the results of various researchers.

5.5 ICH Segmentation

Hssayeni et al. implemented a U-Net-based architecture for segmentation of ICH regions in head CT [87]. They achieved high accuracy, high sensitivity, and a low Dice score of 0.31 owing to false-positive segmentation near bones. They applied fivefold cross-validation on a dataset of 82 subjects obtained from a hospital in Iraq.

Table 1.4 Benchmarking studies in intracranial haemorrhage detection

Study	Dataset size subjects (images)	Dataset	Pre-processing and method	Result
Kuo et al. (2019)	4766	University of California	Skull and face removal, PatchFCN Dilated ResNet38	AUC 0.991 $\pm$ 0.006 Performance >2/4 radiologists Sensitivity 100%, Specificity 87%
Watanabe et al. (2020)	433 (7914)	Osaka University	Cropping, Multiple contrast images, U-Net, Probability heat maps, ML-based false positive removal	**Patient-based** AUC 0.949, Sensitivity 91.7% Specificity 81.2%, Accuracy 85% **Lesion-based** AUC 0.938, Sensitivity 89.6%, Specificity 81.2%, Accuracy 87.5% **Using CAD** Accuracy 89.7%, FoM 0.82, Reading time 43 s **Without CAD** Accuracy 83.7%, FoM 0.78, Reading time 68 s
Chang et al. (2018)	11,021 (536,266)	University of California Irvine Medical Center	Axial soft-tissue reconstruction, Resizing, Clipping Rescaling, maskROI-based CNN	Accuracy 0.975, AUC 0.983 Sensitivity 0.971, Specificity 0.975, PPV 0.793, NPV 0.997 **Dice score** IPH 0.931, Epidural/subdural 0.683, SAH 0.772
Arab et al. (2020)	55 subjects 57,671,680 voxels 780,894,208 labelled voxels per CT scan	Fraser Health, British Columbia	CNN-DS	Dice score 0.84 $\pm$ 0.06 Recall 0.83 $\pm$ 0.07 Average runtime 0.74 $\pm$ 0.07 s
Ye et al. (2019)	2836 (76,621)	Asian population from three hospitals	Resampling to 512 $\times$ 512, Downsampling to 256 $\times$ 256,	**Two-type classification** AUC $\geq$ 0.98

(continued)

Table 1.4 (continued)

Study	Dataset size subjects (images)	Dataset	Pre-processing and method	Result
			Slice normalization with three intensity ranges, CNN-RNN	**Five-type classification** AUC > 0.8
Chilamkurthy et al. (2018)	313,318 scans **Qure25k dataset** 21,095 scans **CQ500 dataset** 214 + 277 scans	Across 20 centres in India	Deep learning algorithms	**AUC in Qure25k dataset** ICH 0.92, IPH 0.90, IVH 0.96 Subdural 0.92, Extradural 0.93 Subarachnoid 0.90 **AUC in CQ500 dataset** ICH 0.94, IPH 0.95, IVH 0.93 Subdural 0.95, Extradural 0.97 Subarachnoid 0.96
Danilov et al. (2020)	674.258 DICOM and 752,807 DICOM Real-world clinical dataset 300 CT	N.N. Burdenko Neurosurgery Centre Kaggle data	Rescaled window level and window width set, ResNexT architecture, Adam optimizer	Logarithmic loss 0.05 Accuracy IPH 83.5% IVH 89.3% Subdural 81.8% Extradural 82.8% Subarachnoid 82%
Arbabshirani et al. (2018)	46,583 scans	Centers in Geisinger	Resampling to 24 image slices, Resizing 256 x 256, Deep CNN	Median time to diagnosis 512 to 19 min, AUC ICH 0.846, Specificity 0.80, Sensitivity 0.73
Majumdar et al. (2018)	134 subjects 4300 images	Boston University Medical Center	Data augmentation Left-right flipping Random rotation ± 10°, CNN	Sensitivity 81% Specificity 98%
Cho et al. (2019)	135,974	Kyungpook National University Hospital Chilgok	Window level Window width set, Cascade of CNN and FCN	Sensitivity 97.9%, Specificity 98.76%, Precision 80.19%, Recall 82.15% Binary classifier Accuracy 98.28%
Ko et al. (2020)	5,244,234 subjects	ASNR and RSNA	Window width and window level set, Rescaling,	Logarithmic loss 0.07528

(continued)

Table 1.4 (continued)

Study	Dataset size subjects (images)	Dataset	Pre-processing and method	Result
			Rotation, Flipping, Data balancing, Resizing, CNN-LSTM, Xception-based CNN	Balanced data Accuracy 93% Unbalanced data Accuracy 89%
Lee et al. (2019)	904 scans	Department of Radiology, Massachusetts General Hospital	Geometric transformation Nonlinear denoising filter, Multiwindow Slice-level interpolation, Deep CNN pre-trained on ImageNet, Atlas creation module Prediction-basis detection	Mean average precision 0.85 Sensitivity >92% Specificity >92% Localization accuracy of attention maps Overlap 78.1%
Ker et al. (2019)	399 volumetric brain data 12,000 images	National Neuroscience Institute, Singapore	Thresholding, 3D CNN	Binary classification with thresholding $F1_{score}$ 0.706 to 0.902 without thresholding $F1_{score}$ 0.919 to 0.952 Four class classification $F1_{score}$ 0.684

However, the method failed to localize ICH regions in subtle IPH subjects. Zhao et al. proposed a reliable DL algorithm no-new Net (nnU-Net) for the evaluation of ICH, IVH, and PHE [88]. The nnU-Net is a cascade of several types of U-net architectures. They reported Dice scores of 0.92, 0.79, and 0.71 for lesion segmentation; PPVs of 0.92, 0.76 and 0.69; and sensitivities of 0.93, 0.88, and 0.81 respectively on a dataset of 460 subjects. The multiresolution algorithm took only 15 s for analysis compared to 540 s for the manual segmentation, a 97% improvement in processing time. Xu et al. trained a DL-based model using binary cross-entropy for pixel-wise segmentation [89]. The method omitted data augmentation and dropout but applied binary cross-entropy loss; managed Dice scores of 0.89–0.95 and identified non-hemorrhagic scans with an accuracy of 96.5%. Analysis of a single-CT took only 5 s enabling its application for clinical applications. Ironside et al. applied U-Net-based CNN architecture with 50% dropout and L2 regularisation for automatic segmentation in ICH [90]. The method was accurate and faster than traditional segmentation approaches. ICH segmentation algorithms based on U-Net are summarized in Table 1.5.

Table 1.5 Benchmarking studies in intracranial haemorrhage segmentation

Study	Dataset size subjects (images)	Dataset	Pre-processing	Method	Result
Hssayeni et al. (2020)	82 (2491)	Al Hilla Teaching Hospital-Iraq	Removal of 5 pixels from the image border	U-Net	Jaccard index 0.21 Dice score 0.31 Sensitivity 97.2% Specificity 50.4% Accuracy 82.5%
J. Xu et al. (2021)	3297 images	Beijing Tiantan Hospital, QingPu Branch of Zhongshan Hospital	Normalization	Dense U-Net	Dice coefficient ICH 0.90 ± 0.06 EDH 0.88 ± 0.12 SDH 0.82 ± 0.16
Ironside et al. (2019)	300 (397) 12,968 image slices	Intracerebral Haemorrhage Outcomes Project	Windowing, Thresholding, Normalization, Denoising, Closing, Data augmentation	CNN U-Net	Dice similarity Manual 0.894 ± 0.264 Semi-automated 0.905 ± 0.254

6 Challenges

Multiple challenges are described in the application of DL algorithms for medical data. In retinal fundus images, scientists have reported the scarcity of a large annotated dataset for vessel segmentation [36, 37, 57]. Popular datasets such as the DRIVE and High-Resolution Fundus (HRF) Image Database used to study classification algorithms lack sufficient variance [37]. Further, the thin and irregular vessel profiles in these scans create additional burden in segmentation [37]. Densely connected CNN [53], and deep supervised CNN [54] achieve >95% accuracy. However, these cascaded architectures lead to vanishing gradients. Further, imbalanced data owing to inadequate representations of data representing each class leads to overfitting. Weight adjustments, data augmentation, and data management are applied to improve performance [60, 62]. Moreover, a standalone implementation of an automated system is deferred due to class imbalance [64].

In ICH detection, semantic segmentation is preferred owing to the small dataset and haemorrhage variability [81]. Head CT contains a variable number of image slices owing to the variability in head size, slice thickness, and contrast. Further, interslice dimensionality variations are observed and standardizations are performed before applying to DL algorithms [73]. The slices are low-contrast images and "windowing" is applied for improving the contrast. Another principal challenge is the localization of the haemorrhage. Most algorithms detected the haemorrhage but lesion localization is a challenge predominantly due to the lack of annotated data and the computational burden to process 3D voxels [72].

To summarize, major challenges in the application of DL in biomedical images are:

1. The availability of good quality annotated datasets [63].
2. The inherent variability in arteries, tissue, and acquisition techniques (modality) in the case of biomedical images.
3. The vanishing gradient problem in cascaded architectures.
4. Overfitting due to fewer data representations in each class.
5. Class imbalance between abnormal and normal classes.

7 Conclusion

This chapter summarizes about the application of deep learning on biomedical images. Often medical evaluation is time-sensitive and DL algorithms achieved a significant reduction in analysis time. Workflow optimization and triage alteration are suggested as patients benefitted from computer-aided diagnosis. Several algorithms benefitted from subjective pre-processing, transfer learning, and ensemble approaches. In situations where early diagnosis is crucial, integrating DL algorithms to the clinical workflow reduced diagnosis time and improved diagnostic accuracy. Moreover, abnormality detection and disease staging improved significantly on the application of deep CNN, suggesting its use as a second medical opinion.

Recently, DL-based automated diagnosis is gaining traction. In a patient acceptability study for screening diabetic retinopathy (DR) the mean assessment time improved and participants preferred the automated method over the traditional method. There are several challenges involved in making the DL-based automated algorithms a part of the clinical routine. It is difficult to apply a generalization to the training data owing to the variation in ethnicity, modality, equipment, and resolution. Thus, algorithms are fine-tuned with proper data samples before deploying. Biomedical images are highly heterogeneous across the modality, protocol, shape, size, and internal structure of objects. Further, there are inter-subject variations (person to person) and intra-subject variations (same person at different times). Another challenge is the delineation of objects in biomedical images owing to the representation of object boundary. Finally, the robustness of the automatic algorithm used for medical image processing is also significant. Importantly, when applied in a clinical routine these algorithms should never fail or produce false results.

References

1. Loan NA, Parah SA, Sheikh JA, Akhoon JA, Bhat GM (2017) Hiding Electronic Patient Record (EPR) in medical images: a high capacity and computationally efficient technique for e-healthcare applications. J Biomed Inform 73:125–136. https://doi.org/10.1016/j.jbi.2017.08.002
2. Kaw JA, Loan NA, Parah SA, Muhammad K, Sheikh JA, Bhat GM (2019) A reversible and secure patient information hiding system for IoT driven e-health. Int J Inf Manag 45:262–275
3. Gull S, Mansour RF, Aljehane NO, Parah SA (2021) A self-embedding technique for tamper detection and localization of medical images for smart-health. Multimed Tools Appl 80(19): 29939–29964
4. Parah SA, Sheikh JA, Ahad F, Loan NA, Bhat GM (2017) Information hiding in medical images: a robust medical image watermarking system for E-healthcare. Multimed Tools Appl 76(8):10599–10633. https://doi.org/10.1007/s11042-015-3127-y
5. Shah AA, Parah SA, Rashid M, Elhoseny M (2020) Efficient image encryption scheme based on generalized logistic map for real time image processing. J Real-Time Image Proc 17(6): 2139–2151. https://doi.org/10.1007/s11554-020-01008-4
6. Jan A, Parah SA, Hussan M, Malik BA (2021) Double layer security using crypto-stego techniques: a comprehensive review. Heal Technol 12:1–23
7. Gull S, Parah SA, Khan M (2020) Reversible data hiding exploiting Huffman encoding with dual images for IoMT based healthcare. Comput Commun 163:134–149
8. Parah SA, Sheikh JA, Bhat GM (2015) Hiding in encrypted images: a three tier security data hiding system. Multidim Syst Sign Process 28:549–572
9. Friston KJ, Jezzard P, Turner R (1994) Analysis of functional MRI time-series. Hum Brain Mapp 1(2):153–171. https://doi.org/10.1002/hbm.460010207
10. Rashid TA, Zhao J (2020) Remote tracking of Parkinson's Disease progression using ensembles of Deep Belief Network and Self-Organizing Map. Expert Syst Appl 159:113562. https://doi.org/10.1016/j.eswa.2020.113562
11. Rashid M, Singh H, Goyal V (2021) Efficient feature selection technique based on fast Fourier transform with PSO-GA for functional magnetic resonance imaging. In: 2021 2nd International conference on computation, automation and knowledge management (ICCAKM). IEEE, New York, pp 238–242
12. Jamthikar A, Gupta D, Khanna NN, Araki T, Saba L, Nicolaides A, Sharma A, Omerzu T, Suri HS, Gupta A, Mavrogeni S, Turk M, Laird JR, Protogerou A, Sfikakis PP, Kitas GD, Viswanathan V, Pareek G, Miner M, Suri JS (2019) A special report on changing trends in preventive stroke/cardiovascular risk assessment via B-mode ultrasonography. Curr Atheroscler Rep 21(7):25. https://doi.org/10.1007/s11883-019-0788-4
13. Wyawahare MV, Patil PM, Abhyankar HK (2009) Image registration techniques: an overview. Int J Sign Process Image Process Pattern Recogn 2(3):11–28
14. Lo SCB, Lou SLA, Chien MV, Mun SK (1995) Artificial convolution neural network techniques and applications for lung nodule detection. IEEE Trans Med Imaging 14(4):711–718. https://doi.org/10.1109/42.476112
15. Lecun Y, Bottou L, Bengio Y, Haffner P (1998) Gradient-based learning applied to document recognition. Proc IEEE 86(11):2278–2324. https://doi.org/10.1109/5.726791
16. Russakovsky O, Deng J, Su H, Krause J, Satheesh S, Ma S, Huang Z, Karpathy A, Khosla A, Bernstein M, Berg AC, Fei-Fei L (2015) ImageNet large scale visual recognition challenge. Int J Comput Vis 115(3):211–252. https://doi.org/10.1007/s11263-015-0816-y
17. Kumar I, Alshamrani SS, Kumar A, Rawat J, Singh KU, Rashid M, AlGhamdi AS (2021) Deep learning approach for analysis and characterization of COVID-19. Comput Mater Cont 70:451–468
18. Anthimopoulos M, Christodoulidis S, Ebner L, Christe A, Mougiakakou S (2016) Lung pattern classification for interstitial lung diseases using a deep convolutional neural network. IEEE Trans Med Imaging 35(5):1207–1216. https://doi.org/10.1109/TMI.2016.2535865

19. Song W, Li S, Liu J, Qin H, Zhang B, Zhang S, Hao A (2019) Multitask cascade convolution neural networks for automatic thyroid nodule detection and recognition. IEEE J Biomed Health Inform 23(3):1215–1224. https://doi.org/10.1109/JBHI.2018.2852718
20. Sun W, Tseng TLB, Zhang J, Qian W (2017) Enhancing deep convolutional neural network scheme for breast cancer diagnosis with unlabeled data. Comput Med Imaging Graph 57:4–9. https://doi.org/10.1016/j.compmedimag.2016.07.004
21. Wang Z, Li M, Wang H, Jiang H, Yao Y, Zhang H, Xin J (2019) Breast cancer detection using extreme learning machine based on feature fusion with CNN deep features. IEEE Access 7: 105146–105158. https://doi.org/10.1109/ACCESS 2019.2892795
22. Farooq A, Anwar S, Awais M, Rehman S (2017) A deep CNN based multi-class classification of Alzheimer's disease using MRI. In: IST 2017 - IEEE international conference on imaging systems and techniques, Proceedings, 2018-January, pp 1–6. https://doi.org/10.1109/IST.2017.8261460
23. Anwar SM, Majid M, Qayyum A, Awais M, Alnowami M, Khan MK (2018) Medical image analysis using convolutional neural networks: a review. J Med Syst 42:226
24. Ravi D, Wong C, Deligianni F, Berthelot M, Andreu-Perez J, Lo B, Yang GZ (2017) Deep learning for health informatics. IEEE J Biomed Health Inform 21(1):4–21. https://doi.org/10.1109/JBHI.2016.2636665
25. Chollet F (2017) Xception: deep learning with depthwise separable convolutions. In: 2017 IEEE conference on computer vision and pattern recognition (CVPR), pp 1800–1807. https://doi.org/10.1109/CVPR.2017.195
26. Mondal S, Agarwal K, Rashid M (2019) Deep learning approach for automatic classification of X-ray images using convolutional neural network. In: Proceedings of the IEEE international conference image information processing, 2019-November, pp 326–331. https://doi.org/10.1109/ICIIP47207.2019.8985687
27. Szegedy C, Ioffe S, Vanhoucke V, Alemi AA (2017) Inception-v4, Inception-ResNet and the impact of residual connections on learning. Proc AAAI Conf Artif Intell 31(1):1602.07261
28. Rudyanto RD, Kerkstra S, van Rikxoort EM, Fetita C, Brillet PY, Lefevre C, Xue W, Zhu X, Liang J, Öksüz IL, Ünay D, Kadipaşaoğlu K, Estépar RSJ, Ross JC, Washko GR, Prieto JC, Hoyos MH, Orkisz M, Meine H, van Ginneken B (2014) Comparing algorithms for automated vessel segmentation in computed tomography scans of the lung: the VESSEL12 study. Med Image Anal 18(7):1217–1232. https://doi.org/10.1016/j.media.2014.07.003
29. Jia T, Zhang H, Meng H (2014) A novel lung nodules detection scheme based on vessel segmentation on CT images. Biomed Mater Eng 24(6):3179–3186. https://doi.org/10.3233/BME-141139
30. Korfiatis PD, Kalogeropoulou C, Karahaliou AN, Kazantzi AD, Costaridou LI (2011) Vessel tree segmentation in presence of interstitial lung disease in MDCT. IEEE Trans Inf Technol Biomed 15(2):214–220. https://doi.org/10.1109/TITB.2011.2112668
31. Guo W, Gu X, Fang Q, Li Q (2020) Comparison of performances of conventional and deep learning-based methods in segmentation of lung vessels and registration of chest radiographs. Radiol Phys Technol 2020:0123456789. https://doi.org/10.1007/s12194-020-00584-1
32. Keel S, Lee PY, Scheetz J, Li Z, Kotowicz MA, MacIsaac RJ, He M (2018) Feasibility and patient acceptability of a novel artificial intelligence-based screening model for diabetic retinopathy at endocrinology outpatient services: a pilot study. Sci Rep 8(1). https://doi.org/10.1038/s41598-018-22612-2
33. Günthner R, Henner H, Christine H, Susanne A, Georg L, Stephan K, Julia M et al. (2019) Impaired retinal vessel dilation predicts mortality in end-stage renal disease. Circulation research 124(12):1796–1807
34. Miri M, Amini Z, Rabbani H, Kafieh R (2017) A comprehensive study of retinal vessel classification methods in fundus images. J Med Sign Sens 7(2):59–70. https://doi.org/10.4103/2228-7477.205505

35. Yan Z, Yang X, Cheng KT (2019) A three-stage deep learning model for accurate retinal vessel segmentation. IEEE J Biomed Health Inform 23(4):1427–1436. https://doi.org/10.1109/JBHI.2018.2872813
36. Girard F, Kavalec C, Cheriet F (2019) Joint segmentation and classification of retinal arteries/veins from fundus images. Artif Intell Med 94(December 2017):96–109. https://doi.org/10.1016/j.artmed.2019.02.004
37. Hemelings R, Elen B, Stalmans I, Van Keer K, De Boever P, Blaschko MB (2019) Artery–vein segmentation in fundus images using a fully convolutional network. Comput Med Imaging Graph 76:101636. https://doi.org/10.1016/j.compmedimag.2019.05.004
38. Lahiri A, Roy AG, Sheet D, Biswas PK (2016) Deep neural ensemble for retinal vessel segmentation in fundus images towards achieving label-free angiography. In: Proceedings of the annual international conference of the IEEE engineering in medicine and biology society, EMBS, 2016-October, pp 1340–1343. https://doi.org/10.1109/EMBC.2016.7590955
39. Birenbaum A, Greenspan H (2016) In: Carneiro G, Mateus D, Peter L, Bradley A, Tavares JMRS, Belagiannis V, Papa JP, Nascimento JC, Loog M, Lu Z, Cardoso JS, Cornebise J (eds) Longitudinal multiple sclerosis lesion segmentation using multi-view convolutional neural networks, vol 10008. Springer International Publishing, New York, pp 58–67. https://doi.org/10.1007/978-3-319-46976-8_7
40. Aslani S, Dayan M, Storelli L, Filippi M, Murino V, Rocca MA, Sona D (2019) Multi-branch convolutional neural network for multiple sclerosis lesion segmentation. NeuroImage 196:1–15. https://doi.org/10.1016/j.neuroimage.2019.03.068
41. Aslani S, Dayan M, Murino V, Sona D (2019) Deep 2D encoder-decoder convolutional neural network for multiple sclerosis lesion segmentation in brain MRI. In: Lecture notes in computer science (including subseries lecture notes in artificial intelligence and lecture notes in bioinformatics), 11383 LNCS, pp 132–141. https://doi.org/10.1007/978-3-030-11723-8_13
42. Rashid M, Singh H, Goyal V (2020) The use of machine learning and deep learning algorithms in functional magnetic resonance imaging—a systematic review. Expert Syst 37(6):1–29. https://doi.org/10.1111/exsy.12644
43. Suk HI, Lee SW, Shen D (2015) Latent feature representation with stacked auto-encoder for AD/MCI diagnosis. Brain Struct Funct 220(2):841–859. https://doi.org/10.1007/s00429-013-0687-3
44. Liu W, Wang Z, Liu X, Zeng N, Liu Y, Alsaadi FE (2017) A survey of deep neural network architectures and their applications. Neurocomputing 234:11–26. https://doi.org/10.1016/j.neucom.2016.12.038
45. Salakhutdinov R, Hinton G (2009) Deep Boltzmann machines. In: Artificial intelligence and statistics
46. Shen D, Wu G, Suk HI (2017) Deep learning in medical image analysis. Annu Rev Biomed Eng 19:221–248. https://doi.org/10.1146/annurev-bioeng-071516-044442
47. Cheng JZ, Ni D, Chou YH, Qin J, Tiu CM, Chang YC, Huang CS, Shen D, Chen CM (2016) Computer-aided diagnosis with deep learning architecture: applications to breast lesions in US images and pulmonary nodules in CT scans. Sci Rep 6(1):1–13. https://doi.org/10.1038/srep24454
48. Qadri SF, Ahmad M, Ai D, Yang J, Wang Y (2018) Deep belief network based vertebra segmentation for CT images. Commun Comput Inf Sci 875:536–545. https://doi.org/10.1007/978-981-13-1702-6_53
49. Ahmad M, Ai D, Xie G, Qadri SF, Song H, Huang Y, Wang Y, Yang J (2019) Deep belief network modeling for automatic liver segmentation. IEEE Access 7:20585–20595. https://doi.org/10.1109/ACCESS.2019.2896961
50. Nilashi M, Ahmadi H, Sheikhtaheri A, Naemi R, Alotaibi R, Abdulsalam Alarood A, Munshi A, Rao B, Zohrabian V, Cedeno P, Saha A, Pahade J, Davis MA (2021) Utility of artificial intelligence tool as a prospective radiology peer reviewer—detection of unreported intracranial haemorrhage. Acad Radiol 28(1):85–93. https://doi.org/10.1016/j.acra.2020.01.035

51. Ronneberger O, Fischer P, Brox T (2015) In: Mori K, Sakuma I, Sato Y, Barillot C, Navab N (eds) U-Net: convolutional networks for biomedical image segmentation, vol 8150. Springer, Berlin, pp 234–241. https://doi.org/10.1007/978-3-319-24574-4_28
52. Braun G, Hafner B, Königstein K, Infanger D, Klenk C, Rossmeissl A, Schmidt-Trucksäss A, Hanssen H (2018) Association of cardiorespiratory fitness with retinal vessel diameters as a biomarker of cardiovascular risk. Microvasc Res 120:36–40. https://doi.org/10.1016/j.mvr.2018.06.001
53. Liu Z-F, Zhang Y-Z, Liu P-Z, Zhang Y, Luo Y-M, Du Y-Z, Peng Y, Li P (2018) Retinal vessel segmentation using densely connected convolution neural network with colorful fundus images. J Med Imag Health Inform 8(6):1300–1307. https://doi.org/10.1166/jmihi.2018.2429
54. Fu H, Xu Y, Lin S, Wong DWK, Liu J (2016) Deepvessel: retinal vessel segmentation via deep learning and conditional random field. In: Lecture notes in computer science (including subseries lecture notes in artificial intelligence and lecture notes in bioinformatics), 9901 LNCS(DI), pp 132–139. https://doi.org/10.1007/978-3-319-46723-8_16
55. Lepetit-Aimon G, Duval R, Cheriet F (2018) Large receptive field fully convolutional network for semantic segmentation of retinal vasculature in fundus images. In: Lecture notes in computer science (including subseries lecture notes in artificial intelligence and lecture notes in bioinformatics), 11039 LNCS, pp 201–209. https://doi.org/10.1007/978-3-030-00949-6_24
56. Xu X, Ding W, Abràmoff MD, Cao R (2017) An improved arteriovenous classification method for the early diagnostics of various diseases in retinal image. Comput Methods Prog Biomed 141:3–9. https://doi.org/10.1016/j.cmpb.2017.01.007
57. Li K, Qi X, Luo Y, Yao Z, Zhou X, Sun M (2020) Accurate retinal vessel segmentation in color fundus images via fully attention-based networks. IEEE J Biomed Health Inform 25(6): 2071–2081. https://doi.org/10.1109/jbhi.2020.3028180
58. Li X, Wang W, Hu X, Yang J (2019) Selective kernel networks. ArXiv:510–519
59. Luong MT, Pham H, Manning CD (2015) Effective approaches to attention-based neural machine translation. In: Conference proceedings - EMNLP 2015: conference on empirical methods in natural language processing, pp 1412–1421. https://doi.org/10.18653/v1/d15-1166
60. Roy S, Butman JA, Reich DS, Calabresi PA, Pham DL (2018) Multiple sclerosis lesion segmentation from brain MRI via fully convolutional neural networks. ArXiv 2013
61. Vaidya S, Chunduru A, Muthuganapathy R, Krishnamurthi G (2015) Longitudinal multiple sclerosis lesion segmentation usign 3{D} convulutional neural networks
62. Valverde S, Cabezas M, Roura E, González-Villà S, Pareto D, Vilanova JC, Ramió-Torrentà L, Rovira À, Oliver A, Lladó X (2017) Improving automated multiple sclerosis lesion segmentation with a cascaded 3D convolutional neural network approach. NeuroImage 155:159–168. https://doi.org/10.1016/j.neuroimage.2017.04.034
63. Jin YW, Jia S, Ashraf AB, Hu P (2020) Integrative data augmentation with U-Net segmentation masks improves detection of lymph. Cancers (Basel) 12(10):2934
64. Steiner DF, Macdonald R, Liu Y, Truszkowski P, Hipp JD, Gammage C, Thng F, Peng L, Stumpe MC (2018) Impact of deep learning assistance on the histopatholcgic review of lymph nodes for metastatic breast cancer. Am J Surg Pathol 42(12):1636–1645. https://doi.org/10.1097/PAS.0000000000001151
65. Vesal S, Ravikumar N, Davari A, Ellmann S, Maier A (2018) Classification of breast cancer histology images using transfer learning. In: Proceedings of 2019 16th international Bhurban conference on applied sciences and technology, IBCAST 2019, pp 328–332
66. Liu Y, Kohlberger T, Norouzi M, Dahl GE, Smith JL, Mohtashamian A, Olson N, Peng LH, Hipp JD, Stumpe MC (2019) Artificial intelligence–based breast cancer nodal metastasis detection: insights into the black box for pathologists. Arch Pathol Lab Med 143(7):859–868. https://doi.org/10.5858/arpa.2018-0147-OA
67. An SJ, Kim TJ, Yoon BW (2017) Epidemiology, risk factors, and clinical features of intracerebral haemorrhage: an update. J Stroke 19(1):3–10. https://doi.org/10.5853/jos.2016.00864

68. Counsell C, Boonyakarnkul S, Dennis M, Sandercock P, Bamford J, Burn J, Warlow C (1995) Primary intracerebral haemorrhage in the Oxfordshire community stroke project: prognosis. Cerebrovasc Dis 5(1):26–34. https://doi.org/10.1159/000107814
69. Zia E, Engström G, Svensson PJ, Norrving B, Pessah-Rasmussen H (2009) Three-year survival and stroke recurrence rates in patients with primary intracerebral haemorrhage. Stroke 40(11): 3567–3573. https://doi.org/10.1161/STROKEAHA.109.556324
70. Kowalski RG (2004) Initial misdiagnosis and outcome after subarachnoid haemorrhage. JAMA 291(7):866. https://doi.org/10.1001/jama.291.7.866
71. Vermeulen MJ, Schull MJ (2007) Missed diagnosis of subarachnoid haemorrhage in the emergency department. Stroke 38(4):1216–1221. https://doi.org/10.1161/01.STR.0000259661.05525.9a10.1109/IBCAST.2019.8667221
72. Watanabe Y, Tanaka T, Nishida A, Takahashi H, Fujiwara M, Fujiwara T, Arisawa A, Yano H, Tomiyama N, Nakamura H, Todo K, Yoshiya K (2020) Improvement of the diagnostic accuracy for intracranial haemorrhage using deep learning–based computer-assisted detection. Neuroradiology. https://doi.org/10.1007/s00234-020-02566-x
73. Arbabshirani MR, Fornwalt BK, Mongelluzzo GJ, Suever JD, Geise BD, Patel AA, Moore GJ (2018) Advanced machine learning in action: identification of intracranial haemorrhage on computed tomography scans of the head with clinical workflow integration. Npj Dig Med 1(1): 9. https://doi.org/10.1038/s41746-017-0015-z
74. Arab A, Chinda B, Medvedev G, Siu W, Guo H, Gu T, Moreno S, Hamarneh G, Ester M, Song X (2020) A fast and fully-automated deep-learning approach for accurate haemorrhage segmentation and volume quantification in non-contrast whole-head CT. Sci Rep 10(1):1–12. https://doi.org/10.1038/s41598-020-76459-7
75. Majumdar A, Brattain L, Telfer B, Farris C, Scalera J (2018) Detecting intracranial haemorrhage with deep learning. In: Proceedings of the annual international conference of the IEEE engineering in medicine and biology society, EMBS, 2018-July, pp 583–587. https://doi.org/10.1109/EMBC.2018.8512336
76. Chilamkurthy S, Ghosh R, Tanamala S, Biviji M, Campeau NG, Venugopal VK, Mahajan V, Rao P, Warier P (2018) Deep learning algorithms for detection of critical findings in head CT scans: a retrospective study. Lancet 392(10162):2388–2396. https://doi.org/10.1016/S0140-6736(18)31645-3
77. Rava RA, Seymour SE, LaQue ME, Peterson BA, Snyder KV, Mokin M, Waqas M, Hoi Y, Davies JM, Levy EI, Siddiqui AH, Ionita CN (2021) Assessment of an artificial intelligence algorithm for detection of intracranial haemorrhage. World Neurosurg 150:e209–e217. https://doi.org/10.1016/j.wneu.2021.02.134
78. Cho J, Park KS, Karki M, Lee E, Ko S, Kim JK, Lee D, Choe J, Son J, Kim M, Lee S, Lee J, Yoon C, Park S (2019) Improving sensitivity on identification and delineation of intracranial haemorrhage lesion using cascaded deep learning models. J Digit Imaging 32(3):450–461. https://doi.org/10.1007/s10278-018-00172-1
79. Ye H, Gao F, Yin Y, Guo D, Zhao P, Lu Y, Wang X, Bai J, Cao K, Song Q, Zhang H, Chen W, Guo X, Xia J (2019) Precise diagnosis of intracranial haemorrhage and subtypes using a three-dimensional joint convolutional and recurrent neural network. Eur Radiol 29(11):6191–6201. https://doi.org/10.1007/s00330-019-06163-2
80. Rao B, Zohrabian V, Cedeno P, Saha A, Pahade J, Davis MA (2021) Utility of artificial intelligence tool as a prospective radiology peer reviewer—detection of unreported intracranial haemorrhage. Acad Radiol 28(1):85–93. https://doi.org/10.1016/j.acra.2020.01.035
81. Kuo W, Häne C, Mukherjee P, Malik J, Yuh EL (2019) Expert-level detection of acute intracranial haemorrhage on head computed tomography using deep learning. Proc Natl Acad Sci U S A 116(45):22737–22745. https://doi.org/10.1073/pnas.1908021116
82. Chang PD, Kuoy E, Grinband J, Weinberg BD, Thompson M, Homo R, Chen J, Abcede H, Shafie M, Sugrue L, Filippi CG, Su MY, Yu W, Hess C, Chow D (2018) Hybrid 3D/2D convolutional neural network for haemorrhage evaluation on head CT. Am J Neuroradiol 39(9): 1609–1616. https://doi.org/10.3174/ajnr.A5742

83. Danilov G, Kotik K, Negreeva A, Tsukanova T, Shifrin M, Zakharova N, Batalov A, Pronin I, Potapov A (2020) Classification of intracranial haemorrhage subtypes using deep learning on CT scans. Stud Health Technol Inform 272:370–373. https://doi.org/10.3233/SHTI200572
84. Ker J, Singh SP, Bai Y, Rao J, Lim T, Wang L (2019) Image thresholding improves 3-dimensional convolutional neural network diagnosis of different acute brain haemorrhages on computed tomography scans. Sensors (Switzerland) 19(9). https://doi.org/10.3390/s19092167
85. Ko H, Chung H, Lee H, Lee J (2020) Feasible study on intracranial haemorrhage detection and classification using a CNN-LSTM network. In: Proceedings of the annual international conference of the IEEE engineering in medicine and biology society, EMBS, 2020-July, pp 1290–1293. https://doi.org/10.1109/EMBC44109.2020.9176162
86. Lee H, Sehyo Y, Mohammad M, Myeongchan K, Shahein HT, Claude EG, Sarah AE et al. (2019) An explainable deep-learning algorithm for the detection of acute intracranial haemorrhage from small datasets. Nature biomedical engineering 3(3):173–182
87. Hssayeni MD, Croock MS, Salman AD, Al-Khafaji HF, Yahya ZA, Ghoraani B (2020) Intracranial haemorrhage segmentation using a deep convolutional model. Data 5(1):1–18. https://doi.org/10.3390/data5010014
88. Zhao X, Kaixing C, Ge W, Guyue Z, Xin Z, Chuanfeng L, Shiman W, Yun C, Guotong X, and Zhenwei Y et al. (2021) Deep learning shows good reliability for automatic segmentation and volume measurement of brain hemorrhage, intraventricular extension, and peripheral edema. European Radiology 31(7):5012–5020
89. Xu J, Rongguo Z, Zijian Z, Chunxue W, Qiang G, Huiling Z, Shuang W et al. (2021) Deep network for the automatic segmentation and quantification of intracranial hemorrhage on CT. Frontiers in Neuroscience 1084
90. Ironside N, Chen CJ, Mutasa S, Sim JL, Marfatia S, Roh D, Ding D, Mayer SA, Lignelli A, Connolly ES (2019) Fully automated segmentation algorithm for hematoma volumetric analysis in spontaneous intracerebral haemorrhage. Stroke 50(12):3416–3423. https://doi.org/10.1161/STROKEAHA.119.026561

Chapter 2
Detection of Breast Cancer Masses in Mammogram Images with Watershed Segmentation and Machine Learning Approach

Amanpreet Kaur, Mamoon Rashid, Ali Kashif Bashir, and Shabir Ahmad Parah

Contents

A. Kaur
School of Computer Science & Engineering, Lovely Professional University, Jalandhar, India

M. Rashid (✉)
Department of Computer Engineering, Faculty of Science and Technology, Vishwakarma University, Pune, India

A. K. Bashir
Department of Computing and Mathematics, Manchester Metropolitan University, Manchester, UK

S. A. Parah
PG Department of Electronics and Instrumentation Technology, University of Kashmir, Srinagar, India

S. A. Parah et al. (eds.), *Artificial Intelligence for Innovative Healthcare Informatics*,
https://doi.org/10.1007/978-3-030-96569-3_2

1 Introduction

In Healthcare systems, the wrong diagnosis of diseases is one of the reasons for increasing death rates in the world. Breast Cancer is one such disease that is a great challenge in healthcare systems at present. According to the reports published by the World Health Organization, 23% growth related cases and 14% of tumors in women occur due to breast malignancy [1]. Mammography is among the most commonly used screening process and analytic software in clinical and scientific fields. Mammography is considered the most widespread verification and analytic resource in specialized medical and clinical fields [2]. To analyze such mammograms that are daily generated in hospitals become a challenge for the radiologists to go through all the images whole day long and can also lead to several errors in diagnosis by a physician, so a computer-aided diagnosis system is developed to reduce the radiologist's diagnosis time and accuracy, thus improving the physician's ability to predict cancer at an early stage and recommending for further biopsies and treatment.

As advances have been made in the medical field, many computational systems have been developed to help healthcare professionals in interpreting the tasks that are related to radiological imaging [3–7]. The development of Computer-Aided Design (CAD) systems contributed to the age of modern medicine and is presently considered an important source of information. These systems helped in achieving higher success rates in the identification of various diseases like breast cancer [8]. For its contributions in detecting breast cancer, Computer-Aided Design (CAD) systems improved images to reduce the unwanted noise particles and enhance an image by improving the contrast and differentiating the foreground and background area thus helping in differentiating benign and malignant lesions. However, the better performance in CAD systems largely depends on the methods and techniques that are applied extracting features and performing its segmentation.

Various research works are present in state-of-art that have contributed to detecting masses in breast cancer from mammogram images. Based on various studies, the major indicators of breast cancer in mammogram images are micro-calcifications and masses. It is always challenging to interpret these abnormalities due to their low commonness [9]. Moreover, due to the large generation of mammogram volume in images, the concerned radiologists get flooded in screening these images with the best performance. Existing research studies suggest that it is more difficult to handle masses in mammogram images than micro-calcifications due to the varying properties of masses. A major challenge in mammogram image masses is their variable nature in terms of size, shape, and margins and as a result, turn into uncertain boundaries [10]. Due to these uncertain boundaries, there are high chances for radiologists to miss portions carrying visible masses.

Machine learning-based approaches are one of the cost-effective and best choices for diagnosing mammographic masses. These approaches first perform segmentation in mammogram images into several regions and then do extraction of features out of these regions. Finally, the extracted features are labeled into masses and normal tissues, and then a machine learning classifier is trained for these features for efficient detection of masses wherever found in images [11]. However, it is often challenging for classifiers to model all masses in training data for feeding all experiences for efficient results. Moreover, the presence of uncertain boundaries is always going to give a challenge for achieving better performance in mass detection. Therefore, there is a need for an efficient machine learning model that will help the healthcare sector in providing solutions for these challenges.

Based on the above challenges, we highlight the main contributions of the chapter as follows:

1. Pre-processing of mammogram images is done using median filter and morphological operations. The enhanced resulting images are passed through contour segmentation where a region of interest is segmented using watershed segmentation technique and then features are extracted using random forest.
2. Proposing a hybrid machine learning classification model based on MLP, J48, and K-Means for the detection of masses in breast cancer with high accuracy.
3. To compare validated results of our model with state of the art for evaluating the performance of our model in terms of Precision, Recall, and F-Measure.
4. To validate results achieved by the proposed model using ANOVA for determining the amount of change.

The rest of the chapter is organized as: Sect. 2 discusses the background that has been carried out in the related work. Further, Sect. 3 includes the methods and materials with dataset description and various segmentation techniques used in this chapter. Section 4 is regarding the proposed work approach that is used to implement this research, Sect. 5 provides us the performance evaluation of the proposed model and the achieved results, and their comparison is given in Sect. 6. Section 7 comes up with a conclusion and future directions.

2 Background

Data preprocessing approaches are used for noise reduction, data normalization, and transformation and outlier detection, etc. and this approach is put in practice before the classification approach [12]. Image segmentation is an important step to assist breast cancer diagnosis or prognosis of breast masses in mammography. Finding contour mass is the key factor for correct mass interpretation. In recent years, numerous studies have aimed to the early prognosis or diagnosis of cancers of the breast via image processing and pattern recognition methods [13]. For mass recognition, detection of suspicious lesion and (ROI) Region of interest is extracted to distinguish ROI between normal, benign and malignant cases. Several types of research have been carried over feature extraction and classification over the years [14]. The framework to build a group of edge-stop characteristics is recommended regarding the edge-based contour model to segment objects along with inadequately defined boundaries [15]. Experiments were conducted on medical images using the distance regularized level set for edge-based active contour models and its effectiveness is measured using k-nearest neighbors and the support vector machine. A marker-controlled segmentation approach is introduced to find breast cancer [16]. Experiments were conducted on the MIAS dataset providing the overall detection accuracy rate of 90% to overcome the limitation of watershed technique i.e. over-segmentation. To overcome this limitation curvelet transform at the pre-processing step is used. A new segmentation technique of single and multi-resolution remote sensing images is proposed [17]. Watershed used to gain the fine details and thus helping to limit. Evaluations results provide through experiments indicate the better and precise accuracy measure of segmentation technique [18]. A neural network model for classification and proper diagnosis of breast cancer and benign disease for breast biopsy is developed to make predictions providing overall 89.64% accuracy [19]. Radial Basis Function Neural Network classification technique is proposed for mammograms to classify normal and abnormal breasts providing an accuracy of 93.98% [20]. A novel machine learning model is proposed for predicting breast cancer metastasis [21]. This research claims that this model has the potential of predicting breast cancer before the timeline of 3 months. An attempt is made to distinguish subtypes in breast cancer molecules using deep learning models [22]. This research concluded that deep learning methods play a vital role in the discovery of radio genomic links in breast cancer. An attempt is made to check whether machine learning will reduce the number of mammograms for helping radiologists in their interpretation [23]. This research concluded that there is a reduction in the number of mammograms with a machine learning approach which is needed for radiologists without affecting the accuracy required for diagnosis. The breast cancer diagnosis model is proposed by combining 12 support vector machines [24]. This research claims that this model of ensemble outperforms other models in its start-of-art. A novel intelligent model is proposed for the diagnosis of breast cancer with the consideration of the misclassification cost of breast cancer [25]. This research shows the efficiency of their model by using Genetic Algorithm wrapper and performed feature selection in terms of the CSSVM method. The classification model is developed for classifying mammograms using SVM Classifier [26]. This research has used a Hough Transform for the feature selection of mammograms. This research further claims that their proposed model is quite effective for an abnormal type of mammogram. The deficiencies in the watershed algorithm for the application of input images are improved by pre-processing this using Curvelet Transform. This transform improves the contrast of images that are usually present in the degraded form [27]. Curvelet Transform-based adaptive algorithm has been proposed for image denoising for the removal of noise from digital images to improve their efficiency and performance. This research claims an increased performance for image denoising of enhanced images by 0.044 for random noise [28]. Different types of classifiers have been applied for mammogram images for raising their accuracy. Classifiers of Decision Trees, Fuzzy K-Nearest Neighbor, Naïve Bayes, Ensemble, and Support Vector Machine are applied for mammogram images. For each kind of classifier, results are shown in terms of sensitivity and specificity [29]. Marker Controlled Watershed method has been used for image segmentation for tracking cell nuclei. This research claims an accuracy of 98.8% for the segmentation process [30]. The breast mass tumor model has been developed with marker-controlled watershed segmentation. This research claims an accuracy of 90% for the detection of mass tumors when applied for the Mammographic Image Analysis Society dataset [31]. Tomosynthesis is combined with mammography for better performance in terms of breast screening [26]. Mammographic Risk Scoring and Segmentation of Breast Density is done with a Deep Learning unsupervised model [32]. Computer-aided detection for mammographic lesions is done with the help of a deep learning model using the Convolutional Neural Network [33]. An attempt is made to predict health care diseases with the help of a hybrid machine learning model and analyze the previous history of patients with diseases for effective solutions [34]. Deep Convolutional Neural Network is used for developing a Computer-Aided Detection System for the prediction of masses in breast images [35–37]. Classification and detection of lesions are done in mammogram images by developing a model in deep learning. This work has achieved high sensitivity with less false positive marks for each image [38–41].

Based on the various studies discussed in this section, we can clearly verify the need of detecting masses in mammogram images of breasts. The use of several machine learning techniques with an emphasis on feature extraction is carried out for improving the tissue characterization and helping in classifying them into normal tissues and masses. So it will be interesting to propose a novel approach for segmenting tissue images for better feature extraction and then classifying them for the detection of masses.

3 Methods and Materials

This section describes the various methods and materials to be used for the proposed methodology. Firstly, the dataset mammogram images are submitted to pre-processing techniques which reduce unwanted distortions using filtering techniques. Next, the features in each region of interest are extracted. Finally, the proposed hybrid classifier is used to train the model for a prepared dataset for the detection of Breast Cancer.

3.1 Dataset

In this work, the authors used the Mammographic mass dataset, taken from the publicly available online database site UCI Machine Learning Repository [35]. This dataset contains mammographic information regarding breast cancer clinical instances, collected at the Institute of Radiology of the University between 2003 and 2006. This database comprises a total of 961 clinical instances, out of which there are 516 benign cases and 445 malignant cases. Among the list of

Table 2.1 Mammographic mass dataset attributes

Attributes	Range
BIRADS	1–5 BIRADS categories ordinal and non-predictive
Age	Patients age
Shape	Round = 1, Oval = 2, Lobular = 3, Irregular = 4
Margin	Circumscribed = 1, Microlobulated = 2, Obscured = 3, Ill-defined = 4, Spiculated = 5
Density	High density = 1, Iso density = 2, Low density = 3, Fat-containing density = 4
Severity	Benign case = 0; Malignant case = 1

961 specialized medical instances, there are a variety of instances with five attributes of shape, density, BIRADS, patient's age, and margin described in Table 2.1.

3.2 Data Preprocessing

A mammographic image is submitted for a pre-processing step to enhance its features. As mammograms take time and effort to interpret, preprocessing will be needed to increase the quality of an image and also to make the feature extraction and segmentation stages easier and reliable. This stage is normally used for noise-reduction to improve image so that we are able to detect the worrisome features more accurately. In this chapter, an efficient median filter is applied to the image for reducing noise and enhancing image features. The flow of pre-processing is summed up in Fig. 2.1.

3.3 Segmentation

Segmentation is the process of dividing the image into smaller parts based on some criteria. The segmentation is performed when it is getting from the previous steps. The aim of segmentation is to assign a value to each pixel.

3.3.1 Morphological Operation

Morphological procedures are related to the form or characteristics of the image. These kinds of procedures rely solely on the ordering of pixel valuations and are therefore suited for binary image evaluation and greyscale images. Consider binary image B (u, v) which is computed using dilation and then subtraction in the form of Eqs. (2.1 and 2.2):

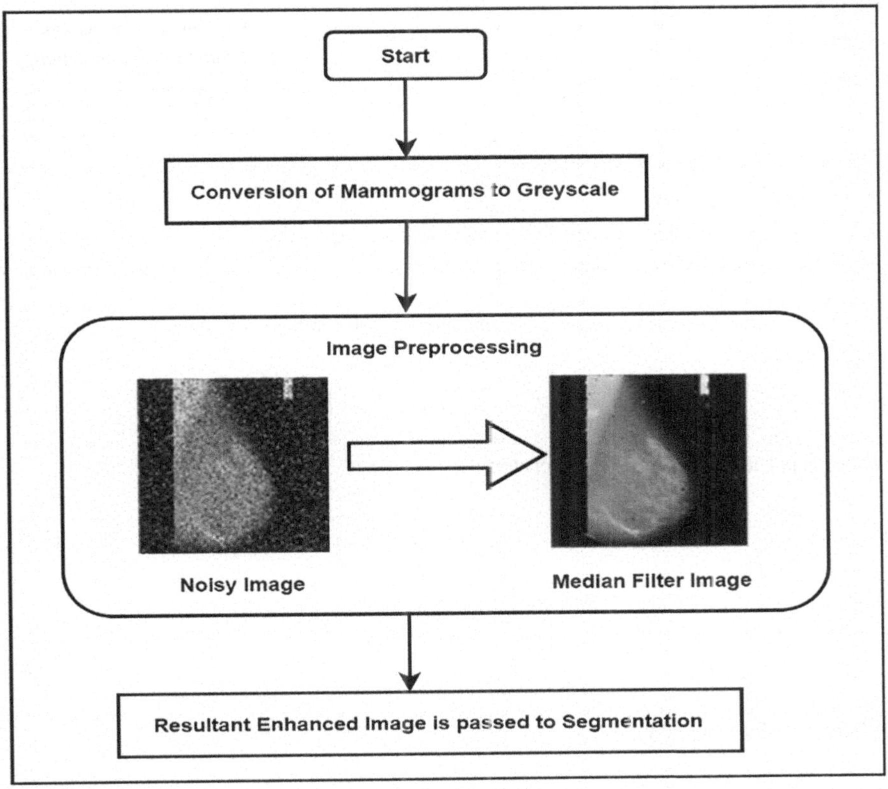

Fig. 2.1 Preprocessing of mammogram images

$$I' = I \ominus H \tag{2.1}$$

$$B\,(u, v) = XOR\,(I'\,(u, v), I\,(u, v)) \tag{2.2}$$

3.3.2 Active Contour Model

Active contour model is energy-based function and is defined in Eq. (2.3) as:

$$E_{snake} = E_{co} + E_{cu} + E_i \tag{2.3}$$

Where E_{co} *and* E_{cu} corresponded to the internal energy, while the E_i corresponded to the external one. The description of parameters used in Eq. (2.3) is given in Table 2.2.

Considering set of snaxels $= \{s_1, s_2, \ldots\ldots\ s_N\}$, the partial energy is given in Eqs. (2.4–2.7) as given below:

Table 2.2 Description of parameters

E_{co}	Contour continuity energy
E_{cu}	Contour curvature energy
E_i	Image energy

Table 2.3 Weight factor descriptions

Parameters	Description
α	Responsible for contour continuity in that a high value
β	Responsible for snake corners in that a high value for a specific snaxel made the angle
γ	Responsible for making snaxels more sensitive to the image energy

$$E_{co} = \left| \overline{\delta} - |s_i - s_{i-1}| \right| \tag{2.4}$$

where $\overline{\delta}$ is the average distance covered.

$$E_{cu} = |s_{i-1} - 2s_i + s_{i+1}|^2 \tag{2.5}$$

And

$$E_i = -|\nabla I|^2 \tag{2.6}$$

Where I is the intensity

$$E_{snake,i} = \alpha E_{cont,i} + \beta E_{curv,i} + \gamma E_{image,i} \tag{2.7}$$

where α, β *and* γ are appropriate weighting factors. The description of these parameters is given in Table 2.3.

3.3.3 Watershed Segmentation

Watershed Segmentation is based on visualizing a gray-level image as a topographic surface with three dimensions: two special coordinates versus intensity and in this segmentation gradient magnitude of the image is to be considered as the topographic surface. It aims to locate regions of high-intensity gradients (watersheds) that divide neighbored local minima (basins). Markers are the local minima with the gradient and this will include the problem of over-segmentation that involves region merging. Over segmentation will be a vital dilemma associated with watershed transformation. To prevent this dilemma, a technique known as marker-controlled watershed segmentation is considered. It is a robust and flexible method for segmenting objects with closed contours. The marker-controlled watershed segmentation is shown in Fig. 2.2.

Marker-Controlled Watershed Segmentation uses the following basic procedure:

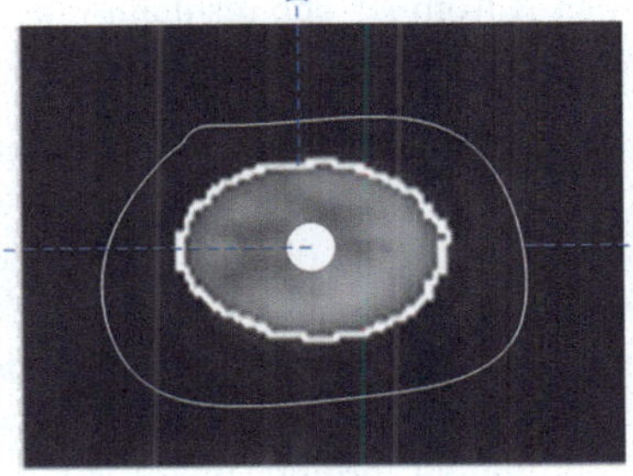

Fig. 2.2 Marker-controlled watershed segmentation

Table 2.4 Gradient parameters

$I_{gradient}$	Gradient magnitude of the image
I	Source image
*	Symbol of the convolution operation

1. Calculate the segmentation function. It deems an impression where darker areas would be the materials which an individual wants to segment. The main purpose of this step is to generate gradient magnitude images that are to be used for later segmentation steps. Gradient magnitude is computed with the original step image which is denoted as $I_{gradient}$. The Sobel operator is utilized to evaluate this gradient within vertical and horizontal directions in terms of Eqs. (2.8–2.10)

$$g_x = \begin{bmatrix} 1 & 0 & 1 \\ 2 & 0 & -2 \\ 1 & 0 & -1 \end{bmatrix} * I \tag{2.8}$$

$$g_y = \begin{bmatrix} 1 & 2 & 1 \\ 0 & 0 & 0 \\ -1 & -2 & -1 \end{bmatrix} * I \tag{2.9}$$

$$I_{gradient} = \sqrt{{g_x}^2 + {g_y}^2} \tag{2.10}$$

   The description of parameters in Eqs. (2.8–2.10) is given in Table 2.4.
2. Determine the foreground markers. They are connected blobs regarding pixels within every single object. The steps are given below:

   (a) First, apply morphological opening to the image I. This step will reduce the additional and preserve the required objects. Denote it with I_o
   (b) Then erosion to the opening image is applied to result in an eroded image I_E. This step will separate all the connected objects as a result.

(c) Reconstruct the image taking I_E as a marker and I_o as a mask. The resultant image will be denoted as I_r
(d) Subtract I_r from I_o. The resultant image will be I_s.

3. Next, the morphological dilation operation is performed on the eroded image I_E denoted as I_D. The result acquired can be considered internal markers that have marked almost all of the objects and are denoted as I_{in}.
4. Next, evaluate external markers from the image I_{in}. Exterior marker (EM) represents the background surrounding spot whose purpose is to limit affected areas and specific zones of the inner marker. The actual EM can be immediately bought through firstly computing a Euclidean long-distance transform with the binary IM of picture B and then putting on watershed transform towards the long-distance transform of B. External indicators are computed from a result of watershed rigid lines.

$$D(x_i, y_i) = 0, \text{If } O(x_i, y_i) = 1 \tag{2.11}$$

$$D(x_i, y_i) = \sqrt{\left[(x_i - x_j)^2 + (y_i - y_j)^2\right]}, \text{If } O(x_i, y_i) = 0 \tag{2.12}$$

5. Morphological gradient and Minima imposition: Combine I_{in} with I_{em} and get the final marker image I_{MA}. Now, modified gradient magnitude image I_{Modify} is acquired using minimal imposition technique on $I_{gradient}$. The purpose of minima imposition is to remove false minima. The modified gradient magnitude image I_{Modify} is computed by using Eqs. (2.11–2.13)

$$I_{Modify} = R^{\varepsilon}{}_{\left(I_{gradient}+1\right)\wedge I_M}(I_M) \tag{2.13}$$

Where $R^{\varepsilon}{}_{\left(I_{gradient}+1\right)\wedge I_M}(I_M)$ represents the morphological erosion reconstruction of I_M from ($I_{gradient}$ + 1) ∧ I_M, and symbol ∧ represents point-wise minimum between $I_{gradient}$ + 1 and I_M.

Finally, after applying the watershed transform to I_{Modify} reasonably segmented phase image I_{obj} is obtained.

4 Proposed Approach

This section includes a description of the proposed methodology.

1. Firstly, pre-processing of mammogram images is done using median filter and morphological operations. The enhanced resulting images are passed through

contour segmentation where a region of interest is segmented using watershed segmentation technique and then features are extracted using random forest.

2. Secondly, a hybrid machine learning classification model based on MLP, J48, and K-Means is proposed for the detection of masses in breast cancer with high accuracy.
3. Results of our hybrid machine learning model are compared with state-of-the-art for evaluating the performance of our model in terms of Precision, Recall, and F-Measure. Later, Analysis of Variance (ANOVA) is used to evaluate the significant change in performance measures.

4.1 Hybrid K-Mean and J48 Based Classification

The steps involved in clustering the Mammogram images by the k-Means algorithm and Decision Tree Classification Algorithm j48 are given below.

Pseudocode

Load a mammographic mass database

Select the initial partition of the dataset taken into k clusters such that $\{c_1 \ldots\ldots c_k\}$

Evaluate cluster centroids $\overline{w} = \sum_{j=1}^{k_i} w_{ij}$ where

i = 1.....k

For each w_i *in dataset instances do*

Reallocate w_i *to the cluster close to it,* $w_i \in C_s$

And C_s *moved to* C_t , If

$\| w_i - \overline{w_t} \| < \| w_i - \overline{w_j}$, j = 1 ....k and j $\neq$ s

Re-evaluate centroids

Stop once cluster membership is stabilized

Apply Decision tree (C_t, A, T)

If C_t includes the training data evaluation for the same class $s_j \in S$ instances then,

make decision tree T with the same class s_j

Elseif $A = \varnothing$ then

make t_d into a leaf node s_j, the most frequent class in C_t

else

$\rho_0 = \textit{Impurity evaluation} - 1(C_t)$

For all attributes $a_K \in a_1, a_2 \ldots\ldots a_K$ do

$\rho_1 = \textit{Impurity evaluation} - 2(a_k, C_t)$

End

Select $a_g \in a_1, a_2 \ldots\ldots a_K$ providing biggest impurity reduction through $\rho_0 - \rho_1$

If $\rho_0 - \rho_1 < \textit{threshold}$

Make T leaf node label as s_j

Else

Make T a decision node on a_g

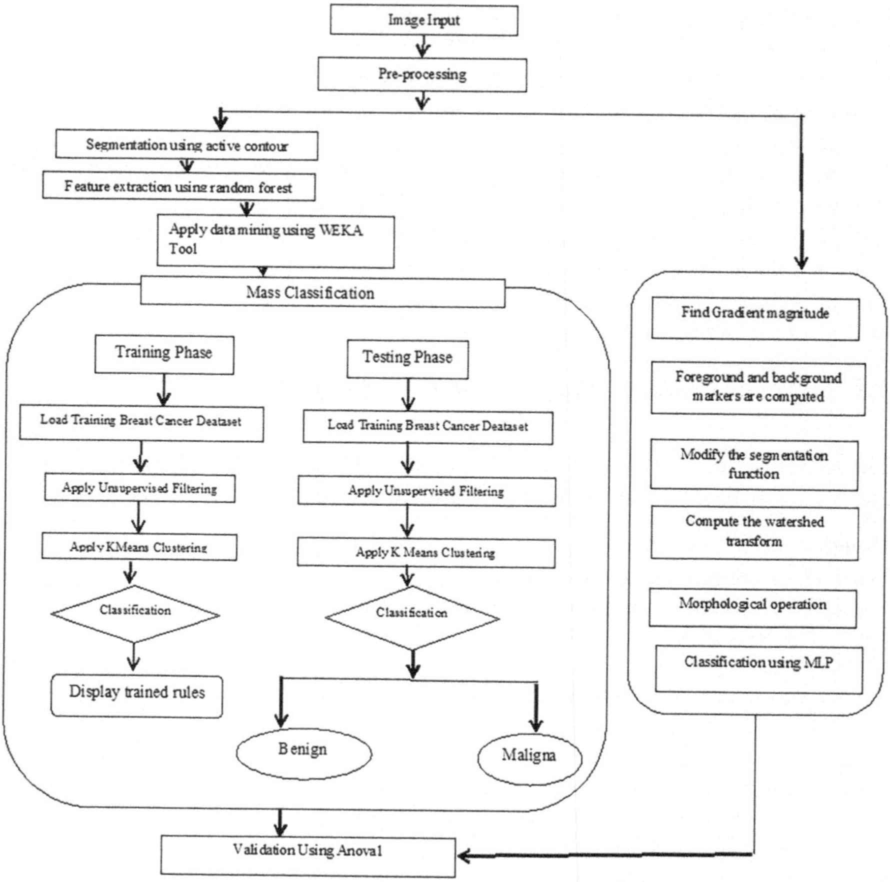

Fig. 2.3 Overall methodology of proposed work for the prediction of breast cancer

$V_1 \quad V_2 \ldots\ldots V_n$ be the possible values of a_g
Divide C_t into n subsets.
Divide to subset $C_{t1} \quad C_{t2} \ldots\ldots C_{tn}$ based on the possible values of a_g
For each C_{tj} *in* $C_{t1} \quad C_{t2} \ldots\ldots C_{tn}$ do
If $C_{tj} \neq \varnothing$ then
Create edge node t_J for v_j as a child node of t_d
Decision tree $(C_{tj}, A - \{a_g\}, t_j)$ // here a_g removed
End
End
End
End

The overall methodology of the proposed work is outlined in Fig. 2.3.

5 Performance Evaluation

The performance of the classifier is shown in the form of a confusion matrix as the output. A confusion matrix encompasses information about actual and forecast classifications done by a cataloging method.

Kappa Statistics Kappa is a quantitative measure of the agreement for chance agreement. Kappa provides a numerical rating of the degree. The actual calculation is usually the good distinction between how many agreements will be found as compared to how much agreement would be in the expected one. Kappa Statistics can be computed with the formula given in Eq. (2.14).

$$k = \frac{p(a) - p(e)}{1 - P(e)} \tag{2.14}$$

The description of parameters in Eq. (2.14) is given in Table 2.5:

Table 2.6 represents the performance evaluation of kappa statistics of multilayer perceptron + feature extraction (FE) using contours, k-mean + j48 + FE using contours, and watershed segmentation with multilayer perceptron (MLP). The results evaluated are tested using anova1. This testing indicates that in terms of significant change, watershed segmentation with MLP indicates that it is significant in terms of kappa statistics as the p-value for these results is less than 0.005.

The Anova Table for Kappa Statistics is given in Table 2.7.

Table 2.5 Kappa statistics parameters

p (a)	Percentage agreement
p (e)	Chance agreement
k = 1	Specify complete agreement
k = 0	Specify chance of agreement

Table 2.6 Evaluation measure of kappa statistics

Images	MLP + FE using contour	Watershed with MLP	k-mean + j48 + FE using contour
Image 1	0.72428	0.81424	0.81416
Image 2	0.70032	0.7657	0.8137
Image 3	0.85922	0.80818	0.88
Image 4	0.658	0.78416	0.80128
Image 5	0.70018	0.8261	0.81428
Image 6	0.66982	0.85588	0.86804
Image 7	0.69464	0.80814	0.77206
Image 8	0.69318	0.82006	0.86814
Image 9	0.66504	0.814	0.84922
Image 10	0.71192	0.8619	0.79608

Table 2.7 Anova table for kappa statistics

Source	SS	DF	MS	F	Prob > F
Columns	0.0875	2	0.04375	**24.22**	0.45377e−007
Error	0.04877	27	0.00181		
Total	0.13628	29			

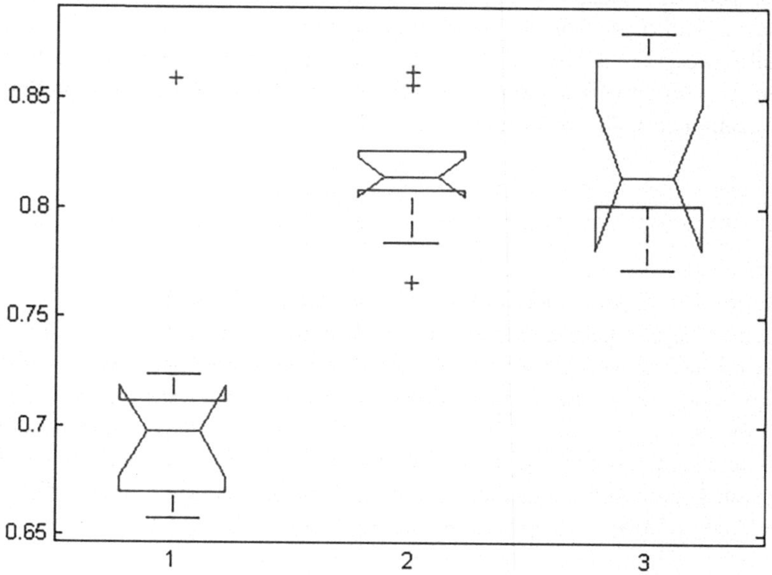

Fig. 2.4 Comparison graph of kappa statistics indicating significant change for different techniques used for evaluation

Table 2.7 represents the ANOVA analysis. The P-value 0.45377e−007 is less than the 5% confidence threshold indicating that the null hypothesis has been refuted. The results of ANOVA testing are visually represented in Fig. 2.4.

Mean Absolute Error The mean absolute error (MAE) is a quantity used to measure predictions of the eventual outcomes. The mean absolute error is given in Eq. (2.15) as

$$\mathrm{MAE} = \frac{1}{n}\sum\nolimits_{i=1}^{n} |f_i - y_i| = \frac{1}{n}\sum\nolimits_{i=1}^{n} |e_i| \tag{2.15}$$

Where $e_i = |f_i - y_i|$ and f_i = prediction, y_i = true value.

Table 2.8 represents the performance evaluation of mean absolute error of multilayer perceptron + feature extraction (FE) using contours, k-mean + j48 + FE using contours, and watershed segmentation with multilayer perceptron (MLP). The results evaluated are tested using anova1. This testing indicates that in terms of

Table 2.8 Evaluation measure of mean absolute error

Images	MLP + FE using contour	Watershed with MLP	k-mean + j48 + FE using contour
Image 1	0.3257	0.29248	0.069
Image 2	0.3211	0.29918	0.0963
Image 3	0.3272	0.29699	0.1197
Image 4	0.32826	0.29786	0.1926
Image 5	0.3187	0.2939	0.08868
Image 6	0.32254	0.29416	0.06804
Image 7	0.27712	0.29736	0.14078
Image 8	0.32438	0.29708	0.0678
Image 9	0.32088	0.29696	0.08308
Image 10	0.32212	0.2925	0.09548

Table 2.9 Anova table for mean absolute error

Source	SS	DF	MS	F	Prob > F
Columns	0.28315	2	0.14157	**237.37**	7.35965e−019
Error	0.0161	27	0.0006		
Total	0.29925	29			

significant change, k-mean + j48 + FE using contour indicates that it is significant in terms of mean absolute error as the p-value for these results is less than 0.005.

The Anova Table for Mean Absolute Error is given in Table 2.9.

Table 2.9 represents the ANOVA analysis. The P-value 7.35965e−019 is less than the 5% confidence threshold indicating that the null hypothesis has been accepted. The results of ANOVA testing is visually represented in Fig. 2.5

Misclassification Error The classification error E_j of an individual program j depends on the number of instances that are incorrectly classified and is represented in Eq. (2.16) as:

$$E_j = \frac{F}{n} \times 100 \qquad (2.16)$$

Where f indicates incorrectly classified cases and n is the total number of cases.

Table 2.10 represents the performance evaluation of misclassification error of multilayer perceptron + feature extraction (FE) using contours, k-mean + j48 + FE using contours, and watershed segmentation with multilayer perceptron (MLP). The results evaluated are tested using anova1. This testing indicates that in terms of significant change that k-mean + j48 + FE using contour indicates that it is significant in terms of misclassification error as the p-value for these results is less than 0.005.

The Anova Table for Misclassification Error is given in Table 2.11.

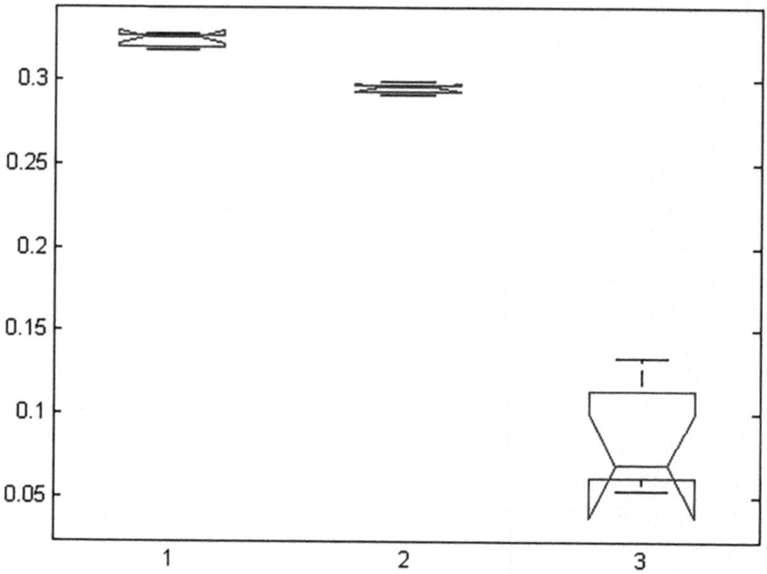

Fig. 2.5 Comparison graph of mean absolute error indicating significant change for different techniques used for evaluation

Table 2.10 Evaluation measure of misclassification error

Images	MLP + FE using contour	Watershed with MLP	k-mean + j48 + FE using contour
Image 1	16	12.4	12.4
Image 2	20	15.6	12.4
Image 3	18	12.8	8
Image 4	22.8	14.4	13.2
Image 5	20	11.6	12.4
Image 6	22	9.6	8.8
Image 7	16	12.4	12.4
Image 8	20.4	12.8	15.2
Image 9	22.4	12.4	10
Image 10	19.2	9.2	13.6

Table 2.11 Anova table for misclassification error

Source	SS	DF	MS	F	Prob > F
Columns	455.851	2	227.925	49.55	9.2076e−010
Error	124.208	27	4.6		
Total	580.059	29			

Table 2.11 represents the ANOVA analysis. The P-value 9.2076e−010 is less than the 5% confidence threshold indicating that the null hypothesis has been refuted. The results of ANOVA testing are visually represented in Fig. 2.6.

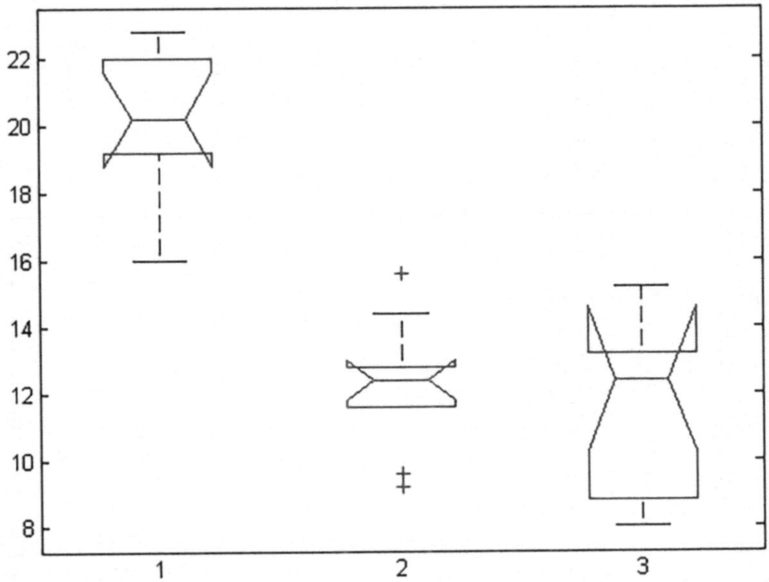

Fig. 2.6 Comparison graph of misclassification error indicating significant change for different techniques used for evaluation

Table 2.12 Evaluation measure of FP rate

Images	MLP + FE using contour	Watershed with MLP	k-mean + j48 + FE using contour
Image 1	0.12	0.0614	0.051
Image 2	0.092	0.0774	0.066
Image 3	0.096	0.0638	0.082
Image 4	0.115	0.0704	0.0678
Image 5	0.0996	0.058	0.0614
Image 6	0.1104	0.0476	0.0436
Image 7	0.1002	0.064	0.0768
Image 8	0.1024	0.0594	0.043
Image 9	0.11	0.0622	0.0514
Image 10	0.0952	0.0464	0.0574

FP Rate The false-positive rate (FP) is the part of negative cases that were inaccurately classified as positive and is calculated using Eq. (2.17) as

$$FP\ Rate = \frac{FP}{FP + TN} \tag{2.17}$$

Table 2.12 represents the performance evaluation of the FP rate of multilayer perceptron + feature extraction (FE) using contours, k-mean + j48 + FE using contours, and watershed segmentation with multilayer perceptron (MLP). The

Table 2.13 Anova table for FP rate

Source	SS	DF	MS	F	Prob > F
Columns	0.01234	2	0.00617	52.44	5.02054e−010
Error	0.00318	27	0.00012		
Total	0.01552	29			

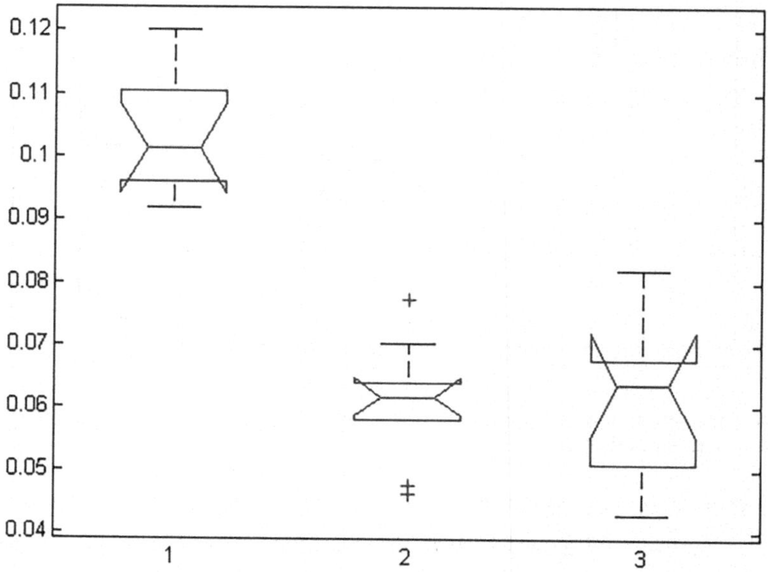

Fig. 2.7 Comparison graph of FP rate indicating significant change for different techniques used for evaluation

results evaluated are tested using anova1. This testing indicates that in terms of significant change, k-mean + j48 + FE using contour indicates that it is significant in terms of FP rate as the p-value for these results is less than 0.005.

The Anova Table for FP is given in Table 2.13.

Table 2.13 represents the ANOVA analysis. The P-value 5.02054e−010 is less than the 5% confidence threshold indicating that the null hypothesis has been accepted widely. The results of ANOVA testing are visually represented in Fig. 2.7.

6 Results and Discussions

In this section, the qualitative feature extraction results of the proposed methodology are shown. An input mammographic image is processed under different stages one by one providing us the enhanced results. Figure 2.8a represents the input image, Fig. 2.8b shows the median filtered image, Fig. 2.8c, d images represent the

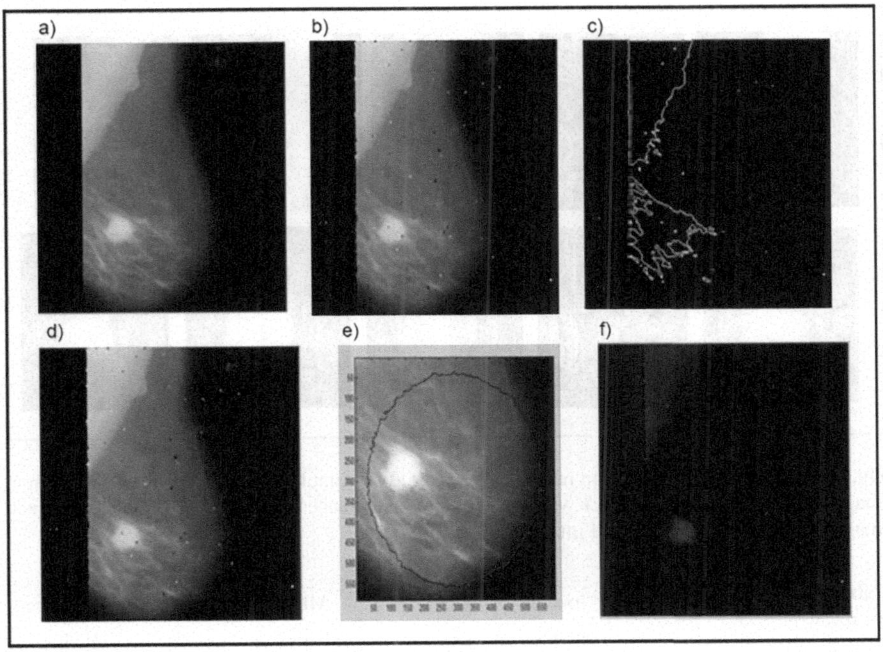

Fig. 2.8 Results evaluated in proposed methodology. (**a**) Input image, (**b**) medium filter image, (**c**) morphological operation, (**d**) morphological operation, (**e**) contour segmentation, (**f**) image with malignant features

morphological operation. These operations describe the pre-processing steps providing an enhanced image. Figure 2.8e represents contour segmentation and Fig. 2.8f represents the image where the malignant features are extracted using decision trees.

The qualitative feature extraction results are shown in Fig. 2.9. Two input mammographic image is processed under watershed segmentation. Figure 2.9a represents an input image, Fig. 2.9b shows the gradient image, Fig. 2.9c represents the watershed of gradient image, Fig. 2.9d represents marker-based region segmented and Fig. 2.9e represents a watershed segmented image.

To evaluate the performance of the results that are obtained for making precise predictions, evaluation criteria in terms of Accuracy, Recall, Precision, and F-measure are considered.

1. **Recall**: Recall deals with the identification of optimistic conditions that suggest the actual percentage with all the different optimistic conditions found and can be computed using Eq. (2.18) as:

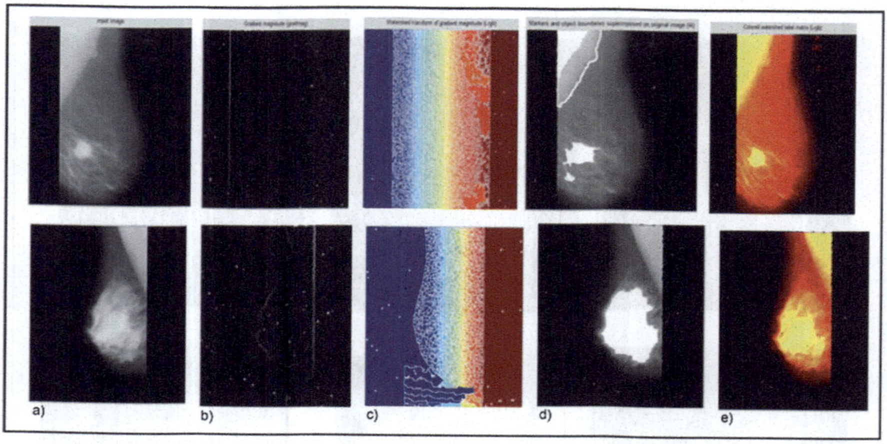

Fig. 2.9 Watershed segmentation results evaluated of two sample mammogram images. (**a**) Input images, (**b**) gradient images, (**c**) watershed of gradient images, (**d**) marked region segmented images, (**e**) watershed segmented images

Table 2.14 Statistical results for recall

Images	MLP	Proposed
Image 1	0.74	0.96
Image 2	0.84	0.9
Image 3	0.76	0.9
Image 4	0.72	0.94
Image 5	0.80	0.92
Image 6	0.72	0.88

$$Re\,call = TP/(TP + FN) \tag{2.18}$$

The evaluation of recall for six images is shown in Table 2.14 and plotted in Fig. 2.10.

2. **Accuracy**: Accuracy deals with the effectiveness of the classifier and is the most commonly used indicator that reflects the precision of results that are predicted and can be computed by Eq. (2.19) as:

$$Accuracy = (TP + TN)/(TP + TN + FP + FN) \tag{2.19}$$

The evaluation of accuracy for six images is shown in Table 2.15 and plotted in Fig. 2.11.

3. **Precision**: Precision, also known as PPV (positive predictive value) deals with the total correct positive predictions divided by the total number of positive predictions as can be computed using Eq. (2.20).

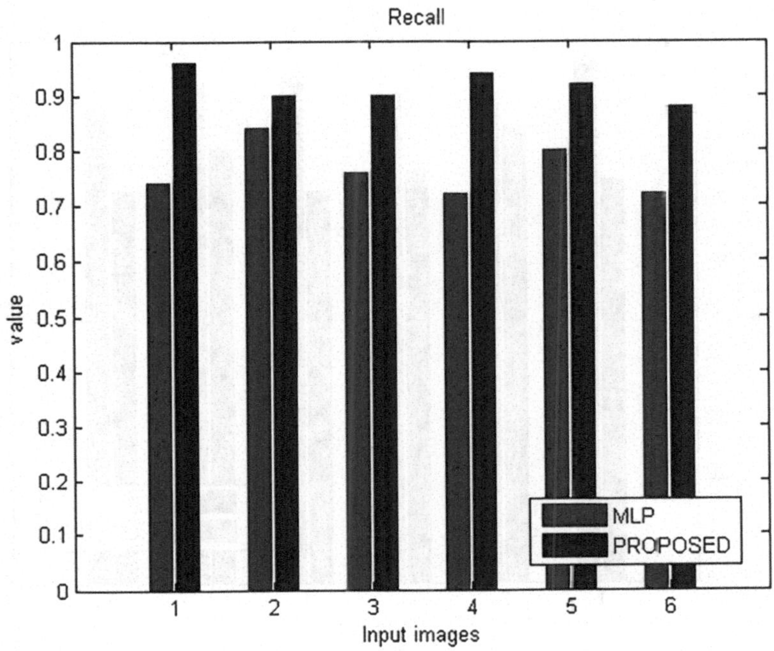

Fig. 2.10 Plot of recall for statistical results of mammogram images

Table 2.15 Statistical results for accuracy

Images	MLP	Proposed
Image 1	74	96
Image 2	84	90
Image 3	76	90
Image 4	72	94
Image 5	80	92
Image 6	72	88

$$Precision = TP/(TP + FP) \tag{2.20}$$

The evaluation of precision for six images is shown in Table 2.16 and plotted in Fig. 2.12.

4. **F-Measure**: The harmonic mean of the recall and precision can be computed by F-measure by Eq. (2.21) as:

$$F\text{-}measure = (2^{*}\mathrm{R}^{*}\mathrm{P})/(\mathrm{R} + \mathrm{P}) \tag{2.21}$$

The evaluation of the F-measure for six images is shown in Table 2.17 and plotted in Fig. 2.13.

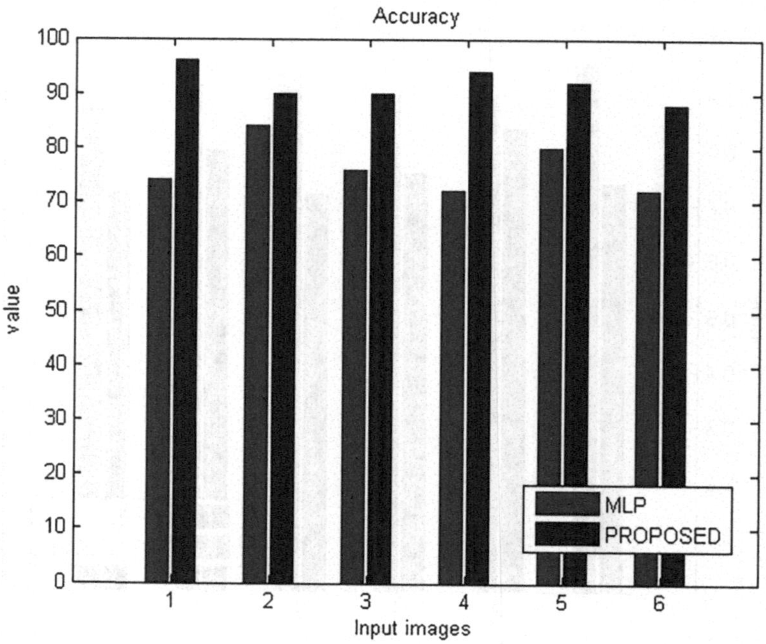

Fig. 2.11 Plot of accuracy for statistical results of mammogram images

Table 2.16 Statistical results for precision

Images	MLP	Proposed
Image 1	0.824	0.96
Image 2	0.85	0.924
Image 3	0.78	0.924
Image 4	0.806	0.949
Image 5	0.847	0.924
Image 6	0.809	0.911

7 Conclusion

Analysis of mammograms is a big challenge for radiologists and often leads to various errors in diagnosis. In this research, the pre-processing mammogram images are done using median filter and morphological operations. The authors used contour segmentation for segmentation of the region of interest using the watershed segmentation technique and then extracted features using random forest. The resultant images are then passed to a hybrid machine learning-based classification model based on Multilayer Perceptron (MLP), Decision Tree (j48), and K-Means for the detection of breast cancer with high accuracy and to eliminate the errors caused due to the manual diagnosis of radiologists. Malignancy is predicted on the mammographic mass dataset containing 961 clinical instances. The comparison of classified

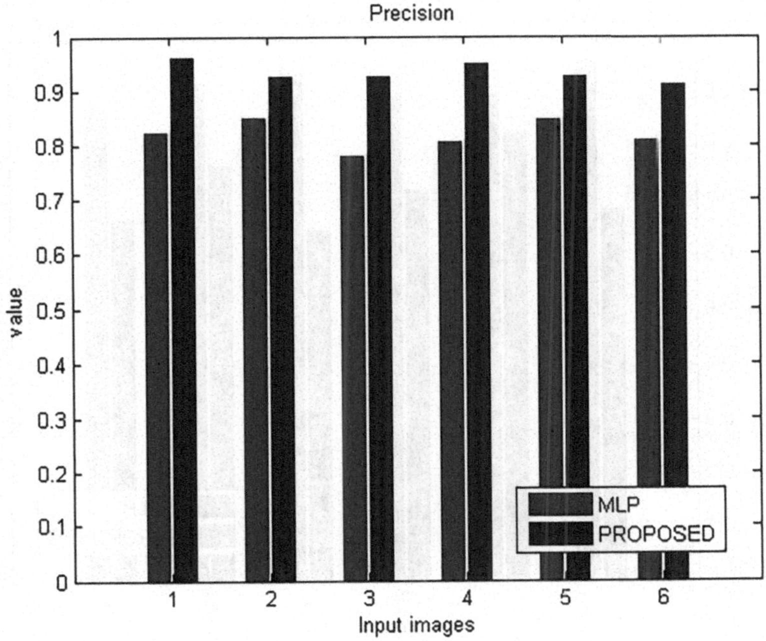

Fig. 2.12 Plot of precision for statistical results of mammogram images

Table 2.17 Statistical results for F-measure

Images	MLP	Proposed
Image 1	0.685	0.96
Image 2	0.828	0.898
Image 3	0.721	0.898
Image 4	0.648	0.939
Image 5	0.768	0.92
Image 6	0.667	0.876

results of watershed segmentation using Multilayer perceptron with results from using active contour segmentation and random forest feature extraction with a classifier such as Multilayer perceptron and hybrid k-mean and J-48 for parameters such as kappa statistics, FP rate, misclassification error, and mean absolute error is evaluated and tested using ANOVA. The performance of the proposed hybrid method provides significant results. This indicates a more effective method for outlier detection. In the future, we can further do the experimental study on the other clustering and classification techniques to make decisions more accurately and less time-consuming for the diagnosis. Furthermore, we can use real-time data that can provide a more precise lesion description that can give rise to deep learning classification.

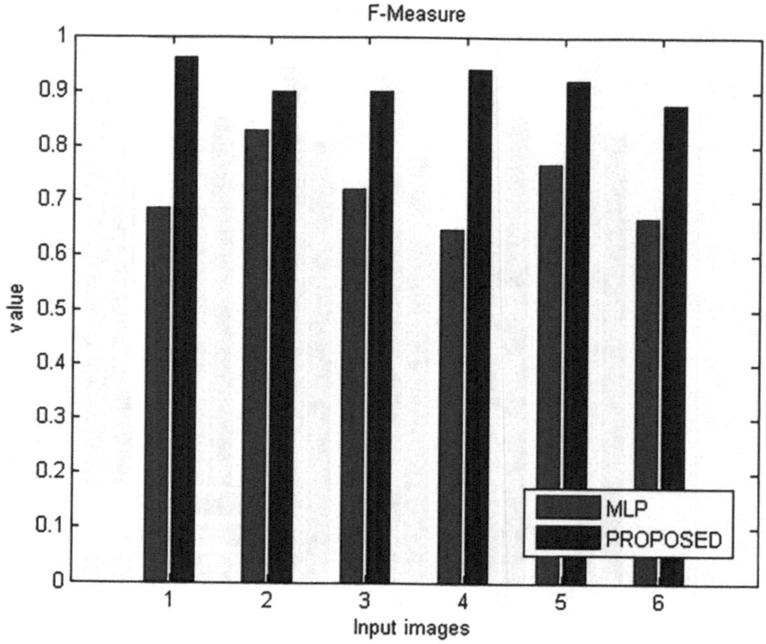

Fig. 2.13 Plot of F-measure for statistical results of mammogram images

References

1. Huang ML, Hung YH, Lee WM, Li RK, Wang TH (2012) Usage of case-based reasoning, neural network and adaptive neuro-fuzzy inference system classification techniques in breast cancer dataset classification diagnosis. J Med Syst 36(2):407–414
2. Luo ST, Cheng BW (2012) Diagnosing breast masses in digital mammography using feature selection and ensemble methods. J Med Syst 36(2):569–577
3. Gull S, Loan NA, Parah SA (2020) An efficient watermarking technique for tamper detection and localization of medical images. J Ambient Intell Humaniz Comput 11:1799–1808
4. Loan NA, Parah SA, Sheikh JA, Akhoon JA, Bhat GM (2017) Hiding Electronic Patient Record (EPR) in medical images: a high capacity and computationally efficient technique for e-healthcare applications. J Biomed Inform 73:125–136. https://doi.org/10.1016/j.jbi.2017.08.002
5. Singh KU, Abu-Hamatta HS, Kumar A, Singhal A, Rashid M, Bashir AK (2021) Secure watermarking scheme for color DICOM images in telemedicine applications. Comput Mater Cont 70(2):2525–2542
6. Iwendi C, Bashir AK, Peshkar A, Sujatha R, Chatterjee JM, Pasupuleti S, Mishra R, Pillai S, Jo O (2020) COVID-19 patient health prediction using boosted random forest algorithm. Front Public Health 8:357
7. Rathour N, Alshamrani SS, Singh R, Gehlot A, Rashid M, Akram SV, AlGhamdi AS (2021) IoMT based facial emotion recognition system using deep convolution neural networks. Electronics 10(11):1289
8. Cheng HD, Shan J, Ju W, Guo Y, Zhang L (2010) Automated breast cancer detection and classification using ultrasound images: a survey. Pattern Recogn 43(1):299–317

9. Birdwell RL (2009) The preponderance of evidence supports computer-aided detection for screening mammography. Radiology 253(1):9–16
10. Rashid M, Singh H, Goyal V (2021) Efficient feature selection technique based on fast Fourier transform with PSO-GA for functional magnetic resonance imaging. In: 2021 2nd International conference on computation, automation and knowledge management (ICCAKM). IEEE, New York, pp 238–242
11. Parah SA, Kaw JA, Bellavista P, Loan NA, Bhat GM, Muhammad K, Victor A (2020) Efficient security and authentication for edge-based internet of medical things. IEEE Internet Things J 8(21):15652–15662
12. Berber T, Alpkocak A, Balci P, Dicle O (2013) Breast mass contour segmentation algorithm in digital mammograms. Comput Methods Prog Biomed 110(2):150–159
13. Giannoglou GD et al (2007) A novel active contour model for fully automated segmentation of intravascular ultrasound images: in vivo validation in human coronary arteries. Comput Biol Med 37(9):1292–1302
14. Pratondo A, Chee-Kong C, Sim-Heng O (2016) Robust edge-stop functions for edge-based active contour models in medical image segmentation. IEEE Signal Process Lett 23(2):222–226
15. Lewis SH, Dong A (2012) Detection of breast tumor candidates using marker-controlled watershed segmentation and morphological analysis. In: 2012 IEEE Southwest symposium on image analysis and interpretation 2012 Apr 22. IEEE, New York, pp 1–4
16. Gaetano R, Masi G, Poggi G, Verdoliva L, Scarpa G (2014) Marker-controlled watershed-based segmentation of multiresolution remote sensing images. IEEE Trans Geosci Remote Sens 53(6): 2987–3004
17. Heidari E, Sobati MA, Movahedirad S (2016) Accurate prediction of nanofluid viscosity using a multilayer perceptron artificial neural network (MLP-ANN). Chemom Intell Lab Syst 155:73–85
18. Miao KH, Miao GJ (2013) Mammographic diagnosis for breast cancer biopsy predictions using neural network classification model and receiver operating characteristic (ROC) curve evaluation. J Select Areas Bioinformatics 3(9)
19. Pratiwi M, Harefa J, Nanda S (2015) Mammogram's classification using gray-level co-occurrence matrix and radial basis function neural network. Proc Comput Sci 59:83–91
20. Tseng YJ, Huang CE, Wen CN, Lai PY, Wu MH, Sun YC, Wang HY, Lu JJ (2020) Predicting breast cancer metastasis by using serum biomarkers and clinicopathological data with machine learning technologies. Int J Med Inform 128:79–86
21. Zhu Z, Albadawy E, Saha A, Zhang J, Harowicz MR, Mazurowski MA (2019) Deep learning for identifying radiogenomic associations in breast cancer. Comput Biol Med 109:85–90
22. Kyono T, Fiona JG, Mihaela VS (2019) Improving workflow efficiency for mammography using machine learning. J Am Coll Radiol 17(1 Pt A):56–63
23. Wang H, Zheng B, Yoon SW, Ko HS (2018) A support vector machine-based ensemble algorithm for breast cancer diagnosis. Eur J Oper Res 267(2):687–699
24. Liu N, Qi ES, Xu M, Gao B, Liu GQ (2019) A novel intelligent classification model for breast cancer diagnosis. Inf Process Manag 56(3):609–623
25. Vijayarajeswari R, Parthasarathy P, Vivekanandan S, Basha AA (2019) Classification of mammogram for early detection of breast cancer using SVM classifier and Hough transform. Measurement 146:800–805
26. Hamdi MA (2014) Modified algorithm marker-controlled watershed transform for image segmentation based on curvelet threshold. Middle-East J Sci Res 20(3):323–327
27. Youssif AA, Darwish AA, Madbouly AM (2010) Adaptive algorithm for image denoising based on curvelet threshold. Int J Comput Sci Netw Secur 10(1):322–330
28. Kamalakannan J, Thirumal T, Vaidhyanathan A, MukeshBhai KD (2015) Study on different classification technique for mammogram image. In: 2015 International conference on circuits, power and computing technologies. IEEE, New York, pp 1–5

29. Yang X, Li H, Zhou X (2006) Nuclei segmentation using marker-controlled watershed, tracking using mean-shift, and Kalman filter in time-lapse microscopy. IEEE Trans Circuits Syst I Regular Pap 53(11):2405–2414
30. Lewis SH, Dong A (2012) Detection of breast tumor candidates using marker-controlled watershed segmentation and morphological analysis. In: 2012 IEEE Southwest symposium on image analysis and interpretation. IEEE, New York, pp 1–4
31. Friedewald SM, Rafferty EA, Rose SL, Durand MA, Plecha DM, Greenberg JS, Hayes MK, Copit DS, Carlson KL, Cink TM, Barke LD (2014) Breast cancer screening using tomosynthesis in combination with digital mammography. JAMA 311(24):2499–2507
32. Kallenberg M, Petersen K, Nielsen M, Ng AY, Diao P, Igel C, Vachon CM, Holland K, Winkel RR, Karssemeijer N, Lillholm M (2016) Unsupervised deep learning applied to breast density segmentation and mammographic risk scoring. IEEE Trans Med Imaging 35(5):1322–1331
33. Kooi T, Litjens G, Van GB, Gubern-Mérida A, Sánchez CI, Mann R, den Heeten A, Karssemeijer N (2017) Large scale deep learning for computer aided detection of mammographic lesions. Med Image Anal 35:303–312
34. Rashid M, Singh H, Goyal V (2020) The use of machine learning and deep learning algorithms in functional magnetic resonance imaging—a systematic review. Expert Syst 37(6):e12644
35. Mondal S, Agarwal K, Rashid M (2019) Deep learning approach for automatic classification of x-ray images using convolutional neural network. In: 2019 Fifth international conference on image information processing (ICIIP). IEEE, New York, pp 326–331
36. Gull S, Mansour RF, Aljehane NO, Parah SA (2021) A self-embedding technique for tamper detection and localization of medical images for smart-health. Multimed Tools Appl 80(19): 29939–29964
37. Sethi GK, Ahmad N, Rehman MB, Dafallaa HMEI, Rashid M (2021) Use of artificial intelligence in healthcare systems: state-of-the-art survey. In: 2021 2nd International conference on intelligent engineering and management (ICIEM). IEEE, New York, pp 243–248
38. Ribli D, Horváth A, Unger Z, Pollner P, Csabai I (2018) Detecting and classifying lesions in mammograms with deep learning. Sci Rep 8(1):4165
39. Shah AA, Parah SA, Rashid M, Elhoseny M (2020) Efficient image encryption scheme based on generalized logistic map for real time image processing. J Real-Time Image Process 17(6): 2139–2151
40. Khan AA, Shaikh AA, Cheikhrouhou O, Laghari AA, Rashid M, Shafiq M, Hamam H (2021) IMG-forensics: multimedia-enabled information hiding investigation using convolutional neural network. IET Image Process. https://doi.org/10.1049/ipr2.12272
41. Rashid M, Singh H, Goyal V (2020) Analyzing functional magnetic resonance brain images with opencv2. In: 2020 Sixth international conference on parallel, distributed and grid computing. IEEE, New York, pp 451–454

Chapter 3
Cloud-Based Glaucoma Diagnosis in Medical Imaging Using Machine Learning

R. Dhanalakshmi, Jose Anand, K. Poonkavithai, and V. Vijayakumar

Contents

1 Introduction

ML is a subset of Artificial Intelligence (AI) that gives computers the ability to learn from the data that is fed into it. The data is analyzed to find a specific pattern using a learning algorithm. The learning algorithm makes data-driven predictions or recommendations by creating a model from sample inputs which are generally huge

R. Dhanalakshmi (✉)
Department of Computer Science and Engineering, KCG College of Technology, Chennai, India

J. Anand
Department of Electronics and Communication Engineering, KCG College of Technology, Chennai, India

K. Poonkavithai
Department of Computer Science and Engineering, Hindustan Institute of Science and Technology, Chennai, India

V. Vijayakumar
School of Computer Science and Engineering, The University of New South Wales, Sydney, NSW, Australia

S. A. Parah et al. (eds.), *Artificial Intelligence for Innovative Healthcare Informatics*,
https://doi.org/10.1007/978-3-030-96569-3_3

[1]. ML has been applied in several domains and industries like Retail-Automobiles, Life Sciences-Agriculture, Health Care-Breast cancer prediction, Network Security-Malware, etc. [2]. ML used in health care is one of the most challenging as the machine is being used to make a recommendation from the health condition of human beings. In literature few smart applications and recommendations on other ailments have been done using ML [3, 4]. Many times ML is confused with data mining. While ML focuses more on the computational statistic that enables the machine to learn and find a correlation/pattern to find meaningful inferences on the data [5].

Glaucoma is a complex eye disease, the damage in the optic nerve that happens due to pressure and/or other influencing factors leads to progressive, irreversible vision loss. There are three different types of Glaucoma. However, the most popular one tends to be hereditary and may not show up until later in life. The optic nerve is responsible for transmitting images to the brain. When the intraocular pressure increases the optic nerve gets damaged. This damage increases and can lead to permanent vision loss. Early detection is inevitable in glaucoma to avoid permanent blindness within a few years. The mild or no symptoms during the early stages make early detection of Glaucoma very challenging [6]. The aqueous humor is the fluid that supports the lens structure in the eye. A mesh-like channel in the eye keeps this liquid intact. When this channel gets blocked, the liquid secretion inside the eye becomes more. This excessive liquid is the main reason for glaucoma. The root cause for the blockage is unknown to clinicians. However, over years it's been observed that this disease is of heredity type. Very rarely a blunt force trauma affects the eye, an infection that affects the eye severely, blockage of blood vessels inside the eye, and some inflammatory conditions could also cause Glaucoma [7].

There are two major types of glaucoma. Primary Open-Angle Glaucoma is the most common type. Nearly three million Americans get affected by this type of glaucoma. The eye's drainage canals get blocked due to some reason and hence the eye becomes clogged over time. This excessive fluid increases the eye pressure and hence leads to damage of the optic nerve. The affected person never faces any kind of discomfort in terms of pain or eyesight. People who have sensitive optic nerves that get affected by fluctuations in pressures are more prone to get affected by glaucoma. Regular eye check-ups are important to detect early symptoms [8]. Angle-closure glaucoma happens when a person's iris is not as wide and open as it should be when the pupil enlarges too much and too quickly. This displacement of the iris blocks the fluid drainage. It is as simple as something very small and thin membrane sliding over a drainage canal. When the drainage angle gets completely blocked, eye pressure rises very quickly. This type of glaucoma is also referred to as "closed-angle glaucoma" or "narrow-angle glaucoma" [9].

According to World Health Organization (WHO), glaucoma is the second greatest cause of vision loss worldwide. Glaucoma is known as the "silent thief of sight," mainly because there are no early symptoms to detect this disease. It just silently blocks the canal, initially tampers the side vision first, and then, over time, completely makes the victim feel like looking through a narrow tunnel, and finally, takes away vision altogether [10]. It affects more than 60 million people globally.

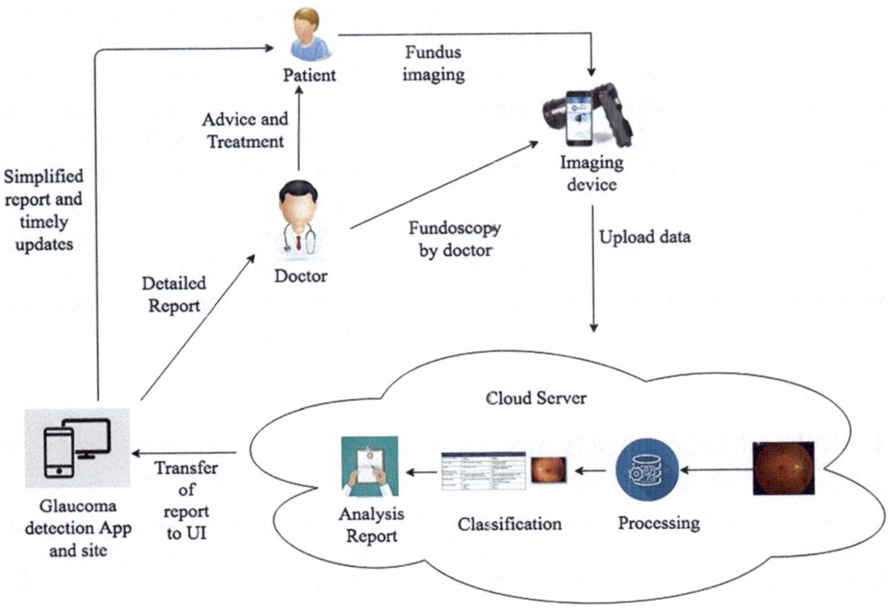

Fig. 3.1 Glaucoma indication diagram

When unchecked, this disease will completely reduce the vision and the loss of vision is irreparable. Early detection, through regular and complete eye check-ups, is very important in avoiding damage caused by glaucoma. Though five tests can easily detect glaucoma, there is no cure. Few doctors suggest laser treatment that may lessen the scarring that will damage central vision by sealing the leaky blood vessels and destroying abnormal vessels [11]. Figure 3.1 shows the architecture diagram of the entire structure.

1.1 Scope of the Work

The main scope of this article is to facilitate the early detection of Glaucoma. Since Glaucoma has no symptoms initially, detection of the disease at an early stage is very difficult. The only cure for Glaucoma patients is a lifelong treatment. When the intraocular pressure increases Ocular hypertension occurs. Glaucoma could be caused by ocular hypertension too; however, there are other influencing factors too. Based on the feed obtained from the funduscopic device that captures the structural integrity and damages in the eye, the presence or absence, current stage of the disease, etc. can be analyzed. This is done by detecting cup to disc ratio from the obtained image from the funduscopic device or the user's mobile phone with the aid of an ophthalmology lens. By implementing the concept of machine learning, the analyzed data can be automatically drawn to a conclusion with a reasonable level of accuracy, thereby finding a solution. The results are highly personalized and the system will be equipped to provide timely updates and instruction to the patient to ensure that proper care is given to the eye preventing the horrific effects that glaucoma can bring about. By using this method, if Glaucoma is detected at early stages, it will be helpful to the doctors to treat the patients effectively. If the proposed system is implemented, it will reduce the damages done by Glaucoma on a large scale.

The rest of the chapter is structured as follows. Section 1.1 describes the scope of the article and Sect. 2 gives a review of the related literature. Section 3 details the structure of cloud-based Glaucoma diagnosis. Section 4 illustrates the analysis of results and discussions. Finally, the conclusion is given in Sect. 5.

2 Related Literature Study

This section explains the various related articles published in the field of medical image processing, glaucoma image analysis, and detection, and finally about image tapering and the Internet of Things (IoT) with interference in a cloud environment.

2.1 Feature Extraction and Tomography

In the literature, three methods are used in the detection of glaucoma presence with image process applications with feature extractions such as CDR and RDR, and classification such as Support Vector Machine (SVM), decision tree or K nearest ML concepts, and Convolutional Neural Network (CNN) on the Bin Rushed database [12]. An annotated benchmark dataset needed for efficient detection of glaucoma using ML is used to diagnose fundoscopy. The optical coherence tomography in retinal layers and optic nerve head are also fed into the computer-aided diagnostic system to help in the early detection of glaucoma in the patient. The annotations feed is taken from multiple ophthalmologists to measure the accuracy of the proposed algorithm [13].

2.2 Image Retrieval and Testing

An image retrieval method using a grey level co-occurrence matrix and shaping feature on content-based image retrieval to obtain perfect results noted with a reduced computational time is discussed using a color histogram-based approach with K-means, to obtain high accuracy [14]. A method for detection of glaucoma by analyzing structural and non-structural features of the retina is proposed and is analyzed based on its cup, disc, and their ratio as well as other features like intensity, texture, and so on. In the initial stages of Glaucoma, few structural changes happen in the retina. If those changes are identified through some means it would aid ophthalmologists to detect glaucoma at an early stage. The clinician can provide medicines to stop its progression. This evaluation is made by comparing the historical data of 100 patients' fundus images and obtaining the average sensitivity and specificity [15]. Analyzing the structural features are observed by visual field testing using Optical Coherence Tomography and fundus images are used in medical imaging for early glaucoma detection [16].

2.3 Automatic Feature Learning

A biometric authentication system using medical imaging is developed. The system can recognize the patients and also verify their proximity to losing vision by using template matching techniques [17]. An Optical Coherence Tomography technique is used in glaucoma detection systems to detect glaucoma at an early stage for treatment and to identify the mature level using fundus images was proposed. A hybrid feature set that consists of a structure of medical images and texture detail of retinal images has been used in this technique [18]. CNN has been used on colored retinal fundus images. Automatic feature learning is done using deep learning techniques, the handcrafted optic disc features are fed into the system as input, and additional features are extracted automatically from the raw images. This proposed system demonstrated accuracy, specificity, and sensitivity at a considerably lower computational cost [19]. A technique to find the cup to disc ratio using k-means clustering algorithm by Region of Interest method to identify Glaucoma which causes elevated intraocular pressure. That pressure would cause gradual vision loss which eventually leads to blindness. The structural damage to the retina is diagnosed by examining the optic disc and optic cup on a few parameters like size, shape, etc. [20].

2.4 Glaucoma Image Analysis

The classification of glaucoma existing images from an unidentified set is achieved by processing the image inhomogeneities and vessel structures and applying the resulting image to the classifier and the vessel-free images and intermediate results are the most important set of data for the doctors. These details provide a better perspective to better understand glaucoma with a success rate [21]. Using vector imaging and edge mapping, the boundary of the aortas is detected in cardiovascular magnetic resonance. The performance of this technique is compared with the active contour model. The edge vector and edge map-based boundary detection approach proves to outperform the active contour-based technique in medical imaging [22]. Glaucoma detection using fundus images and optical coherence tomography with structural features of the retina is analyzed using retinal layer analysis and optic nerve head analysis with concluding that combining structural features from both images would result in more accurate glaucoma assessment [23]. Automated detection of glaucoma using SVM to detect the disease by performing Principal Component Analysis technique is used. A performance analysis was done compared with other existing techniques available for the detection of glaucoma. The nonlinear transformation of the support vectors is used and classification of the images is done. The system will take analyze images and recommend clinical findings of glaucoma. The accuracy of the recommendation made by this proposed classifier is analyzed based on computational time and space factors. The fused method and SVM by morphological-based image classification proved to be better in all the factors considered [24].

2.5 *Glaucoma Detection*

A smartphone-based visual clinical device is developed using a deep learning system for glaucoma detecting system "iGlaucoma" which is a cloud-based application that is tested with several samples for sensitivity and specificity [25]. The disc and cup features are fed into the CNN by brute force. The deep machine-learning system uses segmentation and features extraction techniques to detect glaucoma. Several layers of neurons in the neural network get trained and their results are combined to improve glaucoma detection [26]. In this paper, a detailed discussion on the evolution of glaucoma detection techniques has been analyzed, then the study of medical images, in general, is detailed out. The usage of ML systems and their capability of automatically extracting the necessary characteristics to make a correct diagnosis is presented [27]. Feature engineering is the most important step in machine learning. The raw data is pre-processed and then the right choice to the neural network architecture is chosen. During the training stage with historical medical images are used. The ML algorithm is applied to the eye images of the fundus to predict the presence of glaucoma. This work is produced accuracy better than the one obtained by classical diagnostic systems [28].

2.6 *Image Tampering and IoT*

A deep learning Xception model was used to diagnose chest X-ray images and predict the different diseases from chest X-rays. Since glaucoma is a rare disease, the proposed work uses only an ML algorithm [29]. An efficient image encryption algorithm using permutation technique based on a modular logistic map with a 192-bit key which proves to be secure from statistical and differential attacks is proposed [30]. A watermarking technique was proposed to detect tamper in medical images. This helps to enhance the most wanted details in the medical images [31–

34]. RIM-One V3, DRISHTI, and DRIONS datasets were combined. Segmentation methods were applied on the huge dataset using a cloud-based architecture which results in demonstrating the feasibility of applying the mechanism to glaucoma detection [35]. A device to monitor asthma patients using a cloud platform and a mobile application-based device to display human physiological parameters are developed and tested with a prototype model [36]. An IoT and cloud-based feature extraction and classification model for the detection of glaucoma automatically using the classifier approach for the identification from the color fundus images and bilateral filtering techniques are used to discard the noise that exists in the image which is tested with DRISHTI-GS fundus images [37]. Glaucoma is a rare disease and the images about it are less in volume. A deep learning architecture would be consuming more computational resources for a smaller size of data. The weights and parameters were learned from the formerly hidden layer and used in the next layer to increase the accuracy of prediction [38]. Studies on interferences with cloud environments are discussed in [39].

3 Proposed Cloud-Based Glaucoma Diagnosis

Glaucoma is an eye disease that is one of the most inevitable reasons for blindness worldwide. It is infamously renowned as the "Silent thief of sight". Being an initially unnoticeable disorder, glaucoma will cause an irreversible vision loss by the time it is realized by the patient through vision difficulties. Glaucoma has no symptoms during its early stages which makes it more dangerous. The contemporary system to detect glaucoma, with a series of tests, is complicated and, weighs economically on the patient. This makes it difficult for many to detect glaucoma in its early state. The removal of such complexity from the system will prove to be a valuable contributor to the increase in the number of patients in whom glaucoma is detected in its early stages. This will help reduce the continued expenditures on medication on the condition getting worse and also will prevent the eye from losing sight permanently. This article aims at introducing ML to detect the disorder in its early stage. If the disease is detected in its early stage, the appropriate medication can be prescribed effectively to prevent it from causing more damage to the patient's vision.

The proposed system model consists of a mobile app that deals with all the front-end processes and functionalities of the system. Initially, the patient's retinal image, also known as the fundus image, is obtained using a fundoscopy machine by an ophthalmologist. The captured fundus image is uploaded to the cloud by the ophthalmologist to carry out basic processing like noise removal. Later the image is analyzed to detect the disc structure and is cropped on the borders of the disc. Following it, the cup structure is analyzed and is cropped accordingly. With the obtained cropped images, the cup-to-disc ratio is determined with the diameters of both the images and finding their ratio. With the CDR value, the classification process is carried out by applying the CDR value to the highly trained classifier. Linear Regression is the algorithm in use, to train the classifier as it has the highest accuracy of all. The classifier gives the analysis for glaucoma in a detailed manner to the doctor and abstracted version to the user. The output is forwarded to the app and thus the patient obtains the result. Based on the result, the patient can seek a doctor's advice and follow medication.

Language Specification The programming language used to develop most of the modules in Python. Since python is simple and efficient with several libraries and compatibility factors, it tends to be the best fit for this purpose. Python is used in the image processing module to program ROI to crop the required region of the subject image and also to calculate the C to D Ratio. In the ML module, it is used to import the dataset, pre-process the data, split the dataset into train and test sets, and train the classifier. With that, the required result is predicted for the respective input given. Android app is an essential component of this project and is developed using java and XML. The reason is that the developed app works best and will be lightweight and agile if it's a native app instead of a hybrid version. HTML is used along with some popular frameworks like bootstrap and jQuery to develop an interactive web portal.

Server Django framework is used to establish and develop the server. This is a powerful and efficient web framework developed in python and follows the model-view-template architectural pattern that enables developers to create highly able and feature-rich web applications with the east. It also has well-defined libraries that allow for extensive development by reducing the need to have redundant code written. Django is used to develop the application server to be deployed in the cloud in a Virtual Private Server, making it accessible by all and eventually qualifying it as SaaS. The web page is essentially a web app that is an integrated part of the many functions of Django. The application server will then perform actions like user creation, handling requests, saving images, maintaining the database, performing image analysis, ML through regression, and sending out the result to the app and web page. All under the single environment created through Django.

Database In this system development, the database used is MySQL. It is connected to the Django server using the mysqlclient, a package in python. The database serves to be the pivotal point of coordination among various modules. It holds in it, an intermediate result that acts as input later on. It saves the user details for validation and authentication, saves locations of fundus images, records the CDR values of the patient with their details and the image detail, and finally saves the result of the linear regression module with correspondence to the user.

Use Cases Table 3.1 gives the use cases used for the development of the cloud-based system.

The objective is to recommend symptoms of Glaucoma at its early stage. It is created for the user who is the patient to get the results of the analysis of his/her Glaucoma test and also access the records. For a doctor, it is used to analyze the patient data and get the results. Later the doctor prescribes medication accordingly. The system consists of the following modules.

Table 3.1 Use cases

Use case UC 1	
Scope	Glaucoma Application
Level	User goal
Primary Actor	User
Preconditions	The user is identified and authenticated.
Success Guarantee	The user can access the patient records and perform the analysis with the input image as well.
Main Success Scenario	The user has to register or log in with the required credentials. The doctor is allowed to capture the image and then it is input. The input is uploaded to the server. The analysis runs in the cloud environment and the result is sent back to the application. The result is displayed to the user.
Extensions	If the password is invalid, the application shows a message "password invalid". If the user is patient, the user cannot capture the image.
Technology Used	Android studio is used to develop the mobile application.
Frequency of Occurrence	As per user request.

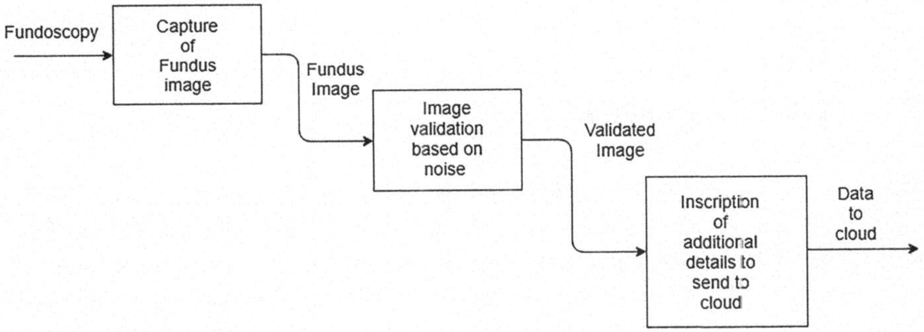

Fig. 3.2 Image Capturing and validation

1. Image Capture and Validation
2. Image Pre-processing
3. CDR Determination
4. Analysis

3.1 Image Capture and Validation

The Image Capture and Validation are shown in Fig. 3.2 is the first module in the system. The image of the patient's retina is being captured by the fundoscopy device. It is handled by the doctor or technician. The captured image is called the fundus image which is then checked if suitable to conduct further analysis. If it satisfies the conditions, then it is said to be valid and that concludes the validation part. The resultant image is forwarded to the following phase of Image Pre-Processing.

3.2 Image Pre-processing

The next phase in the system is Image Pre-processing which is shown in Fig. 3.3. In the image pre-processing module, the image obtained from the previous phase is given as input and is processed for further analysis. Here, the obtained image is converted into a binary image which is made of just black and white pixels. Loop is run from the left pixel towards the border of the disc. The retinal part has two circular structures which play a key role in the determination of glaucoma. They are the cup and the disc. The disc is the outer circle which encircles the cup which is in the shape of a cup. When the loop stops at the appropriate pixel, it is noted. Similarly, another loop from the right is run to find the right side border. Then the image is cropped at the borders. The same process is repeated for the cup and the image is cropped. Thus two images are obtained, one of the discs and another cup. Both the images are forwarded to the next phase where the CDR is determined.

3.3 CDR Determination

The two images are obtained after being processed at the previous phase. Those images are considered to determine the CDR which is also called as Cup-to-Disc Ratio. The CDR is determined using the following steps. The width of the image of Disc is found. The width is the same value as that of the diameter of the disc. Similarly, the diameter of the cup is determined using the width value of the cup

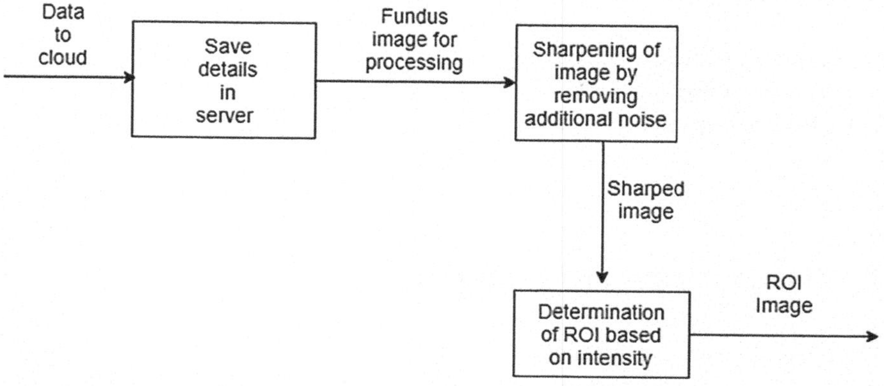

Fig. 3.3 Image pre-processing

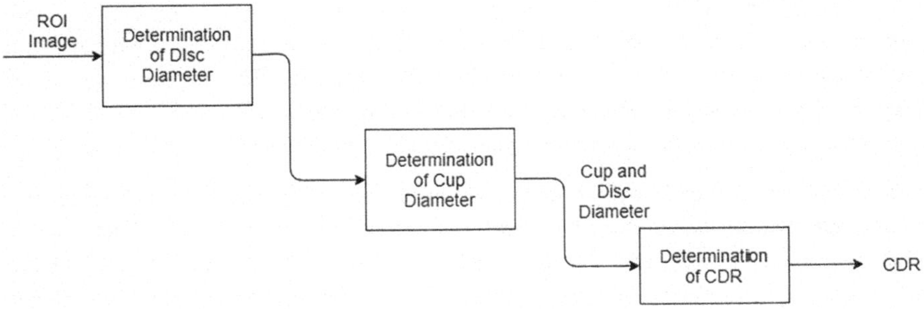

Fig. 3.4 CDR determination

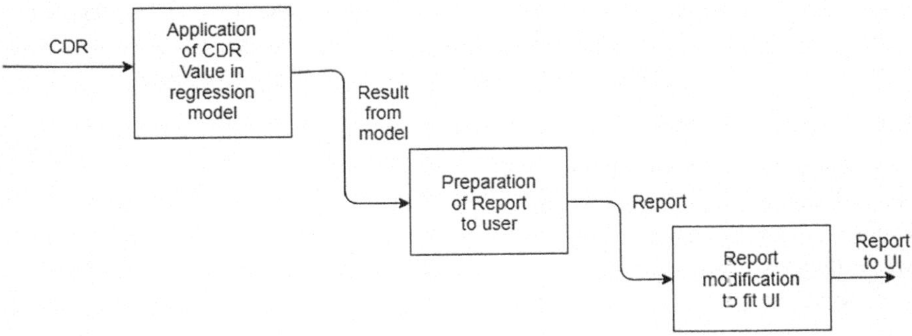

Fig. 3.5 Analysis

image. After obtaining both the values, they are applied to the following formula to determine the CDR value as shown in Fig. 3.4. Here the diameter of the cup is divided by that of the disc and a ratio value of two decimal places is obtained. Thus CDR value is determined. The CDR plays a key role in the determination of Glaucoma and has a vital part in the system. It is based on the CDR value. Thus, glaucoma's existence, as well as severity is determined.

3.4 Analysis

The last module of the system is Analysis which is shown in Fig. 3.5. The analysis phase involves machine learning. In this, an ML classifier is trained using a huge dataset and is trained to the best accuracy. The classifier is trained using Linear Regression. When the CDR value of a patient is obtained, it is applied to the classifier. The classifier based on its accuracy gives a solution. Thus the output is obtained along with the severity of glaucoma. A raw report is prepared and is optimized according to the UI. Later the obtained report is forwarded to the application for the users to access it.

Use Case Diagram The use case diagram portrays how users use the system. Here the different possible scenarios along with the impact on the database are depicted. It describes the functional aspects of the system from the user. The use cases have their properties and constraints that have to be fulfilled by the user to access the database. The sequence of events between user and database is pictured as use cases.

Class Diagram The class diagram is used to visualize the different aspects/features of the application that is built to detect anomalies in the human eye. The systems classes, their attributes, and the relationships between those attributes are evident from this class diagram. The classes in this diagram represent both the main objects and or interactions of the user and database.

Activity Diagram The complete working of the system from the new user registration to the passing messages to the user from another mobile is graphically represented with step-wise activities and actions. The flow of activities involving the conditions of whether to do or not to do an action is also explained.

Cup-to-Disc Determination

Determine the cup diameter w1
w1 = float (p_img.width)
Determine the disc diameter w2
w2 = float (p_img1.width)
Determine the ratio
ratio = round (w1/w2,2)

- Obtain the fundus image from the project directory using Image.open (Path_of_the _image) in the img variable
- Convert img to black and white using img.convert()
- Trim the image to the first white pixel on either side from the center and obtain the width of the image using img.width(), to get the width of the disc.
- From the trimmed image perform the same operation to get the width of the cup
- Determine the CDR using the ratio of the width of the two images as given in Eq. (3.1).

$$\mathrm{CDR} = \frac{Diameter\ \ of\ \ cup}{Diameter\ \ of\ \ disc} \tag{3.1}$$

Analysis

- Obtain the .csv file containing the CDR value and severity values, using the read_csv() function.
- Segregate the obtained dataset into test and train set using train_test_split() of sklearn library.
- X_train,X_test,Y_train,Y_test = train_test_split(X,Y,train_size,random_state) regressor = LinearRegression( ) regressor.fit(X_train, Y_train)

- Predict the severity for CDR using, y = B0 + B1 * x, the value of B0 and B1 are given in Eqs. (3.2) and (3.3) respectively.

$$B0 = \text{mean}(y) - B1^{*}\text{mean}(x) \tag{3.2}$$

$$B1 = \frac{sum((xi - mean(x)) * (yi - mean(y)))}{sum\left((xi - mean(x))^{2}\right)} \tag{3.3}$$

Where,

x is the input, independent variable (CDR)
y is the dependent variable that is being predicted (Severity)
B0 is the intercept
B1 is the slope
xi and yi are the ith value of x and y

- Print the Predicted Value

Operation The model consists of a mobile app that deals with all the front-end processes and functionalities of the system as shown in Fig. 3.6. Initially, the patient eye is being captured using fundoscopy by the doctor. The captured input image is forwarded to the cloud to carry out basic processing. Later the image is analyzed to detect the disc structure and is cropped on the borders of the disc. Following it, the cup structure is analyzed and is cropped accordingly. With the obtained cropped images, the cup-to-disc ratio is determined with the diameters of both the images and finding their ratio. With the CDR value, the classification process is carried out by applying the CDR value to the highly trained classifier. The classifier gives out the result as output with its level of accuracy. Normally Linear Regression is the preferred algorithm to train the classifier as it has the highest accuracy of all. The output is forwarded to the app and thus the patient obtains the result. Based on the result, the patient can seek a doctor's advice and follow medication.

4 Results and Discussions

The various test cases carried out for the evaluation process and their details are mentioned in Tables 3.2, 3.3, 3.4, and 3.5.

The user upon accessing the web application is required to enroll into the system either as a patient or as a doctor as per their qualification. This is a single-point authentication for the system and does not include any other authentication down the line. Once the user has enrolled he is eligible to access the service. The user is then authenticated with the respective credentials provided at the time of signup and is directed to their respective dashboards. Once the authentication is done, the doctor is required to upload the image of the patient's fundus image to the cloud for processing and prediction of CDR value for obtaining the severity and the presence

Fig. 3.6 Working diagram

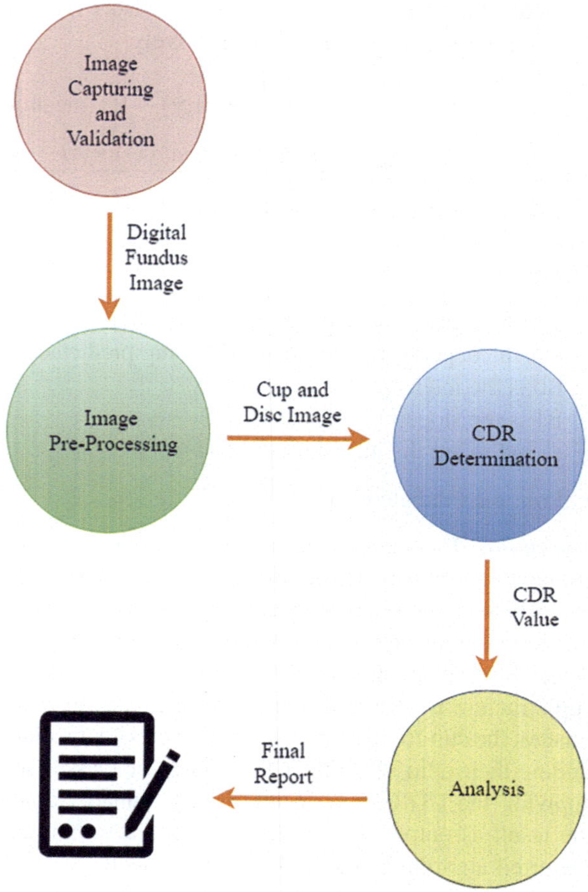

Table 3.2 Test case for image pre-processing

Project Name: cloud Based Detection of Glaucoma using Machine Learning	
Test Case Id: <01>	Test Designed by: Balasubramaniam T
Test Priority: High	Test Designed on: 14-02-2018
Module Name: Image Pre-Processing	Test Executed by: Ashwath S
Test Title: Extraction of Cup and Disc from Fundus image	Test Executed Date: 19-02-2018
Description: To Extract the Cup and Disc from Fundus image using ROI Technique.	
Pre-condition: User need to log in before uploading an image for Pre-processing	

of glaucoma. It is at this point the image is sent to the Django server to be saved in the backend to be processed upon.

The result of that process is obtained on the next page. After the uploading of the fundus image is done, the doctor's dashboard will display a detailed report. The

Table 3.3 Test case for image pre-processing

Step	Test step	Test data	Expected result	Actual result	Status
1	Converting to Black and white image	Digital Fundus image	Black and white image	Black and white image	Pass
2	Locating the Cup and Disc Border	Black and White Image	White pixel Point on the Border of Cup and Disc	A white pixel point on the Border of the cup and disc	Pass
3	Cutting the Cup and Disc portion	Black and white image with White pixel	Cup and Disc processed image	Cup and Disc Processed image	Pass
4	Determine CDR Value	Cup and Disc	CDR value	CDR value	Pass

Table 3.4 Test case for machine learning module

Project Name: cloud Based Detection of Glaucoma using Machine Learning	
Test Case Id: <02>	Test Designed by: Ashwath S
Test Priority: High	Test Designed on: 04-03-2018
Module Name: Cup-to-Disc Determination	Test Executed by: Balasubramaniam T
Test Title: Prediction of severity for input CDR	Test Execution Date: 08-03-2018
Description: Obtaining the best-fitting line for the training data set and thus predicting the severity for the unknown value.	
Pre-Condition: CDR Value must be determined.	

Table 3.5 Test case for cup-to-disc determination

Step	Test step	Test data	Expected result	Actual result	Status
1	Obtain the dataset from the system	CSV file containing the dataset	Transfer of dataset into an object	Transfer of dataset into an object	Pass
2	Splitting the dataset into test and train set	Object containing dataset	Two datasets, namely test, and train	Two datasets, namely test, and train	Pass
3	Train the regression model using the training dataset	Train dataset	Trained module with best-fitting line	Trained module with best-fitting line	Pass
4	Predict the Severity for the Test dataset	Test dataset	The severity of the input CDR	The severity of the input CDR	Pass

report will have in it the fundus images the patient's name and id along with the date of the test. It'll also have the CDR value, the severity and will state whether glaucoma is present or not. These values are discrete to the doctor. That being said, it's served only to the doctor as it is a detailed version of the report. These details make more sense at the hands of the doctor over the patient. The patient receives a more abstracted result on the web app.

The proposed system is a holistic solution for both patients and doctors. The preliminary interaction between the patient and the doctor happens through the web app. If the patient needs physical observation, then he/she meets the doctor. The details that the doctor needs are all fetched from the cloud. The medical images are stored in the cloud to reduce the storage dependency. Moreover, the medical images of new patients are made use of in the ML process to improvise the accuracy of prediction. The doctors feed in the consultation in the system to enable automatic medication recommendations in the future.

The unique feature of the proposed work, when compared to the existing work, is the holistic nature and usage of the cloud. The existing works concentrate on the ML algorithms and the proposed work has built an appropriate user interface for both doctors and patients.

5 Conclusion

Glaucoma is a deadly disease, which has the potential to cause permanent blindness can ruin lives if left undetected and untreated. Enormous numbers of patients are sufferings due to this disease which has been recorded around the globe. Therefore, the proposed model will be of great use to the patients as well as the doctors and on the whole, in the field of medicine. The system has societal causes in it and that it helps improve the standards of people. With early detection, the disorder can be well treated and the consequences can be mitigated well in advance.

References

1. Tong Y, Lu W, Yu Y, Shen Y (2020) Application of machine learning in ophthalmic imaging modalities. Eye Vision 7:1–15
2. An G, Omodaka K, Hashimoto K, Tsuda S, Shiga Y, Takada N, Nakazawa T (2019) Glaucoma diagnosis with machine learning based on optical coherence tomography and color fundus images. J Healthc Eng 2019:4061313
3. Sarah I, Soundarya K, Tamil Thendral S, Dhanalakshmi R, Deenadayalan T (2020) DYS-I-CAN: an aid for the dyslexic to improve the skills using mobile application. In: 2020 International conference on system, computation, automation, and networking (ICSCAN). IEEE, New York, pp 1–5. https://doi.org/10.1109/ICSCAN49426.2020.9262375
4. Kumar VA, Sharmila S, Kumar A, Bashir AK, Rashid M, Gupta SK, Alnumay WS (2021) A novel solution for finding postpartum hemorrhage using fuzzy neural techniques. Neural Comput Applic 2021:1–14
5. Rashid M, Singh H, Goyal V (2020) The use of machine learning and deep learning algorithms in functional magnetic resonance imaging-a systematic review. Expert Syst 37(6):e12644
6. Tham YC, Li X, Wong TY, Quigley HA, Aung T, Cheng CY (2014) The global prevalence of glaucoma and projections of glaucoma burden through 2040: a systematic review and meta-analysis. Ophthalmology 121(11):2081–2090
7. https://www.insightvisioncenter.com/treating-and-controlling-glaucoma/

8. Shafiq M, Tian Z, Bashir AK, Du X, Guizani M (2020) CorrAUC: a malicious bot-IoT traffic detection method in IoT network using machine-learning techniques. IEEE Internet Things J 8(5):3242–3254
9. Kim YK, Jeoung JW, Park KH (2017) Inferior macular damage in glaucoma: its relationship to retinal nerve fiber layer defect in macular vulnerability zone. J Glaucoma 26(2):126–132
10. Ramakrishnan N (2020) An intelligent system for early detection of eye diseases that lead to irreversible vision loss
11. Jiang F, Jiang Y, Zhi H, Dong Y, Li H, Ma S, Wang Y (2017) Artificial intelligence in healthcare: past, present, and future. Stroke Vasc Neurol 2(4)
12. Pandey A, Patre P, Minj J (2020) Detection of glaucoma disease using image processing, soft computing, and deep learning approaches. In: 2020 Fourth international conference on I-SMAC (IoT in social, mobile, analytics, and cloud) (I-SMAC). IEEE, New York, pp 1–7
13. Salam AA, Akram MU, Arouj A, Basit I, Shaqur T, Javed H, Wazir K (2017) Benchmark data set for glaucoma detection with an annotated cup to disc ratio. In: 2017 International conference on signals and systems (ICSigSys). IEEE, New York, pp 227–233
14. Devi TS, Dhanalakshmi R, Sankar S (2020) An improved framework for sentiment analysis for college reviews. Int J Adv Trends Comput Sci Eng 9(2):1959–1963, 162.
15. Salam AA, Khalil T, Akram MU, Jameel A, Basit I (2016) Automated detection of glaucoma using structural and non-structural features. Springerplus 5(1):1–21
16. Salam AA, Akram MU, Wazir K, Anwar SM (2015) A review analysis on early glaucoma detection using structural features. In: 2015 IEEE international conference on imaging systems and techniques (IST). IEEE, New York, pp 1–6
17. Anand J, Flora TA, Philip AS (2013) Finger-vein-based biometric security system. Int J Res Eng Technol. eISSN: 2319-1163
18. Rashid M, Singh H, Goyal V (2021) Efficient feature selection technique based on fast Fourier transform with PSO-GA for functional magnetic resonance imaging. In: 2021 2nd International conference on computation, automation and knowledge management (ICCAKM). IEEE, New York, pp 238–242
19. Al-Bander B, Williams BM, Al-Taee MA, Al-Nuaimy W, Zheng Y (2017) A novel choroid segmentation method for retinal diagnosis using deep learning. In: 2017 10th International conference on developments in esystems engineering (DeSE). IEEE, New York, pp 182–187
20. Ayub J, Ahmad J, Muhammad J, Aziz L, Ayub S, Akram U, Basit I (2016) Glaucoma detection through the optic disc and cup segmentation using K-mean clustering. In: 2016 International conference on computing, electronic and electrical engineering (ICE Cube). IEEE, New York, pp 143–147
21. Bock R, Meier J, Michelson G, Nyúl LG, Hornegger J (2007) Classifying glaucoma with image-based features from fundus photographs. In: Joint pattern recognition symposium. Springer, Berlin, pp 355–364
22. Kumaran N, Rangaraj V, Siva Sharan S, Dhanalakshmi R (2020) Intelligent personal assistant–Implementing voice commands enabling speech recognition. In: 2020 International conference on system, computation, automation and networking (ICSCAN), pp. 1–5, https://doi.org/10.1109/ICSCAN49426.2020.9262279
23. Nawaldgi S (2016) Review of automated glaucoma detection techniques. In: 2016 International conference on wireless communications, signal processing and networking (WiSPNET). IEEE, New York, pp 1435–1438
24. Thangaraj V, Natarajan V (2017) Glaucoma diagnosis using support vector machine. In: 2017 International conference on intelligent computing and control systems (ICICCS). IEEE, New York, pp 394–399
25. Li F, Song D, Chen H, Xiong J, Li X, Zhong H, Ting DS (2020) Development and clinical deployment of a smartphone-based visual field deep learning system for glaucoma detection. NPJ Dig Med 3(1):1–8

26. Civit-Masot J, Domínguez-Morales MJ, Vicente-Díaz S, Civit A (2020) Dual machine-learning system to aid glaucoma diagnosis using disc and cup feature extraction. IEEE Access 8: 127519–127529
27. Ker J, Wang L, Rao J, Lim T (2017) Deep learning applications in medical image analysis. IEEE Access 6:9375–9389
28. Asri H, Mousannif H, Al Moatassime H, Noel T (2016) Using machine learning algorithms for breast cancer risk prediction and diagnosis. Proc Comput Sci 83:1064–1069
29. Civit-Masot J, Luna-Perejon F, Vicente-Diaz S, Corral JMR, Civit A (2019) TPU cloud-based generalized U-Net for eye fundus image segmentation. IEEE Access 7:142379–142387
30. Mondal S, Agarwal K, Rashid M (2019) Deep learning approach for automatic classification of x-ray images using convolutional neural network. In: 2019 Fifth international conference on image information processing (ICIIP). IEEE, New York, pp 326–331
31. Gull S, Loan NA, Parah SA (2020) An efficient watermarking technique for tamper detection and localization of medical images. J Ambient Intell Human Comput 11:1799–1808
32. Shah AA, Parah SA, Rashid M, Elhoseny M (2020) Efficient image encryption scheme based on the generalized logistic map for real-time image processing. J Real-Time Image Proc 17(6): 2139–2151
33. Gull S, Mansour RF, Aljehane NO, Parah SA (2021) A self-embedding technique for tamper detection and localization of medical images for smart-health. Multimed Tools Appl 80(19): 29939–29964
34. Hussan M, Parah SA, Gull S, Qureshi GJ (2021) Tamper detection and self-recovery of medical imagery for smart health. Arab J Sci Eng 46(4):3465–3481
35. Rashid M, Singh H, Goyal V (2019) Cloud storage privacy in health care systems based on IP and geo-location validation using K-mean clustering technique. Int J E-Health Med Commun 10(4):54–65
36. Aljuaid H, Parah SA (2021) Secure patient data transfer using information embedding and hyperchaos. Sensors 21(1):282
37. Anandh R, Indirani G (2020) IoT and cloud-based feature extraction and classification model for automatic glaucoma detection. Int J Emerg Technol 11(2):13–18
38. Sarosh P, Parah SA, Bhat GM, Heidari AA, Muhammad K (2021) Secret sharing-based personal health records management for the Internet of health things. Sustain Cities Soc 74: 103129
39. Dhanalakshmi R, Sridevi T (2020) Adaptive cognitive intelligence in analyzing employee feedback using LSTM. J Intell Fuzzy Syst 39(6):8069–8078

Chapter 4
Leukocytic Cell Nucleus Identification Using Boundary Cell Detection Algorithm with Dilation and Erosion Based Morphometry

Ishfaq Majeed Sheikh and Manzoor Ahmad Chachoo

Contents

1 Introduction

The important component of the human body is the immune system. It is the biological defence system that protects our body from different types of vulnerabilities: virus, bacteria, fungi, parasites and other pathogens. The immune system performs its function by the following components, cells (RBC (Red Blood Cells), WBC'S, T and B lymphocytes), organs and lymphoid tissue. Figure 4.1 describes the structure of the different cell types present in the human body. The cells of the immune system that defends the body from foreign substances are the leukocytes. The WBC'S help in fighting infections, killing harmful bacteria and defend the body from irrelevant substances by creating antibodies. They originate from the soft fatty fluid of the bone called the bone marrow. This process of generating cells in the bone marrow is called hematopoiesis. These cells grow from a hematopoietic stem where

I. M. Sheikh (✉) · M. A. Chachoo
PG Department of Computer Science, University of Kashmir, Srinagar, India
e-mail: ishfaqmajeed.scholar@kashmiruniversity.net

S. A. Parah et al. (eds.), *Artificial Intelligence for Innovative Healthcare Informatics*,
https://doi.org/10.1007/978-3-030-96569-3_4

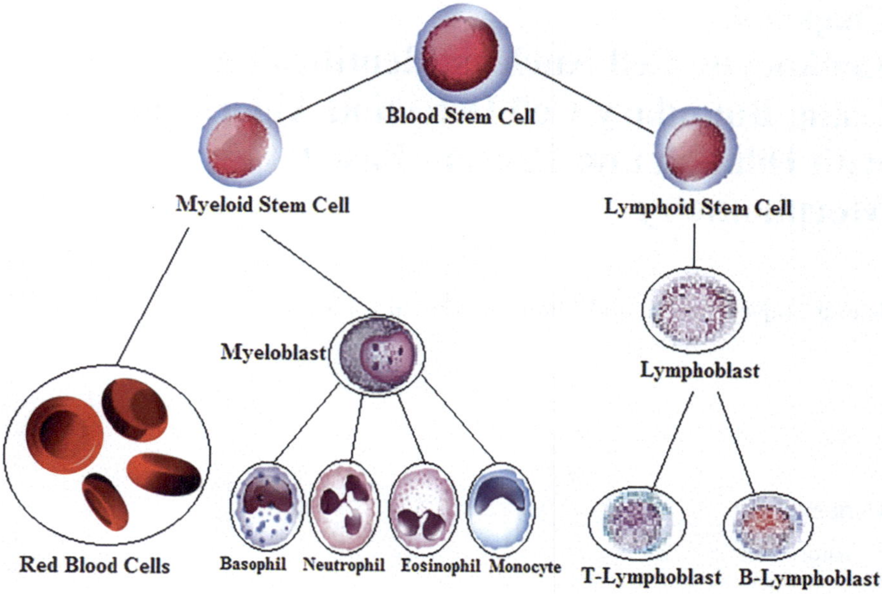

Fig. 4.1 Different types of cells in the human body

we discriminate them at the different stages, this is shown in Fig. 4.2. Different types of leukocytes perform several functions for maintaining the norm in the human body.

1.1 Types of WBC'S

- **Neutrophils**: About 50% of the WBC belongs to the Neutrophil class. The function of the neutrophil cell is to fight foreign invaders. It also communicates with the rest of the immune system to respond to the infection. They are the first in the group to perform their functions by sending biological signals. Around a hundred billion of these cells are released by the bone marrow per day but their normal life span is only 8 h.
- **Eosinophils**: They account for only 5% of the total WBC content in the human body but a major portion of these cells, are present in the digestive system. They also play an important role in fighting bacteria and attacking parasites. When the range of these cells goes out of limits, they may act as the cause for producing allergic symptoms.
- **Basophils**: The component corresponds to only 1% of the portion of leukocytes. The basophils can act as the source for controlling asthma and generates the response to pathogens. The stimulation of these cells releases histamine which may result in inflammation.

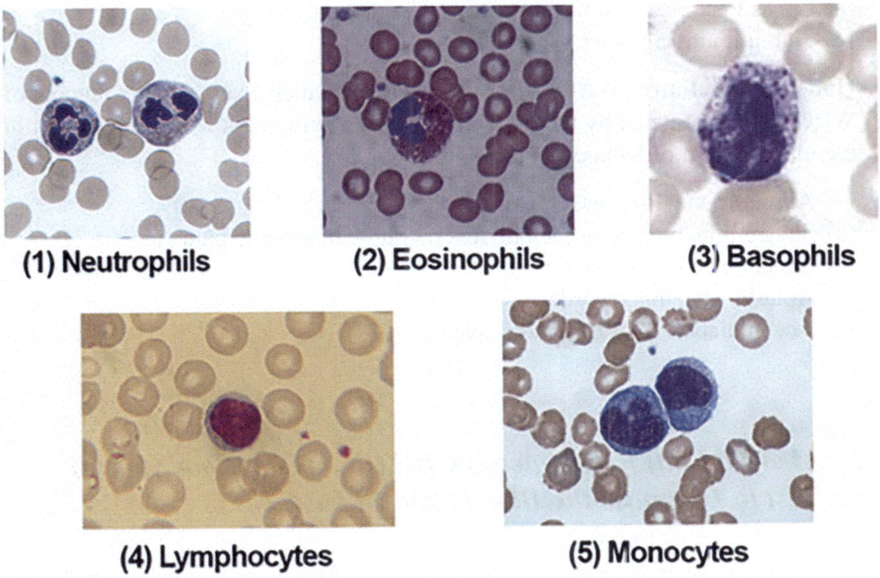

Fig. 4.2 Different types of WBC'S

- **Lymphocytes (B and T)**: The lymphocytic cell system consists of two subtype cells B and T lymphocytes. The T lymphocyte plays the main role indirectly killing most of the foreign invaders whereas B lymphocytes control humoral immunity and is also used to know the efficacy of most of the vaccines.
- **Monocytes**: They comprise around 5–12% of the leukocytes in the human immune system. They perform the function of cleaning the dead cells, also named as garbage trucks of the human immune system.

The leukocytes have a certain range in which they remain beneficial to human health. Within their specified limits they perform the optimal function for the human immune system. If there is any deviation of the leukocytes from the normal limits, overproduction or underproduction of these cells, from the bone marrow. They affect the human body in a harmful way.

1. **Overproduction of WBC'S**: It is the case in which the bone marrow produces an enormous number of WBC'S that grow above the normal limits. This increased growth interrupts the function of the normal flow of the human body. There are multiple causes for this elevated blood cell growth either the bone marrow produces too many cells at the early stage or of the following symptoms.
   (a) Cancer of type leukaemia, in which a large number of abnormal cells are made in the bone marrow.
   (b) Infection.
   (c) Asthma.

(d) Stress may also lead to the increased growth of cells.
(e) Autoimmune disorder.

2. **Under production of WBC'S**: This is the case in which a very smaller number of WBC'S, are produced by the bone marrow. The symptoms which may result in the undergrowth of leukocytes are as follows.

   (a) Autoimmune diseases.
   (b) Severe infections may include fever, cough, diarrhoea, pain etc.
   (c) Cancer of type metastatic.
   (d) Aplastic anaemia disorder.
   (e) Accumulation of WBC in the spleen.

1.2 Medical Staff Recommends CBC (Complete Blood Count) Test to Diagnose the Blood-Related Diseases

To test a wide range of disorders, present in the human body doctors follow a commonly recommended test called CBC that evaluates overall health performance [1–6]. It measures several components RBC, WBC, haemoglobin and platelets. Usually, doctors prescribe this test to analyze one or the combination of the following disorders anaemia, infection and leukaemia. In Table 4.1 we have depicted the result of the CBC for the normal patient. Medical experts recommend this test for the following reasons.

Table 4.1 Normal blood count of the healthy person

Blood component	Range of values
Haemoglobin	Male: 13.2–16.6 g/dL[a] (132–166 g/L) Female: 11.6–15 g/dL (116–150 g/L)
Hematocrit	Male: 38.3–48.6% Female: 35.5–44.9%
White blood cell count	3.4–9.6 billion cells/L (3400–9600 cells/μL)
Red blood cell count	Male: 4.35–5.65 trillion cells/L[b] (4.35–5.65 million cells/μL[c]) Female: 3.92–5.13 trillion cells/L (3.92–5.13 million cells/μL)
Platelet count	Male: 135–317 billion/L (135,000–317,000/μL) Female: 157–371 billion/L (157,000–371,000/μL)

[a]dL = deciliter
[b]L = liter
[c]μL = microliter

- **To review the health performance of the patient**: The doctors usually judge the health of the patient, by analyzing the range of different blood components present in the human body, so that we can get information regarding the different disorders (allergy, infection, anaemia and leukaemia). These measures can be collected using CBC to monitor the overall health information of the patient.
- **To diagnose a related disease**: If somebody experiences a feeling of fever, weakness, inflammation, bleeding and infection. The doctors advise the CBC to the patients for knowing the cause for the related symptoms.
- **Treatment for the disease**. It can also be used to monitor the effect of the desired treatment method. That is related to the counting of blood cells. By doing CBC doctors can get information regarding the perfect medication required for the particular type of symptom.

1.3 Automatic Disease Detection Approach

Automatic detection of the blood disorder can be achieved by using machine learning analysis of the microscopic blood sample images. That can characterize different components of the blood sample image efficiently at the earliest stages. This will aid the medical staff in the treatment of blood-related diseases. Artificial Intelligence has already revolutionized the modern world with the development of powerful machine learning models. For driving autonomous cars, weather forecast prediction, intelligent agents, natural language processing, vision, biometrics etc. know it is time to shift our efforts towards the healthcare system, by developing an automatic disease diagnosing system that will ease the process of the treatment methods. The data which is generated by the medical staff has too much complexity and volume in its nature. The source of information is heterogeneous. The data exist in different format of X-rays, chest images, knee images, blood images, bone marrow, DNA (deoxyribonucleic acid) microarray and RNA (ribonucleic acid) sequencing. In recent, the procedure of analyzing this volume of information has been relying solemnly on the expert of medical staff. Which is complex, time-consuming, and prone to errors. Also, a large portion of the information is not explored because of the negligence of the medical staff this requires the need for intelligent machine learning models to find the meaningful patterns in this vast amount of data.

In the past decade machine learning has been explored in the field of medical sciences to find automatic identification of most of the challenging diseases in the healthcare system like leukaemia, prostate cancer, colon cancer, cardiovascular disease, diabetes, Alzheimer's disease etc. For some of the diseases, automatic drugs have been discovered. That will improve the speed up of the treatment methods. Among the mentioned disease cancer has been observed as the deadliest disease with a maximum number of average deaths per year. Research data has shown that on average around 17 million cancer cases are diagnosed each year and there is the possibility that the average number of cases may go up, to the number of

27 million by the year 2040. Every type of cancer is born from the cells [5, 6]. Which originate from the soft fatty fluid from the bone. These abnormal cells show an unstoppable growth and they live beyond the normal period of life. Which results in the disruption to the flow of normal cells. Usually, cancers are treated with the following methods of treatment as transplantation of bone marrow, radiations, molecular therapies (imatinib, dasatinib and nilotinib), and immunotherapy. These modes of treatment are suggested by the medical expert, based on accurate disease identification. It has been observed in patients about the consequences of these modes of treatment in the form of hair loss, infertility and change of skin colour. The cause behind this was that the medical staff has not utilized the patient's data efficiently, accurate treatment of the disease is only possible, once we can perfectly identify the disease. This identification of the disease can be done by using a machine learning-based solution. It has the potential to explore a vast number of meaningful possibilities from the highly complex structure of the patient's gene data. For some of the diseases, intelligent models have been developed. Consider the case of cardiovascular disease factors that influences the patient's personal life were collected by the risk assessment approach. Then the suggestions of the treatment method were made at the next level. The genetic information of the patient (genes that could cause obesity) was utilized in the development of an intelligent system for type 1 diabetes.

In recent research, we have found most of the diseases are related to the abnormal growth of the different types of WBC'S. Considering this in mind we have picked our objective of analyzing the leukocytic cells from the blood image data content. Features of blood images can only be extracted optimally once; we can properly discriminate multiple components of the blood-related data content. This requires the need for a robust methodology at the segmentation phase because the other phases like the extraction of features and their classification depend upon the accurate segmentation of the multiple blood sub-structures. Keeping this in consideration we have relaxed our objective for sub-segmenting the blood smears using robust methodology with dilation and erosion-based morphology. Our work, will not only have a focus on finding and analyzing the challenges in recent literature but also address some of the challenges in the current methodology.

To analyse the WBC'S automatically, we need to understand the structure of the leukocytic cell system. This can be done, by first segmenting the blood image into several distinct components (WBC, RBC, Platelets and Background). Among the multiple components, present in the blood image only the leukocytes are responsible for different types of blood disorders. This simplifies our machine learning approach because we need to focus only on a single component from the number of blood image data components. Most of the information related to WBC'S are stored in the nucleus of its cell. Keeping this in consideration, we need to divide the cell pattern into two sub-components i.e., the nucleus and the cytoplasm. This has further simplified the direction of our work towards the extraction of cell nucleus pattern because it acts as the main reservoir of the information in the cell body.

2 Literature Review

There is vast literature available on the segmentation of medical blood images. Most of it has thrown light on the boundary cell detection-based approach. It has a focus on retaining the nucleus of different leukocytic cells. The approach extracts the nucleus by identifying discontinuities between different blood components. This is done by computing gradients that show a directional shift in the change of intensities. This procedure is simple. The pattern-based approach performs the segmentation of data points based on their distance to the nearest mean. The data points are grouped into k number of clusters. Each data point belongs to the group with the highest membership value. In [7] the authors have segmented different types of WBC'S from the fluorescent biomedical images. They have divided their work into three stages. In the initial, they have generated L*a*b colour space from the given blood images, as this colour space suits best with the vision and perception. Next, they have utilized an unsupervised machine learning algorithm (k-means) for clustering of the data points based on the Euclidian distance measures between the nearest data points. In the end, they have done morphological processing on the connected data components of the resulting binary image. Even though, the authors claim that the model has generated promising results with a sensitivity of 96.49% and a precision of 98.3584%. There were certain problems with the concerned methodology because the model has highlighted some of the non-WBC components in the leucocyte class.

Liu Y. et al. [8] has proposed an advanced approach for WBC segmentation. The approach has a two-phase process. In which the model first detects the WBC location by the multi-window and multiscale methods. It fits leukocytes with different sizes. Once the model has successfully identified different locations of the WBC, then the authors have done final segmentation of the identified regions by using iterative Grab Cut. The performance of the proposed methodology was evaluated, on the two challenging datasets CellaVision and jiashan. Even though the authors have reported around 98% precision and recall on the mentioned datasets, they were unable to find the optimal parameter values, thus they have manually set the values of the parameters for adjustment of different types of datasets. In [9] the authors have extended the Otsu thresholding algorithm to compute different threshold values for each of the fractal regions in the leukocytic blood image. This has been done to extend the approach to biological images, where a single global threshold value is not sufficient to distinguish different classes of pixel values. However, the model needs improvement in its methodology (inertia weighting, adaptability parameter) to perform robust discrimination of different subcomponents. In [10] NIOA (Nature Inspired Optimization algorithms) is utilized to prevent false positiveness of the segmented data points that belongs to different components of the cell image.

In [11], on blood leukaemia smear images optimal thresholding and morphological operations were performed to generate the texture features. Later supervised and unsupervised classification of the features was done by many of the supervised and unsupervised classifiers to accurately classify the data. Thresholding based methodology was adopted in [12], where the authors had dealt with the k number of thresholds in the binary image. In which, the object is assigned to the positive region if its value is greater than k otherwise the object is treated as non-relevant content of the data. The approach does not work with variate types of illuminations in the input image. The region growing method is proposed in [13] that treats data objects as seeds. Depending upon the size of the seed the model decides whether pixels needed to be added or eroded. To extract cells from the blood image the authors have utilized features like illumination, shape and texture of the blood sample images. Erosion based morphological blood cell analysis was also performed in [14]. The authors have modelled the problem by combining region extraction with erosion-based limits to segment the overlapping leukocytic substructures. The region-based watershed segmentation was adopted on grey level intensities with graph-based manifold learning [15]. The concerned approach has many drawbacks of over or under segmentation of the data. Also, some of the blood cells were not identified in the blood image.

Vonn Vincent Quiñones et al. [16] applied basic grey level boundary cell operations on the blood image. The approach consists of the following steps conversion of RGB (Red Green Blue) blood image to HSV (Hue Saturation Value) and grayscale colour space, component differentiation, binarization and blob detection. The approach does not work appropriately on different types of blood images. Bilkis Jamal Firdosi et al. [17] has done pattern-based clustering on L*a*b colour space by using k-means. The model has not performed appropriately on different WBC types. Also, it has highlighted non-WBC blood components from the blood image. Rosyadi et al. [18] has retained the circularity feature of the blood images by applying Otsu for segmentation, and K-Means for clustering.

Garcia-Lamont et al. [19] has surveyed the most common recent approaches, for the segmentation of biomedical images. The colour of the biomedical image acts as the base for discrimination of sub-components. The authors have put their focus on the grey-level and colour based segmentation approach. The techniques that they have utilized are; boundary cell detection using thresholding, region growing, watershed segmentation for catchment basins supervised and unsupervised segmentation using clustering-based approaches, and some deep learning solutions. To identify leukocytes more appropriately. Anil-Kumar et al. [20] has done a review, on the recent segmentation methods used for the detection of leukaemia. The authors have highlighted most of the automatic disease detection-based approaches. The methods were categorized based on the procedure followed for the segmentation of biomedical images. Wang and Cao [21] propose a quick leukocyte nucleus segmentation method based on the component difference in RGB colour space (B-G), because this difference of the colour components (B and G) is very large in the leukocytes and platelets. Next, they retain the value of the WBC nucleus, by setting a filter that removes the content of platelets. In [22–27] the authors have modelled the problem, by applying the pattern-based segmentation methods on the characteristics of the biomedical images. The objective was to diagnose leukaemia. We have implemented many algorithms from the existing literature for segmentation but we have found some problems associated with ML (Machine Learning) methods that extract the nucleus from the blood image while removing the rest of the content as the image noise.

3 Methodology

Nowadays, in the advent of technology research efforts are being made for the development of computer-aided solutions that will do the automatic analysis on the biomedical image data. The automatic system can be utilized to aid the oncologist in diagnosing the different types of diseases, related to blood disorders. The CAD (Computer Aided Developed) solution, can predict the disease at a very fast rate with high accuracy. The solution comprises some set of steps from the image acquisition to the appropriate leukocytic cell identification. The layout of the CAD architecture is depicted in Fig. 4.3. To diagnose the disease, the oncologist has to only look towards the results where he can get the information about the type and number of WBC cells in the blood image. There are different types of WBC'S (Basophil, Eosinophil, Monocyte, Lymphocyte and Neutrophil) with little variation of parameters (perimeter, eccentricity, intensity etc.) between these cell types moreover, the blood components are congested in nature. This induces complexity in data thus requires the need for efficient machine learning methodology.

Appropriate discrimination of objects in the cell image can be performed, by understanding the structure of sub-components. This can be done by picking the robust method for segmenting the blood sample sub-components. Our work has a focus on the segmentation of microscopic blood image samples. There are two approaches through which we can perform the segmentation of the leukocytic cell nucleus. One is based on leukocytic cell boundary detection that deals with grey level intensities of different blood components, whereas the other has a focus on the pattern-based characterization of the blood samples that use different types of distance measures (Euclidian distance, Manhattan distance, Minkowis distance) to minimize the dissimilarity within the pattern of intraclass sub-segments. We have followed the boundary-based cell detection approach, with dilation and erosion of seed object. It is used to address some of the challenges in the recent literature. The pseudo-code of our model is depicted in Algorithm 4.1.

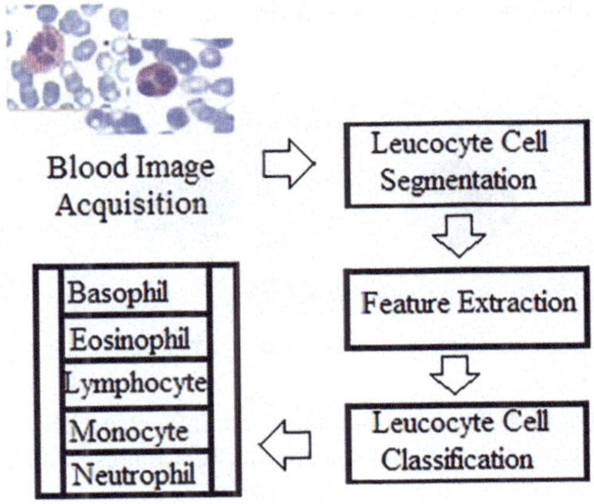

Fig. 4.3 Leucocyte subtype classification

3.1 Formulation of Our Developed Approach

- **Conversion of the RGB blood image to the number of grey levels**: Conversion of the true colour blood image to the grayscale image. The greyscale image does not contain the complexity of large colour variation and it simplifies the differentiation of the leukocytic cell nucleus from the rest of the blood image content. The conversion retains only the luminance information to get a brighter nucleus spot. The result is depicted in Fig. 4.4b with reduced hue and saturation information. We represent the pixels of a given grayscale image in L grey levels [1, 2, 3. . . . L]. Where each of the grey levels has a different set of pixel intensities. The number of pixels at level *I* is denoted by *ni* and the total number of pixels $N = n1 + n2 + n3 + . . + n$.

Algorithm 4.1 Boundary Cell Detection Based Approach

Input: A microscopic blood sample image is read as input.

1. Convert the input image to the number of grey levels.
2. Contrast Enhancement of the number of grey levels for the robust discrimination of blood image substructures.
3. Adjust the selected blood image to the particular image histogram.
4. Choose a global threshold value t that separates Foreground class pixels from background class pixels.
5. Calculate the Variance of Foreground class pixels $V_f = \sigma^2$, Calculate the Variance of Background class pixels $V_b = \sigma^2$, Minimize the within-class variance and maximize the between-class variance.
6. Reduce the damage of the pre-processing steps by applying noise reduction techniques.
7. Segment the processed blood cell image into several regions.
8. Extract the WBC region by choosing the threshold that removes remaining unwanted portions (RBC, Platelets Background and Cytoplasm).
9. Apply dilation and erosion operation to retain the actual shape of the WBC.

Output: Segmented WBC nucleus.

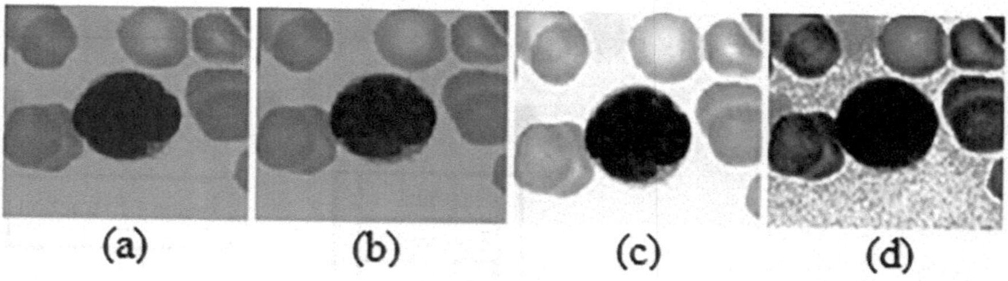

Fig. 4.4 Model results on a test data where labels indicate (**a**) Input blood sample image, (**b**) Discriminated Blood components, (**c**) Contrast adjusted blood image, (**d**) Contrast enhancement by matching **c** to a specified histogram

- **Blood Image Enhancement**: Quality of the blood image is an important factor for leukocytic cell nucleus segmentation, it depends upon the lighting conditions of the surrounding, resolution of the electron microscopic camera, the angle of capturing the blood smear image etc. The received input image at most of the times is of low to medium quality which makes difficulties in discriminating sub-components, thus requires a transformation in quality from the input blood sample quality to the desired level. This is done by the transformation equation that does the enhancement of the blood image, results are depicted in Fig. 4.4c, d.
  - Let x be an input image of dimension $m_i * m_j$ with intensity values between 0 to L − 1. Consider the case of analyzing the blood image, its quality usually falls in the intensity values between 100 and 150 that is enhanced by modifying the values of L to the maximum value i.e., 255. Its objective function is depicted in (4.1).

$$g(x) = \left(\left(\frac{f-100}{150}\right) * 255\right), \forall 100 \le f \le 150 \tag{4.1}$$

  - Next, we normalize the values of histogram p to the desired intensity levels of L so that the extracted pixel values have a uniform distribution, which is computed from (4.2).

$$p_k = \frac{\textit{Number of pixels with intensity k}}{\textit{Total number of pixels}} \quad \text{where k} = 0, 1, 2, 3 \ldots\ldots, \text{L} - 1, \tag{4.2}$$

  - After applying histogram equalization, we need to round of L to the nearest positive integer by the use of floor functions depicted in (4.3) and (4.4).

$$g_{i,j} = \text{floor}\left((\text{L} - 1) * \sum_{n=0}^{f_{i,j}} p_n\right) \tag{4.3}$$

$$T(K) = \text{floor}\left((\text{L} - 1) * \sum_{n=0}^{k} p_n\right) \tag{4.4}$$

- **Global Optimal Threshold *t* selection**: To do robust subcomponent segmentation we have divided the blood cell image components into two classes of pixels, Foreground (WBC Nucleus), the important component and Background (RBC Platelets Cytoplasm and Noise), non-required part. These two classes of pixel levels were separated by computing the optimal threshold levels, using the Otsu threshold algorithm. It is the global optimal threshold algorithm. It works by,

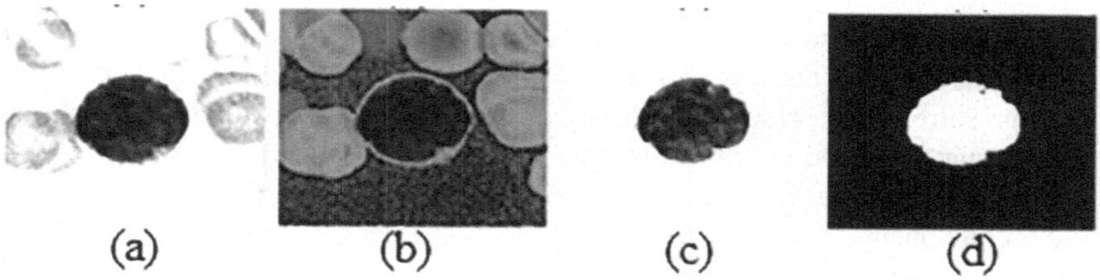

Fig. 4.5 Model results on test data during the nucleus extraction process where labels indicate (**a**) Brightened blood components (RBC, Platelets and Background), (**b**) Highlighted WBC nucleus with some noise, (**c**) Extracting WBC cell with minimum distortion to the nucleus, (**d**) The output of the shape-based Thresholding algorithm was between-class variance is high and within-class variance is low

maximizing the variation between the irrelevant class values and minimize the variation within the relevant pixel class values. Its pseudo-code is depicted in Algorithm 4.2, and results are depicted in Fig. 4.5a. We have represented foreground class pixels by V_f and background class pixels by V_b. These two classes are separated by an optimal global pixel intensity threshold value t were levels $V_b = 0, 1, 2. \ldots. t$ and $V_f = t + 1, t + 2. \ldots. L - 1$.

- **Restoration**: Due to the pre-processing done on blood cell images we are causing some form of damage to the blood image subcomponents, in the form of multiple sources of noise. We need to reverse the effect of the noise by setting filters that will reduce the impact on the final segmented blood components. Noise arises due to the pattern of low-intensity pixel values that are found around the edges of WBC during the extraction of the nucleus. It can be reduced by keeping a filter that removes abnormalities having pixel value less than the particular t. There are various sources of noise found in the processing of blood cell image data; such as salt-and-pepper noise, Gaussian noise or periodic noise. Results of the operation are depicted in Fig. 4.5a.
- **Region separation**: Segmentation involves dividing a blood cell image into several segments or regions. Microscopic blood cell mainly consists of the segments like WBC, RBC, Platelets and Background. Each segment has a particular structure like Size, Eccentricity, Major-Arc and Minor-Arc. Among the given segments we are interested in extracting the WBC portion for the detection of leukaemia. The result of separated components is depicted in Fig. 4.5b.
- **Thresholding**: It involves converting blood cell image into binary image. It reduces complexity and simplifies component recognition and their classification. The binary version contains essential information about the shape and position of the extracted foreground part i.e., WBC Nucleus. Normally only those black and white pixels of blood cell are retained having pixel intensity that matches the intensity level of WBC nucleus remaining unnecessary portion is discarded. Results are depicted in Fig. 4.5c.

- **Edge Detection**: To retain the shape of the WBC cell nucleus both the Sobel Edge Detection and Canny Edge Detection techniques were applied. Edge detection is the most useful approach for detecting discontinuities in a set of connected pixels that lie on the boundary between different regions of the blood cell image, where a gradient is a directional change in the intensity. Sobel detection computes the approximate absolute gradient magnitude at each point by computing 3 ∗ 3 filters. Canny edge detection first removes noise by applying a low pass filter and then it picks out the best pixel values for edges among the multiple pixel values in a local neighborhood. Results are depicted in Fig. 4.5d.
  - Let the convolution mask g_x estimates the gradient in the x-direction and the g_y estimates the gradient in the y-direction, A is the binarized image and ∗ represents the convolution operator. It is depicted in (4.5).

$$g_x = \begin{bmatrix} -2 & 0 & +2 \\ -1 & 0 & +1 \\ -2 & 0 & +2 \end{bmatrix} * A \text{ and } g_y = \begin{bmatrix} -2 & -1 & -2 \\ 0 & 0 & 0 \\ +2 & +1 & +2 \end{bmatrix} * A \tag{4.5}$$

  - The resulting gradient expression for the Sobel filter is given in (4.6).

$$\sqrt[G]{G_x^2 + G_y^2} \tag{4.6}$$

using this information gradient direction is calculated as,

$$\theta = are \tan \left(\frac{g_y}{g_x} \right)$$

Algorithm 4.2 Computing Global Optimal Thresholding Value

Input: Contrast-enhanced blood sample image

1. Compute the pixel intensity weights for background class:
   (a) Represent the weight of background class by W_b.
   (b) Compute the weight of background pixels, $W_b = \sum_{i=1}^{t} \frac{n_i}{N}$
   (c) Mean background pixel weight $\mu_b, W_b = \frac{\sum_{i=1}^{t} i * n_i}{\sum_{i=1}^{t} n_i}$
   - The variance of the background class, $\sigma_b^2 = \frac{\sum_{i=1}^{t} (i-\mu_b)^2 * n_i}{\sum_{i=1}^{t} n_i}$

2. Computation of foreground, pixel intensity weights:
    (a) Represent the weight of foreground class by W_f.
    (b) Compute the weight of foreground pixels, $W_f = \sum_{i=t+1}^{L} \frac{n_i}{N}$
    (c) Mean foreground pixel weight $\mu_f, W_f = \frac{\sum_{i=t+1}^{L} i*n_i}{\sum_{i=t+1}^{L} n_i}$
    (d) The variance of the foreground class, $\sigma_f^2 = \frac{\sum_{i=t+1}^{L} (i-\mu_b)^2*n_i}{\sum_{i=t+1}^{L} n_i}$

3. Compute the within-class variance $\sigma_w^2 = W_b\sigma_b^2 + W_f\sigma_f^2$, by taking the summation of foreground and background variances, multiplied by their associated weights.

Output: a global threshold that maximizes between-class variance and minimizes within-class variance.

- **Morphological Processing**: Mathematical morphological operation is more suitable for retaining the shape of WBC cells in images. The two main processes that can be used in the retention of WBC structure are dilation and erosion. These involve combining two sets of pixels, where one set consists of an input blood sample image which is to be processed and the other is Structuring Element (SE) which is a small matrix of pixels each with a value of zero or one. The SE is said to fit the image if for each of its entries matches the corresponding entries of image pixels. It is set to hit if at least one of its entries matches the corresponding pixel entries of the blood image. Results are shown in Fig. 4.6.

In dilation, every point in the cell image is superimposed by the SE, with its surrounding pixels. It is also called thickening operation where the operation is controlled by the shape of the SE.

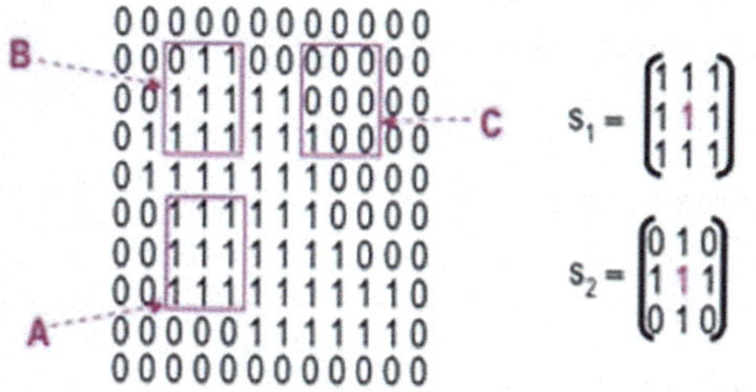

		A	B	C
fit	S_1	yes	no	no
	S_2	yes	yes	no
hit	S_1	yes	yes	yes
	S_2	yes	yes	no

Fig. 4.6 Structuring element fit and hit results

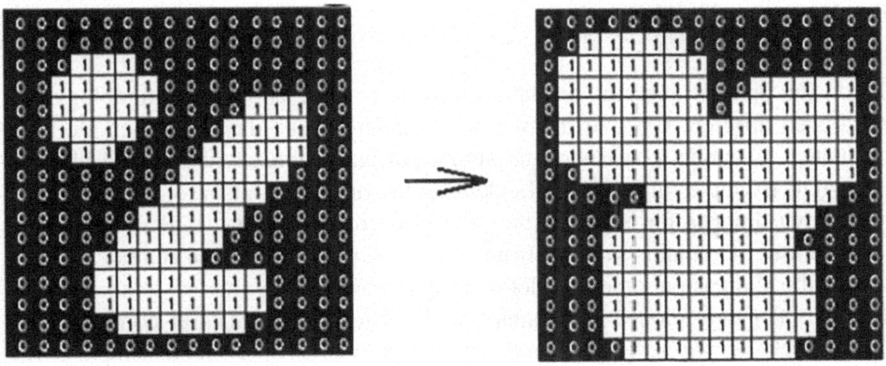

Fig. 4.7 Result of Dilation process on binary Matrix

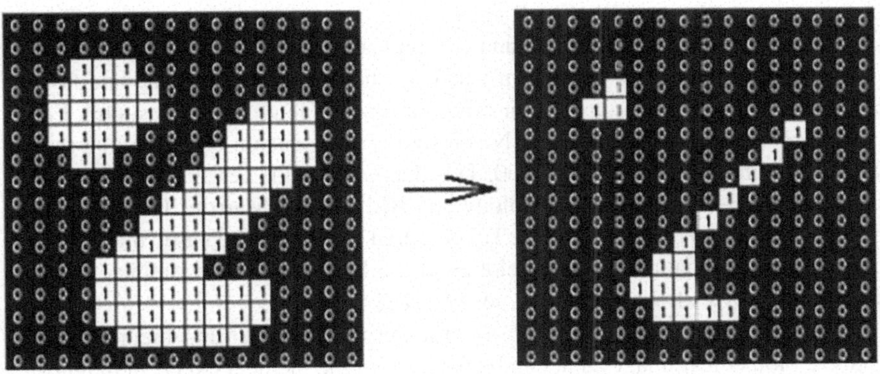

Fig. 4.8 Result of Erosion process on 0,1 Matrix

- The dilation of an image *im* by a structuring element SE (denoted as $im \oplus SE$) produces a new binary image $g = im \oplus SE$ with ones in all locations (*x*, *y*) of blood image at which the SE hits the blood image i.e., $g(x, y) = 1$, if SE hits or fits *im*, otherwise $g(x, y) = 0$ repeating for all pixel coordinates of $g(x, y)$. The effect of dilation is depicted in Fig. 4.7.
- The erosion (opposite of dilation) thins a microscopic cell image *im* with a structuring element SE (denoted as $im \ominus SE$) produces a new binary image $g = im \ominus SE$ places ones in all locations (*x*, *y*) of blood image if and only if the SE fits the blood image i.e., $g(x, y) = 1$ otherwise $g(x, y) = 0$ repeating for all pixel coordinates of $g(x, y)$. The effect of erosion is depicted in Fig. 4.8.

4 Result and Discussions

To do the optimal analysis, on the performance of the adopted methodology, we have used different types of datasets for evaluation. The data on which we have evaluated our model consists of the number of publicly accessible digital libraries ALL-IDB (Acute Lymphoblastic Leukaemia International Database), Kaggle, LISC (Leucocyte Images for Segmentation and Classification). ALL-IDB is the widely used dataset. It contains samples from the leukaemia and non-leukaemia classes in which the dimension of each blood sample image is resampled to the size of 1200*1200 pixels plotted horizontally and vertically. The dataset comprises the two subsets of segmented and non-segmented microscopic blood samples. The segmented set contains around 260 blood images that require only classification and the non-segmented set contains 108 microscopic blood images thus requires segmentation and classification. We have used lymphocytes from both of the subclasses for extraction of WBC cell nucleus and computing their important features for the classification of leukaemia and non-leukaemia cells.

Another public access dataset on which we have evaluated our methodology is the LISC. This dataset contains four different types of leukocytes (Basophil, Eosinophil, Monocyte, Lymphocyte and Neutrophil) the dimension of each blood sample 720*576 with a magnification of 100. This dataset contains nearly 250 colour blood images, collected from the Hematology and BMT (Bone Marrow Transplantation) research centre of the hospital in Tehran, Iran. One more dataset that we have collected for evaluation purpose belongs to the Kaggle. This dataset also contains several leukocytes from different types of WBC cells.

Our main target was to develop an efficient machine learning methodology to analyze biomedical images that can be used to aid the medical expert in diagnosing blood-related disorders. Multiple approaches are used for the identification of WBC cell. The method that extracts these features with minimum distortion is desirable. We have adopted robust methodology with dilation and erosion based morphological operations, to extract the complete leukocytic cell. The work has successfully extracted leukocytic cells, counting their number and computing their basic features. We have depicted results in Fig. 4.9.

Although we have optimally utilized our methodology, to do an automatic analysis of the biomedical image data. Our method mainly concentrates on the retention of the leukocytic cell nucleus, as done by most of the related methods. There exist several new challenges that have been overlooked, by the majority of the recent works. We have observed several new problems while doing experiments in Matlab. To some extent, we have addressed the issues by adopting dilation and erosion-based morphometry. It still needs attention towards the more advanced machine learning models. For that, we are looking for a vision-based solution that will focus on the retention of the complete leukocytic cell, which will do the best characterization of the blood image components. So that, we can easily differentiate various types of leukocytic cells. The challenges are discussed as follows.

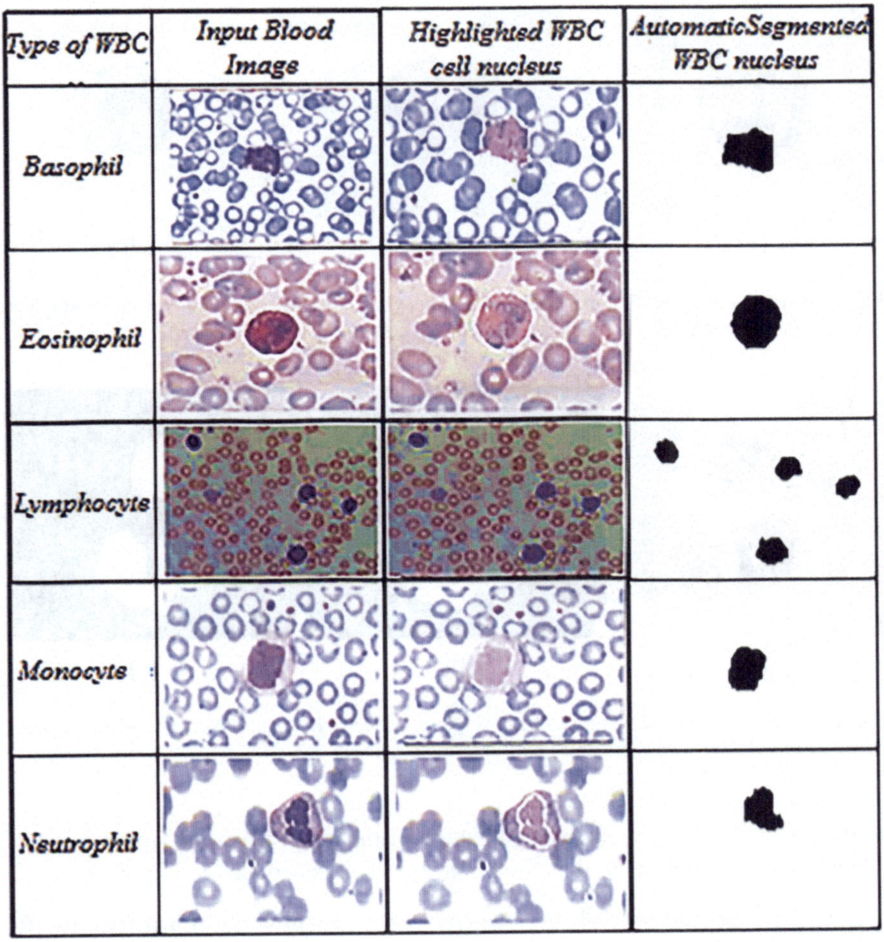

Fig. 4.9 Result of leukocytic cell nucleus extraction on different types of WBC'S

1. **Identify different types of WBC cells**: Every type of leukocytic cell has some specific properties like Eccentricity, size, perimeter, Major-Arc, Minor-Arc etc. that differentiates it from the other types of blood components. All these properties are associated with complete leukocytic cell including cytoplasm. Results have shown that the nucleus extraction process manipulates the size parameter and thus we face difficulty in identifying the type of leukocytic cell. In Fig. 4.10 we have depicted the results.
2. **Counting the leukocytic cells at different stages of maturity**: Leukocytes have been classified into granulocytes and non-granulocytes. The nucleus of the granulocytes gets divided into some segments at the mature stage. Segmenting

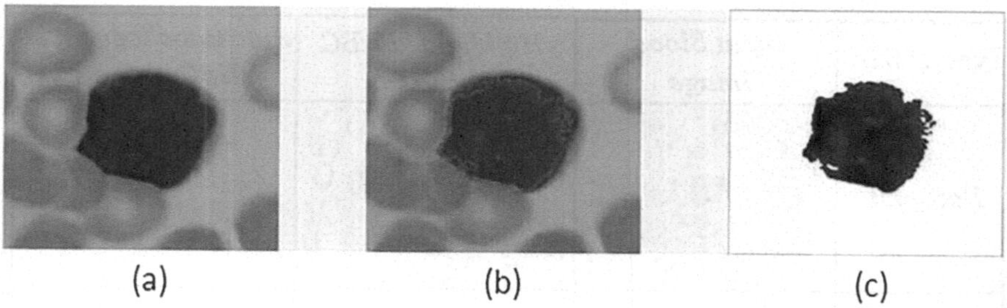

Fig. 4.10 (**a**) Input Blood Sample Image of lymphocytic class. (**b**) Blood Image with Highlighted Nucleus. (**c**) Output WBC cell with size variation in cell size (Neutrophil class)

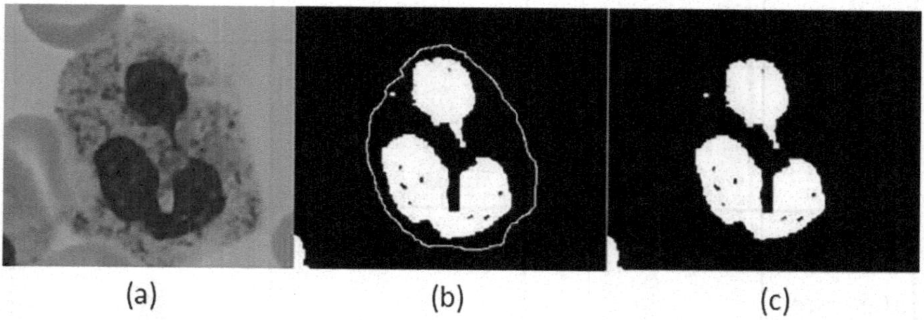

Fig. 4.11 (**a**) Blood image with one object single WBC cell. (**b**) Expected count should be single object. (**c**) Model counted three objects for the single nucleus

the nucleus of the granulocytic cell at the mature stage gives the wrong count of the number of objects in the blood image. Result is depicted in Fig. 4.11.

(a) **Challenge addressed by incorporating morphological process in the methodology**: We have addressed the multiple count problem by utilizing mathematical morphological operations on the divided segments of the single leukocytic cell nucleus. This is an important machine learning tool for analyzing the different types of binary structures in the biomedical image content. This approach can be used for the extraction of leukocytic cell patterns based on the circular structure of the cell and the filtering gradients. There are four operations in the morphological process dilation, erosion, opening and closing. Dilation and closing extend the boundary cell region where ever it finds the hit in the data content of the blood image, we have used these operations for region growing of the cells. Whereas erosion and opening are the reverses of dilation, it shrinks the blood image data content. We have used these two operations to remove the unwanted or irrelevant content (noise) from the blood image. Figure 4.12 shows the results of the morphological processing on the divided or segmented WBC granules. Where, the initial experimental results have shown, the count of three cells, for the single

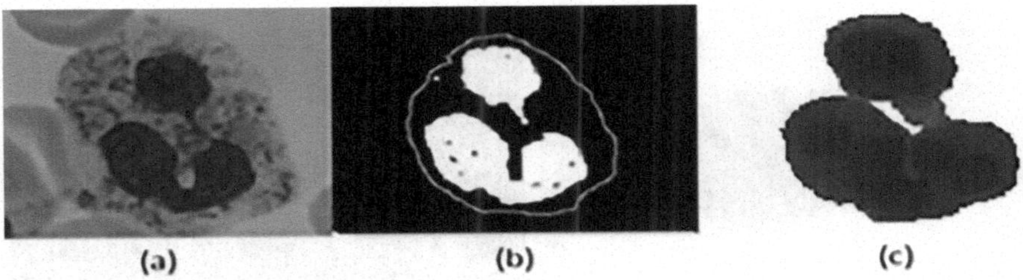

Fig. 4.12 Result of dilation on the microscopic blood sample image, where (**a**) Blood image with one object single WBC cell (**b**) Expected count should be a single object (**c**) Automatic count of a single object

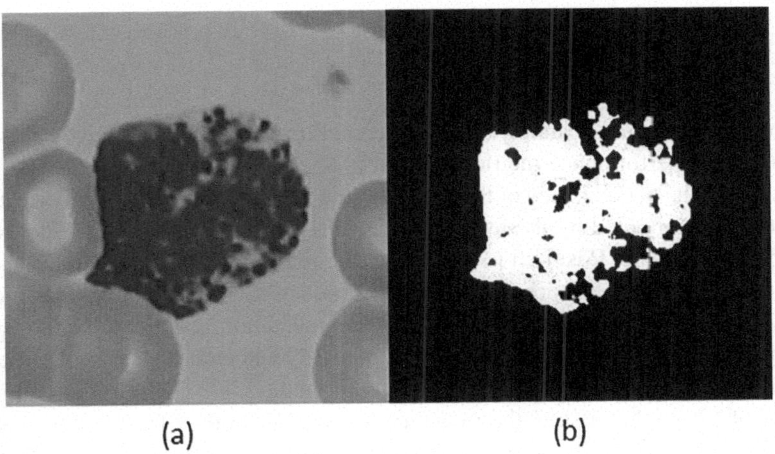

Fig. 4.13 (**a**) Input blood sample image. (**b**) Result of distorted WBC cell nucleus after removing noise from the blood sample image

WBC object cell. After applying morphological processing. We have filled the holes between the granules. It is done by dilating the region, to get the actual result of the single object cell.

3. **Retaining the geometric structure of the leukocytic cells with minimal distortion to the nucleus**: At times noise removal filters distorts the geometric pattern of WBC'S. The filter is a threshold value, and what falls below the value of the filter is removed as noise from the cell image. In Fig. 4.13 the data points of class noise have the same intensity, that matches the pixel intensity of the cell nucleus. Setting the filter of that value removes also the data points of the nucleus. This approach distorts the geometric shape of the cell nucleus.
4. **Handling multiple sources of noise in the data**: Preprocessing leads to small data points, in the form of pixels plotted horizontally and vertically across the blood image. To get a true count of the number of leukocytes noise removal filters are adopted to get rid of the irrelevant content. Figure 4.14 depict its result.

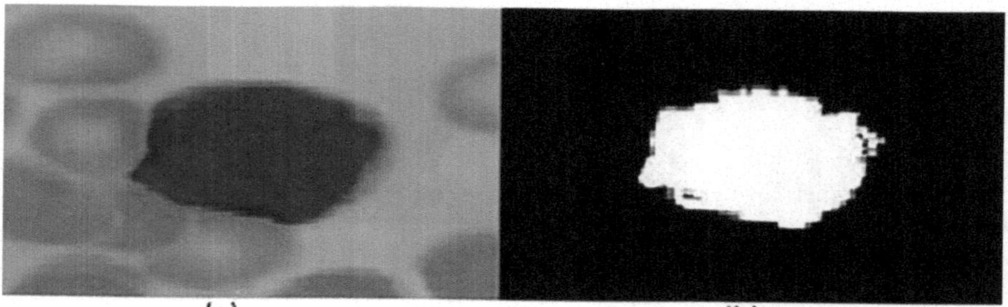

Fig. 4.14 (**a**) Input blood sample image. (**b**) Result of WBC cells

5 Performance Measures

For every successful execution of the concerned methodology, we have calculated the following performance metrics Accuracy, Specificity, Error rate, Precision and Prevalence. The performance of the model on the segmentation of the leukocytic cell nucleus was computed by the following machine learning metrics TP, FP, TN and FN. Where TP (True Positive) is the number of correct predictions. It indicates, the number of leukocytes that are predicted by the model and the same number is present in the blood image. It represents the correct segmentation results by the model. FP (False positive) is the wrong count of the number of leukocytes that are not present in the blood sample image but are counted by our method. FN (False Negative) is the reverse of FP. In this metric, the model does not count some of the leukocytes that are truly present in the blood image. TN (True Negative) is the metric in which the model has not identified the region as the leukocytic cell, and the same region does not belong to that object when counted manually. To evaluate the performance of our method, we have calculated the following performance measures accuracy, sensitivity and precision. The formulation of these measures is depicted in Eqs. (4.7–4.9).

$$Accuracy = \frac{TP + TN}{Total\ data} \tag{4.7}$$

$$Sensitivity = \frac{TP}{TP + FN} \tag{4.8}$$

$$Precision = \frac{TP}{TP + FP} \tag{4.9}$$

The developed approach was tested on some few hundred (250) medical blood images collected from the mentioned datasets in random proportion. We have evaluated the model on different combinations of blood sample images. Figures 4.15 and 4.16 depicts the results of the experiment on the individual and combined subtypes of WBC'S. These blood images were categorized into five different classes (basophil, eosinophil, monocyte, lymphocyte and neutrophil). Table 4.2 represent the result of the confusion metric that is used to evaluate the automatic and manual counting of leukocytic cells.

The approach that we have adopted in our work, has shown comparatively higher performance as compared to some of the proposed methods in the literature. The model has performed best on the segmentation of the lymphocytes, with an average accuracy of 93.1%, which is very high as compared to the segmentation accuracy achieved by Hiren and Velani [24]. They have reported accuracy of 91.07% with an over-segmentation and under-segmentation rate of 6.50% and 6.C4%. The over-segmentation rate has been expressed as the region, which must be included in the background class, the objects were placed in the foreground class of cells. That gives the wrong count of the number of leukocytes. Whereas, the under-segmentation rate is the reverse of over-segmentation, in which multiple cells are counted as a single object. The work of Khalid A. et al. [13] has outperformed our boundary-based cell detection approach, they have achieved the mean best accuracy of 95% on the segmentation of lymphocytes, and 92% on the neutrophils. The model was evaluated

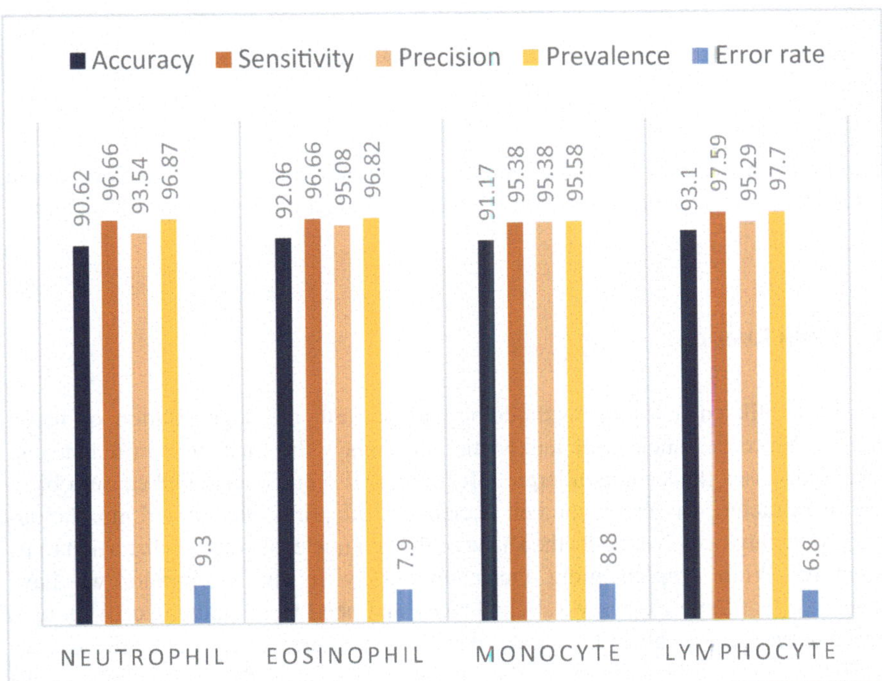

Fig. 4.15 Segmentation performance of the model on different leukocytic cell types

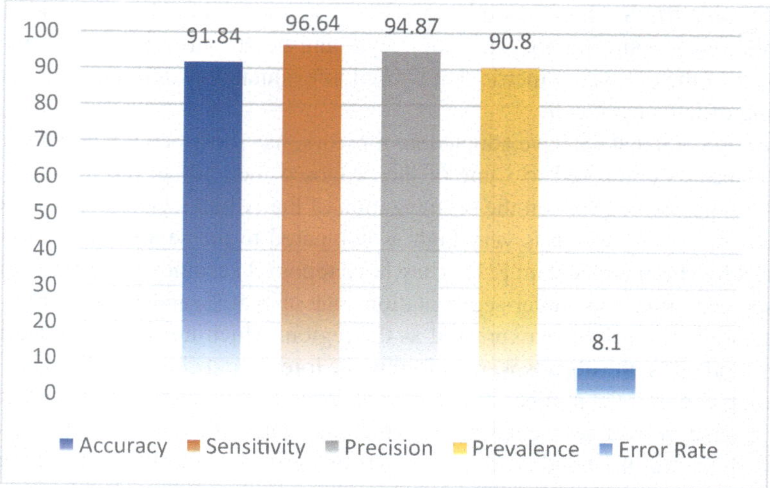

Fig. 4.16 Overall segmentation performance of the model on the combined subtypes of WBC

Table 4.2 Manual and Automatic counting of leukocytes

WBC	Total images	Automatic count	Manual count	TP	FP	FN
Lymphocyte	70	86	87	81	4	2
Monocyte	60	65	68	62	3	3
Eosinophil	60	67	63	58	3	2
Neutrophil	60	50	64	58	4	2
Total	250	268	282	259	14	9

only on the set of 100 samples of microscopic WBC images, which is very less in comparison to our approach, which we have evaluated on 250 blood cell images.

6 Conclusion

We have utilized a robust methodology to perform the segmentation of blood images. Since the nucleus of leukocytic cells, plays the main role in diagnosing several diseases (leukaemia, allergic infections, AIDS). We have picked our objective of extracting the leukocytic cell nucleus, by adopting shape-based morphological processing, which extracts the shape of the cell nucleus with less distortion to its structure. While implementing the methodology in the work-plan, we have observed, that there exist several challenges that need to be addressed. Although, we have perfectly retained the shape of WBC'S appropriately. There still exist the challenges that we have observed during the evaluation of the experiment. So, we come with some new suggestions that needs to be addressed in future.

- For the task of medical blood image analysis, there is a need for a robust method, that should differentiate multiple substructures appropriately.
- While removing other blood components (Cytoplasm, RBC, Platelets, and Background). The methodology for leukocytic cell extraction must focus to retain the geometric structure (cell shape) of the WBC cell.
- To prevent several counts of single WBC. The nucleus extraction process must encompass all the granules of divided WBC inside the curvature cytoplasm, as a single object.

References

1. Vezzoli M, Bonardelli S, Peroni M, Ravanelli M, Garrafa E (2017) A simple blood test, such as complete blood count, can predict calcification grade of abdominal aortic aneurysm. J Vasc Med. https://doi.org/10.1155/2017/1370751
2. Escott-Stump S (2015) Hematology: anemias and blood disorders. Nutr Diagn Relat Care 3(2): 703–748
3. Ferrari D, Motta A, Strollo M, Banfi G, Locatelli M (2020) Routine blood tests as a potential diagnostic tool for COVID-19. Clin Chem Lab Med 58(7):1095–1099. https://doi.org/10.1515/cclm-2020-0398
4. Iv FT, Raess PW, Ang D, Andal JJ, Press R, Tran N (2021) Somatic mutational analysis using next generation sequencing in predicting disease behavior of cytogenetically normal myelodysplastic syndromes. Blood Res Disord. https://doi.org/10.23937/2469-5696/1410063
5. The Leukemia & Lymphoma Society, New York. https://www.ils.org/facts-anstatistics. Accessed 16 Nov 2019
6. Cancer Research UK. http://www.cancerresearchuk.org. Accessed 16 Nov 2019
7. Ferdosi BJ, Nowshin S, Sabera FA, Habiba (2019) White blood cell detection and segmentation from fluorescent images with an improved algorithm using K-means clustering and morphological operators. In: 4th International conference on electrical engineering and information and communication technology, ICEEICT 2018, pp 566–570. https://doi.org/10.1109/CEEICT.2018.8628068
8. Liu Y, Cao F, Zhao J, Chu J (2017) Segmentation of white blood cells image using adaptive location and iteration. IEEE J Biomed Health Inform 21(6):1644–1655. https://doi.org/10.1109/JBHI.2016.2623421
9. Mandyartha EP, Anggraeny FT, Muttaqin F, Akbar FA (2020) Global and adaptive thresholding technique for white blood cell image segmentation. J Phys Conf Ser 1569(2). https://doi.org/10.1088/1742-6596/1569/2/022054
10. Dhal KG, Gálvez J, Ray S, Das A, Das S (2020) Acute lymphoblastic leukaemia image segmentation is driven by stochastic fractal search. Multimed Tools Appl 79(17–18): 12227–12255. https://doi.org/10.1007/s11042-019-08417-z
11. Rawat J, Singh A, Bhadauria HS, Virmani J, Devgun JS (2017) Classification of acute lymphoblastic leukaemia using hybrid hierarchical classifiers. Multimed Tools Appl 76(18): 19057–19085. https://doi.org/10.1007/s11042-017-4478-3
12. Bhavnania LA, Jaliyab UK, Joshib MJ (2015) Blood cell segmentation and counting: a survey. Int J Innov Emerg Res Eng 2(11):21–24
13. Abuhasel KA, Fatichah C, Iliyasu AM (2016) A commixed modified gram-Schmidt and region growing mechanism for white blood cell image segmentation. IEEE, New York
14. Fan J, Zhang Y, Wang R, Li S (2013) A separating algorithm for overlapping cell images. J Softw Eng Appl 2013:179–183

15. Sarosh P, Parah SA, Bhat GM (2021) Fast image encryption framework for medical images. In: 2021 2nd International conference on intelligent engineering and management (ICIEM). IEEE, New York, pp 149–154
16. Quiñones VV, Macawile MJ, Ballado A Jr, Dela Cruz J, Caya MV Leukocyte segmentation and counting based on microscopic blood images using HSV saturation component with blob analysis. In: 2018 3rd International conference on control and robotics engineering
17. Umamaheswari D, Geetha S (2018) Segmentation and classification of acute lymphoblastic leukemia cells tooled with digital image processing and ML techniques. In: Proceedings of the second international conference on intelligent computing and control systems (ICICCS 2018)
18. Rosyadi T, Arif A, Nopriadi, Achmad B, Faridah (2016) Classification of leukocyte images using K-means clustering based on geometry features. In: 6th International annual engineering seminar (InAES), Yogyakarta, Indonesia
19. Garcia-Lamont F, Cervantes J, López A, Rodriguez L (2018) Segmentation of images by color features: a survey. Neurocomputing 292:1–27
20. Anilkumar KK, Manoj VJ, Sagi TM (2020) A survey on image segmentation of blood and bone marrow smear images with emphasis to automated detection of leukemia. Biocybernet Biomed Eng 40(4):1406–1420. https://doi.org/10.1016/j.bbe.2020.08.010
21. Wang Y, Cao Y (2019) Quick leukocyte nucleus segmentation in leukocyte counting. Comput Math Methods Med. https://doi.org/10.1155/2019/3072498
22. Muntasa A, Yusuf M (2019) Modeling of the acute lymphoblastic leukemia detection based on the principal object characteristics of the color image. Proc Comput Sci 157:87–98. https://doi.org/10.1016/j.procs.2019.08.145
23. Acharya V, Kumar P (2019) Detection of acute lymphoblastic leukaemia using image segmentation and data mining algorithms. Med Biol Eng Comput 57(8):1783–1811. https://doi.org/10.1007/s11517-019-01984-1
24. Hiren DV, Velani N (2017) An automated blood cell segmentation using fuzzy based system. In: 8th International conference on computing, communications and networking technologies, ICCCNT 2017. https://doi.org/10.1109/ICCCNT.2017.8203971
25. Gull S, Mansour RF, Aljehane NO, Parah SA (2021) A self-embedding technique for tamper detection and localization of medical images for smart-health. Multimed Tools Appl 80(19): 29939–29964
26. Showkat S, Parah SA, Gull S (2021) Embedding in medical images with contrast enhancement and tamper detection capability. Multimed Tools Appl 80(2):2009–2030
27. Ghayvat H, Pandya SN, Bhattacharya P, Zuhair M, Rashid M, Hakak S, Dev K (2021) CP-BDHCA: Blockchain-based Confidentiality-Privacy preserving Big Data scheme for healthcare clouds and applications. IEEE J Biomed Health Inform. https://doi.org/10.1109/JBHI.2021.3097237

Chapter 5
Effective Prediction of Autism Using Ensemble Method

Siddharaj D. Pujari and K. Anusha

Contents

1 Introduction

ML provides the ability for machines to understand independently on their own based on observations, examining patterns and past experiences from data set. It takes informed decisions based on the available data with the use of various ML algorithms [1–3]. Traditional programming follows the execution of a definite set of instructions. Machine learning is different from traditional programming in such a way that it is based on the input data set and it learns by examining and discovering the relationships between data elements and decides independently based on its learning. Supervised Learning (SL), Unsupervised Learning (UL), and Reinforcement Learning (RL) are three main types of ML [4, 5].

In SL technique, model is trained using the data with known output. The training data contains attributes and corresponding class labels. The input and output are denoted by X and Y respectively. The difference between the predicted value and actual value is known as error, the machine learns by reducing this error. According

S. D. Pujari (✉) · K. Anusha
Vellore Institute of Technology, Chennai, India

S. A. Parah et al. (eds.), *Artificial Intelligence for Innovative Healthcare Informatics*,
https://doi.org/10.1007/978-3-030-96569-3_5

to the error, the factor model is adjusted and implemented. To perform training and testing the whole data is classified as training and testing. To train the model using appropriate algorithm training data is used while for validating the trained model testing data is used. Regression and classification are the two types of SL [6, 7]. Autism is a severe developmental disorder that weakens the ability to interact and communicate [8]. It affects children in many ways and it shows various symptoms and appears in a variety of combinations. It is a common developmental disability in which children may show abnormal behaviors like disability in learning, mental problem, anxiety, motor difficulties, seizures, visual and hearing problems. Some existing systems are available which helps to identify an autistic patient using various visual and facial features and other behavioral data related to them [9, 10].

The classification problem of the SL algorithm is which pre-dictions are in non-continuous form and based on labeled data. The output graph is not-linear and information is not continuous. Classification algorithm examines input data to learn in the training phase and based on this learning, the new data set is classified. Binary classification and multiclass classification are the two types of classification based on the number of output classes [11, 12].

This chapter provides an understanding of various classification techniques that can be used for the prediction of ASD. It also provides a proposed method that is useful in the classification of a patient with ASD or no ASD. The proposed method uses the ensemble classification technique, which is a combination of different classification algorithms. The idea behind using this technique is to improve the accuracy of the proposed model. This chapter aims to help researchers in the selection of effective and appropriate classification techniques to solve prediction problems in their respective applications domains using ML, and to help researchers to understand the concepts and methodology based on ML.

2 Literature Review

In this method, researchers proposed a method for ASD detection using a machine learning model which is a combination of CART and ID3 based on Random Forest. This method is tested against a real autism dataset and results show that the implemented method provides better classification accuracy concerning other algorithms [13–15]. The rules machine learning technique developed by the researchers identifies autistic traits and also provides users knowledge bases in form of rules that can be helpful to experts in their respective domain for identifying the reasons behind the classification process. The experimentation is carried out on the data related to children, adolescents, and adults. The result shows that this approach classifies data with higher predictive accuracy, specificity, sensitivity, and harmonic mean as compared to other algorithms [16–18].

Another classification technique used by researchers is CNN which is based on deep learning, used in various image processing problems. The proposed model contains several layers which are present in CNN. The Matrix Multiplication is used to compute activation, which is followed by a bias offset. The result shows that the prediction model based on CNN works better in terms of accuracy [19]. The study in [20] focuses on ASD detection using eye movement data, using kinematic features, and combined features. Supervised ML techniques have been used to design classification models with feature selection methods. The result shows that using these features accuracy recorded by this model is above 70%. The proposed method in [21] uses a database named Autism Brain Imaging Data Exchange This dataset is applied to nine supervised machine learning methods as part of the implementation. A cross-validation strategy is used in training and testing the machine learning models. The performance is assessed concerning specificity, sensitivity, accuracy, and area under the curve. The result shows that the neural network model performed the best among the rest of the models. In another study, a questionnaire for parents is prepared and responses are recorded in a structured form. Key behaviors are also noted as part of dataset preparation using small home videos of kids. For these two datasets, two separate algorithms are trained and then a combined algorithm is used which combines the results into a single assessment. Feature selection and feature encoding techniques are also used to achieve efficiency among results and testing of performance is carried out with clinical study [22–25].

This research in [26] focuses on finding the effective ML algorithm among various algorithms used in the classification of medical datasets with some pre-processing techniques. It also contains a prediction of the early autism traits in children and adults. The experimentation shows that a combination of appropriate encoding and simple data pre-processing steps with different classifier algorithms like Random Forest, KNN, and logistic regression gives rise to prediction accuracy. The proposed methodology used for the classification of ASD traits contains a combination of various classification models. This technique is used to improve the classification accuracy of weak classifiers. The proposed study contains a combination of the decision tree, SVM, Naïve Bayes and KNN, etc. algorithm. These classifiers accurately classify ASD traits but if it is included as part of the ensemble classification technique then it performs very well and the combined accuracy is much more than the individual classifier.

3 Proposed Method

The proposed method of ASD classification is depicted in Fig. 5.1. It includes various steps such as data pre-processing, train-test split, ensemble classification methods, and classified data as ASD or No ASD.

3.1 Data Pre-processing

This step is used to convert the raw data into a relevant and unambiguous format. Raw data normally contains noise such as incompleteness and inconsistency which may lead to wrong prediction outcomes.

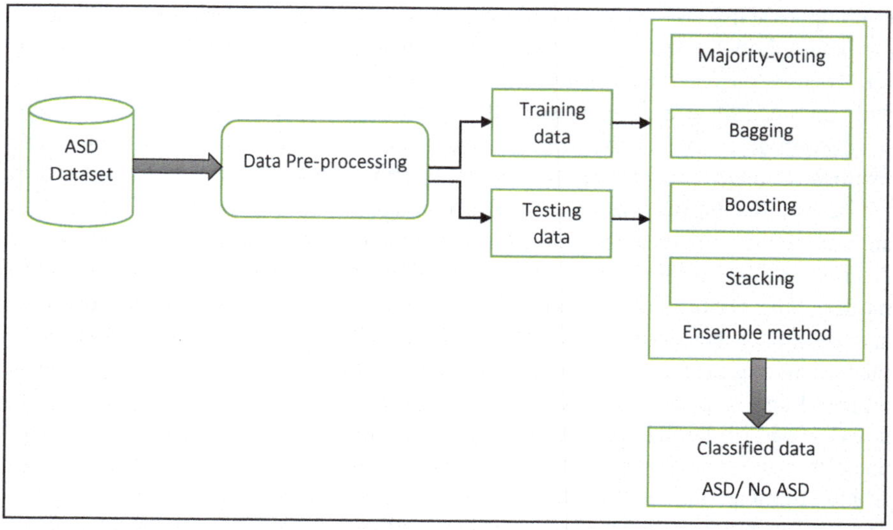

Fig. 5.1 The proposed method for the classification of ASD

In the proposed method pre-processing technique is used in two ways

1. Conversion of textual data into numeric form.
2. Selection of important features and removal of unnecessary features.

In the first method using the label encoding technique, the textual data is converted into a numeric form which is necessary for performing classification tasks using various machine learning algorithms. This process leads to an increase in the total number of features than the original. In another sub-task, the statistical Chi-square test is used which calculates the importance of every feature for the class label. Based on the score obtained using this test top K features were selected for the further classification process.

3.2 Train-Test Split

After data pre-processing, the pre-processed data is divided into 75% and 25% as training and testing data. Training data is used to train the classification model while testing data tests the accuracy of the model.

3.3 Classification Model

The classification model is built using various ML techniques such as Naïve Bayes (NB), K-Nearest Neighbor (KNN), Support Vector Machine (SVM), etc. To enhance classification system accuracy the ensemble technique is used which contains majority voting, weighted averaging, boosting, Bagging, and stacking approaches.

3.3.1 Naïve Bayes

It uses the Bayes theorem as a base for implementation. It assumes that all attributes of the dataset are not related. This classification technique is very easy to build and performs better in terms of accuracy for the very large data set.

The Bayes theorem is as follows

$$P(A/B) = \frac{P\left(\frac{B}{A}\right) * P(A)}{P(B)} \tag{5.1}$$

Here,

P(A/B) = Posterior probability
P(A) = Prior probability of a class
$P\left(\frac{B}{A}\right)$ = Probability of predictor given the class label
P(B) = predictor probability

Working of Naïve Bayes Algorithm

1. Create frequency table from data set by checking attribute values concerning class values.
2. Create a likelihood table by finding probabilities for attribute and class values.
3. To calculate the posterior probability by using the above two values respectively apply the Naïve Bayes formula.

The Naïve Bayes theorem is useful in binary and multiclass classification problems. The selection of the type of Naïve Bayes method is based on the nature of features used and sometimes on the relationship between different features and class labels. This algorithm is easy and fast to predict the class label of any test data. It requires less training data set for training purposes. When it is assumed that features are independent of each other Naïve Bayes performs better.

3.3.2 Support Vector Machine (SVM)

In the SVM classification technique, each data item is represented as a coordinate in N-dimensional space. The classification task includes discovering the line which divides two classes called hyper-plane. Support Vectors are the coordinates. The SVM classifier is a technique that best segregates the two classes. This technique is also used to solve regression problems.

The objective of the SVM algorithm is to separate N-dimensional space into classes by using the hyperplane.

The SVM classifies the data in two ways:

1. Iteratively the SVM generates hyperplanes.
2. Then, it selects the hyperplane that classifies the data for correct classes.

The two types of SVM are as follows

1. **Linear SVM**: Here using a single line data can be separated into two different classes.
2. **Non-linear SVM**: Here if a single straight line cannot classify the data into two classes.

The SVM algorithm uses a kernel that helps to convert input data records into the required form. More dimensions are added to convert non-separable problems into separable problems with help of the kernel. This process makes SVM more powerful, accurate, and flexible.

The types of kernels used by SVM are as follows.

1. **Linear Kernel**

$$\mathrm{K}(\mathrm{y}, \mathrm{yi}) = \mathrm{sum}(\mathrm{y} * \mathrm{yi}) \tag{5.2}$$

2. **Polynomial Kernel**

   It is the generalized linear kernel that is used to differentiate nonlinear input space.

$$\mathrm{k}(\mathrm{Y}, \mathrm{Yi}) = 1 + \mathrm{sum}(\mathrm{Y} * \mathrm{Yi})^{\mathrm{d}} \tag{5.3}$$

   Here, d = degree of polynomial

3. **Radial Basis Function (RBF) Kernel**

$$\mathrm{K}(\mathrm{y}, \mathrm{yi}) = \exp\left(-\mathrm{gamma} * \mathrm{sum}\left(\mathrm{y} - \mathrm{yi}^2\right)\right) \tag{5.4}$$

   Here, the value of gamma is between 0 and 1. The ideal value of gamma is 0.1.

3.3.3 K-Nearest Neighbor (KNN)

K-Nearest Neighbor is one of the simple classification techniques. KNN algorithm is based on distance measure and classification of new data into the class that is closer to the available class. When new test data need to check for classification, KNN easily classifies to a suitable class. It can be used for Regression problems also.

There is no assumption on the data so that it is known as a non-parametric algorithm. It takes time to learn from the training data set so that it is called a lazy learner. At the time of classification, the dataset is stored and then action is performed on the dataset.

The distance measures that are used in KNN classification include Euclidean distance, cosine similarity measure, Minkowsky, correlation, and Chi square

$$d = \sqrt{[(x2 - x1)2 + (y2 - y1)2]} \tag{5.5}$$

Where X1, Y1, and X2, Y2 are the two points in 2-dimensional space.

Working of KNN Algorithm

1. Choose the value of K.
2. Identify the distance between all training data points and new data points.
3. Sort all the training points for their distances with a new data point in ascending order.
4. Choose the 'K' number of nearest neighbors.
5. From these neighbors, identify the number of data points in each class.
6. The new data is assigned to that category for which the number of the neighbor is maximum.

Implementation of the Knn algorithm is simple. And it is not sensitive to the noisy input data. When the training data size is large Knn can be more effective. The Knn requires the calculation of data points with all training data points so that the computation cost is high.

3.4 *Ensemble*

The ensemble technique is used to enhance the efficacy of the weak classifiers and improve the accuracy by combining them with strong classifiers. The merging of different classifiers improves performance to a greater extent than an individual classifier. The types of ensemble methods are discussed below.

1. **Bagging**: This method includes ML classification models of the same type or different types. The random sampling with replacement is used to select data

items from the data set as part of the training data set and send them to an individual classifier for training. The model learns on this data set. As part of testing, the data is passed to all models. By applying majority voting or weighted averaging the final class label is identified. This technique improves the performance of weak models.

2. **Boosting**: It is called sequential learning using ensemble. In this technique, various subsets of the training data set are created. For training, the first model training dataset is used. The second classifier is trained using incorrectly classified data elements by the first model and so on. By using the majority voting or weighted averaging technique the final result is discovered.
3. **Majority Voting**: To identify a final class label of data this technique is used. The majority class label from different classifiers for a specific data item is considered for this purpose. The final class label 'Cj' is defined as

$$\text{Cj} = \text{mode}\{\text{C1}, \text{C2} \ldots \text{Cn}\} \tag{5.6}$$

Where {C1, C2, …, Cn} shows different classifiers used in the classification process.

4. **Stacking**: The stacking method includes the classification of the same dataset on different machine learning models. The different models are used to make a prediction. It contains level-0 and level-1 models. The level-0 (base models) are trained on labeled data (more than one base model can be used) and the result is combined, while the level-1 (metamodel) uses predictions made by base models for their training.

4 Mathematical Measures

Machine learning models are performing various tasks effectively which helps to reduce human efforts numerously. To measure the performance of these models some mathematical measures are used which are accuracy, sensitivity, specificity, f-score, etc. The details are given in the following subsections:

4.1 Accuracy

The accuracy of any machine learning model is nothing but how accurately that model performs its task. Suppose a model is performing a classification task, the

Table 5.1 Confusion matrix

Predicted\Actual	Actual: Yes	Actual: No
Predicted: Yes	TP	FP
Predicted: No	FN	TN

accuracy of that model is defined in terms of no of correctly classified instances from given instances. To understand these terms effectively consider the confusion matrix as given in Table 5.1.

The terms included in the above matrix represents information as:

- True Positive (TP): Actual output is Yes and models Classification is also Yes.
- True Negative (TN): Actual output is No and models Classification is also No.
- False Positive (FP): Actual output is No and models Classification is Yes.
- False Negative (FN): Actual output is Yes and models Classification is No.

Accuracy is calculated as

$$Accuracy = \frac{(TP + TN)}{(TP + \mathrm{TN} + FP + FN)} \tag{5.7}$$

The accuracy of the classification model states the percentage of testing records that are correctly classified for their actual classes.

4.2 *Sensitivity*

Sensitivity or True positive rate (TPR) is a proportion of actual positive records that are correctly identified by the machine learning model.

$$Sensitivity = \frac{TP}{(TP + FN)} \tag{5.8}$$

4.3 *Specificity*

Specificity or True negative rate (TNR) is a proportion of actual negative records that are correctly identified as negative by the classification model.

$$Specificity = \frac{TN}{(TN + FP)} \tag{5.9}$$

4.4 *Efficiency*

The efficiency of a model is calculated as

$$Efficiency = \frac{Sensitivity + Specificity + Accuracy}{3} \tag{5.10}$$

4.5 ROC Curve

The ROC curve is a graph that shows the performance of a classifier. It shows True Positive rate and False Positive rate for different values of threshold.

5 Experimentation

5.1 Dataset

The dataset used in this research work is taken from the UCI Repository which is available publicly and contains behavioral features plus other attributes of individuals that are effective in the detection of ASD. It contains 18 attributes that belong to categorical, continuous, and binary nature. Other information such as gender, age, ethnicity, etc. is also useful to find out ASD.

5.2 Results and Discussion

As part of the implementation, the dataset is used to train and test individual classifiers such as Naïve Bayes, SVM, and KNN and the ensemble methods such as Bagging, Boosting, Stacking, and Majority voting. The results are recorded concerning the accuracy, sensitivity, and specificity. In ensemble method bagging the results are recorded w.r.t KNN (n=5), KNN (n=3), Naïve Bayes, and SVM. In majority voting, the dataset is tested against three individual classifiers. In boosting, the technique Adaboost is used to train and test ASD datasets. In the stacking technique, NB and KNN are used as base classifiers, and SVM is used as meta classifier.

Table 5.2 Accuracy, sensitivity, and specificity measures for various algorithm

Algorithm	Accuracy	Sensitivity	Specificity
Naïve Bayes [7]	93.93	0.9120	0.6693
KNN n=3 [11]	71.59	0.8736	0.8412
KNN n=5 [11]	67.42	0.8846	0.9044
SVC [17]	68.93	1.0	1.0
Bagging Knn(5)	67.42	0.8846	0.9044
Bagging Knn(3)	66.43	0.8846	0.9044
Bagging SVM	69.08	0.8791	0.9142
Bagging NB	93.17	0.9175	0.6706
Boosting (Adaboost)	83.77	0.9285	0.7647
Stacking	93.93	0.9120	0.6693
Voting Ensemble	75.05	0.8846	0.8256

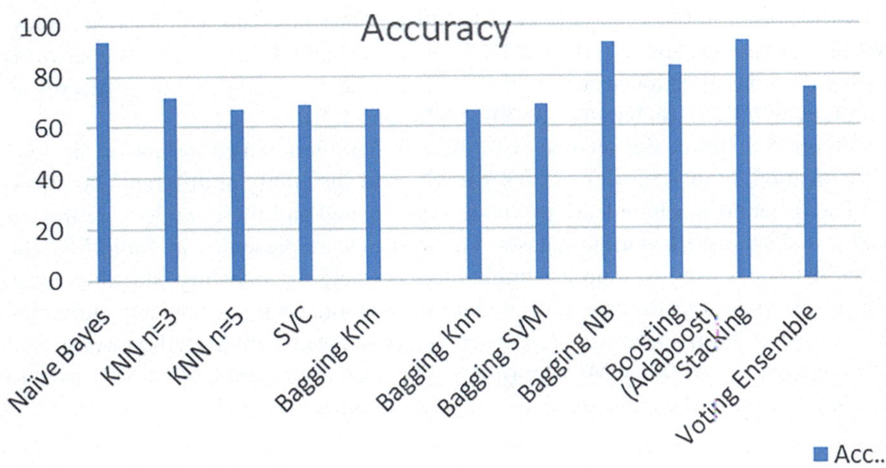

Fig. 5.2 Accuracy of the different classifiers

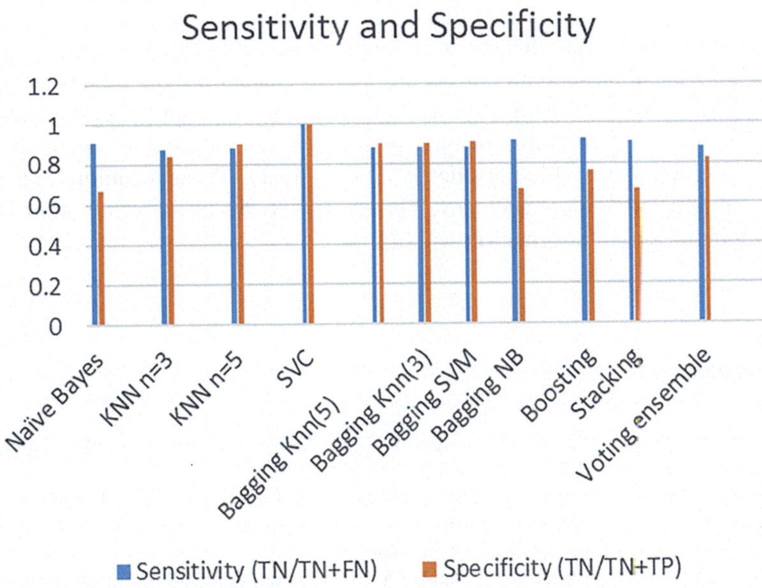

Fig. 5.3 Sensitivity and specificity of the different classifiers

Table 5.2 shows accuracy, sensitivity, and specificity for various machine learning algorithms which are useful in the classification of ASD. The result shows that the Naïve Bayes classifier performs well as compared to SVM and KNN with 93% accuracy when compared as an individual classifier. When bagging is performed with Naïve Bayes as a base classifier it performs well as compared to other base classifiers used in bagging. Adaboost technique classifies data with 84% accuracy. While stacking ensemble (NB and KNN as level-0 and SVM as level 1) performs well with a classification accuracy of 94%. The majority voting technique records an accuracy of 75% (Combination of NB, SVM, and KN).

Figure 5.2 shows the accuracy of different classifiers which are useful in ASD classification. Figure 5.3 shows the sensitivity and specificity of different classifiers.

The different machine learning models are created and these models are trained and tested against the current dataset. The statistics are presented in Table 5.2. The same dataset is used to train ensemble models (bagging, boosting, stacking, etc.). The result shows that the ensemble method shows more accuracy than any individual ML classifier. From these graphs, it is observed that the ensemble method works well as compared to traditional ML algorithms. This technique can be effectively used to predict Autism in the early stage as compared to other classifiers.

6 Conclusion

As machine learning classification techniques impact the decision-making process by providing the highest prediction accuracy. This chapter provides the working and efficiency of existing classification methods that are useful in the classification of **ASD**. The proposed ensemble method performs better in terms of accuracy, simplicity, specificity, etc. which decides ASD effectively. These techniques also give results promptly with more accuracy. This system works as an information system that provides accurate information within time.

References

1. Qayyum A, Qadir J, Bilal M, Al-Fuqaha A (2020) Secure and robust machine learning for healthcare: a survey. IEEE Rev Biomed Eng 14:156–180
2. Küpper C, Stroth S, Wolff N, Hauck F, Kliewer N, Schad-Hansjosten T, Roepke S (2020) Identifying predictive features of autism spectrum disorders in a clinical sample of adolescents and adults using machine learning. Sci Rep 10(1):1–11
3. Gull S, Mansour RF, Aljehane NO, Parah SA (2021) A self-embedding technique for tamper detection and localization of medical images for smart health. Multimed Tools Appl 80(19): 29939–29964
4. Rashid M, Singh H, Goyal V (2020) The use of machine learning and deep learning algorithms in functional magnetic resonance imaging—a systematic review. Expert Syst 37(6):e12644
5. Sarosh P, Parah SA, Bhat GM, Muhammad K (2021) A security management framework for big data in smart healthcare. Big Data Res 25:100225
6. Ahmad MA, Eckert C, Teredesai A (2018) Interpretable machine learning in healthcare. In: Proceedings of the 2018 ACM international conference on bioinformatics, computational biology, and health informatics, pp 559–560
7. Hussan M, Parah SA, Gull S, Qureshi GJ (2021) Tamper detection and self-recovery of medical imagery for smart health. Arab J Sci Eng 46(4):3465–3481

8. Raj S, Masood S (2020) Analysis and detection of autism spectrum disorder using machine learning techniques. Proc Comput Sci 167:994–1004
9. Ray C, Kumar Tripathy H, Mishra S (2019) Assessment of autistic disorder using machine learning approach. In: International conference on intelligent computing and communication. Springer, Singapore, pp 209–219
10. Cantin-Garside KD, Kong Z, White SW, Antezana L, Kim S, Nussbaum MA (2020) Detecting and classifying self-injurious behavior in autism spectrum disorder using machine learning techniques. J Autism Dev Disord 50(11):4039–4052
11. Mondal S, Agarwal K, Rashid M (2019) Deep learning approach for automatic classification of x-ray images using convolutional neural network. In: 2019 Fifth international conference on image information processing (ICIIP). IEEE, New York, pp 326–331
12. Shah AA, Parah SA, Rashid M, Elhoseny M (2020) Efficient image encryption scheme based on the generalized logistic map for real-time image processing. J Real-Time Image Proc 17(6): 2139–2151
13. Omar KS, Mondal P, Khan NS, Rizvi MRK, Islam MN (2019) A machine learning approach to predict autism spectrum disorder. In: 2019 International conference on electrical, computer and communication engineering (ECCE). IEEE, New York, pp 1–6
14. Gull S, Parah SA, Muhammad K (2020) Reversible data hiding exploiting Huffman encoding with dual images for IoMT based healthcare. Comput Commun 163:134–149
15. Rashid M, Yousuf MM, Ram B, Goyal V (2019) Novel big data approach for drug prediction in health care systems. In: 2019 International conference on automation, computational and technology management (ICACTM). IEEE, New York, pp 325–329
16. Thabtah F, Peebles D (2020) A new machine learning model based on induction of rules for autism detection. Health Informatics J 26(1):264–286
17. Sarosh P, Parah SA, Bhat GM, Heidari AA, Muhammad K (2021) Secret sharing-based personal health records management for the Internet of health things. Sustain Cities Soc 74: 103129
18. Rashid M, Singh H, Goyal V (2020) Analyzing functional magnetic resonance brain images with opencv2. In: 2020 Sixth international conference on parallel, distributed and grid computing (PDGC). IEEE, New York, pp 451–454
19. Bhola J, Jeet R, Jawarneh MMM, Pattekari SA (2021) Machine learning techniques for analysing and identifying autism spectrum disorder. In: Artificial intelligence for accurate analysis and detection of autism spectrum disorder. IGI Global, Hershey, PA, pp 69–81
20. Bilgen I, Guvercin G, Rekik I (2020) Machine learning methods for brain network classification: application to autism diagnosis using cortical morphological networks. J Neurosci Methods 343:108799
21. Ruggieri V, Gómez JL, Martínez MM, Arberas C (2019) Aging and autism: understanding, intervention, and proposals to improve quality of Life. Curr Pharm Des 25(41):4454–4461
22. Abbas H, Garberson F, Glover E, Wall DP (2018) Machine learning approach for early detection of autism by combining questionnaire and home video screening. J Am Med Inform Assoc 25(8):1000–1007
23. Kumar I, Alshamrani SS, Kumar A, Rawat J, Singh KU, Rashid M, AlGhamdi AS (2021) Deep learning approach for analysis and characterization of COVID-19. Comput Mater Cont 70:451–468
24. Jha N, Prashar D, Rashid M, Shafiq M, Khan R, Pruncu CI, Saravana Kumar M (2021) Deep learning approach for discovery of in silico drugs for combating COVID-19. J Healthc Eng 2021:6668985
25. Devika Varshini G, Chinnaiyan R (2020) Optimized machine learning classification approaches for prediction of autism spectrum disorder. Ann Autism Dev Disord 1(1):1001
26. Gull S, Loan NA, Parah SA (2020) An efficient watermarking technique for tamper detection and localization of medical images. J Ambient Intell Human Comput 11:1799–1808

Part II
Artificial Intelligence (AI) Classification Models for COVID-19 Pandemic

Chapter 6
Automatic Classification of COVID-19 Infected Patients Using Convolution Neural Network Models

Suhail Nazeer, Parsa Sarosh, and Shabir A. Parah

Contents

1 Introduction

The World Health Organization (WHO) declared COVID-19 as a public health emergency in January 2020 [1]. There have been 231,916,063 cases recorded to date and the number of deaths is a whopping number at 4,751,607. The pandemic has affected more than 200 countries and has impacted all the major walks of life. The impact of COVID-19 is more on people that have some identified co-morbidities like heart disease, blood pressure, etc. [2]. The COVID-19 infection has a broad range of symptoms like headache, fever, cough, Acute Respiratory Distress Syndrome (ARDS) and in some cases can also lead to pneumonia and death of the patient. The diagnosis of COVID-19 is done using the antibody test or the RT-PCR. The RT-PCR is time-consuming as it is a manual testing method and has a high false-negative rate [3]. It requires time for manual sample collection, and transportation, sophisticated laboratory equipment, Personal Protective Equipment (PPEs), and testing swabs in huge numbers. As the identification of COVID-19 patients is

S. Nazeer · P. Sarosh · S. A. Parah (✉)
PG Department of Electronics and Instrumentation Technology, University of Kashmir, Srinagar, India

S. A. Parah et al. (eds.), *Artificial Intelligence for Innovative Healthcare Informatics*,
https://doi.org/10.1007/978-3-030-96569-3_6

inefficient because of the high false-negative rate of RT-PCR, there is an increased spread of the virus and an overall increase in the number of cases and deaths [4, 5]. According to the WHO the radiological examination using Chest X-Ray or CT images of patients is the most efficient method to diagnose pneumonia and can help in timely and effective triage and treatment of the patient. COVID-19 affects the lungs causing Ground-Glass Opacities (GGO), crazy paving patterns, and pulmonary consolidation. Monitoring the effect of COVID-19 on the epithelial cells of the respiratory tract can help in the early identification of the disease. Recently the use of Deep learning has been identified for the COVID-19 management finding applications in COVID-19 diagnosis, contact tracing, forecasting, and vaccine development. The use of X-Ray images for the early screening and triage of COVID-19 patients can help to contain the virus. The X-Ray images can be generated at any low-end medical facility with less complicated technological equipment [6, 7]. Most of the medical centers have the setup required to generate the X-Ray images and proves less expensive for the patients as well [8, 9]. Although X-Rays do not provide a detailed 3D-pulmonary view however they can assist the radiologist by providing a preliminary visual tool for the diagnosis of COVID-19 pneumonia [10, 11].

Many pre-trained models like AlexNet, VGG19, ResNetV2, and InceptionV3 have been trained using X-Ray images and demonstrate accuracy values up to 98%. However, these models exhibit a high level of computational complexity. I. D. Apostolopoulos and Mpesiana [12] demonstrate a transfer learning based-method for COVID-19 detection. They train models like VGG19, Xception, ResNetV2, MobileNet, and Inception models and conclude that VGG19 and MobileNet can achieve the highest level of accuracy. They utilized 1427 images with 224 COVID-19 positive, 700 Common pneumonia, and 504 normal category images. The VGG19 and MobileNet models achieve 97.8% accuracy in the classification task. K. H. Shibly et al. [13] propose a method to detect COVID-19 from X-Ray images using the Faster R-CNN object detection model. Their method uses a custom dataset of 5450 X-Ray images obtained from the RSNA pneumonia dataset and Cohen et al.'s Chest X-Ray dataset. R. Sethi et al. [14] demonstrate the use of four different CNN architectures like InceptionV3, ResNet50, MobileNet, and Xception pre-trained on the ImageNet dataset and shortlisting MobileNet as the most efficient. M. M. Taresh et al. [15] present an assessment to evaluate different state-of-the-art pre-trained CNN models for COVID-19 detection using X-Ray images. They attempt to identify the best pre-trained model by fine-tuning to increase the detection accuracy. They perform transfer learning by making use of a Chest X-Ray dataset containing 1200 images of patients having COVID-19, 1345 images of viral pneumonia patients, and 1341 images of healthy individuals. They conclude that VGG16 has the best performance with accuracy, sensitivity, specificity, and F1 score of 98.72%, 98.78%, 98.70%, and 97.59 respectively. A. K. Das et al. [16] present a solution for COVID-19 detection using the CNN models. They train multiple CNN networks like ResNet50V2, DenseNet201, and InceptionV3 for individual predictions and then combine the models using the weighted average ensembling technique for classification. The model has been trained on 538 images of COVID-19 positive cases and 468 images of healthy individuals and reports a classification accuracy of 91.62%.

Furthermore, several researchers have developed their models like COVID-Net, COVIDX-Net, CoroNet, and M-Inception among others to detect COVID-19, and have also exhibited high levels of accuracy. A. I. Khan et al. [17] propose a model called CoroNet for COVID-19 detection using X-Ray images. They have used Xception architecture as a base model pre-trained on the ImageNet dataset and subsequently perform training on Chest X-Ray images. They use images of patients having COVID-19, Bacterial Pneumonia, Viral Pneumonia, and Normal classes. The model exhibits an accuracy of 89.6% for the 4-class classification. It shows an accuracy of 95% for the 3-class classification having categories like COVID-19- vs. Normal vs. Pneumonia. The dataset contains 1251 images with 310 for normal, 330 for Bacterial, 284 for COVID-19, and 327 for viral pneumonia. H. Panwar et al. [18] propose a model called nCOVnet to detect COVID-19 from X-Ray images. The model uses an augmented dataset and has 24 layers including convolution, pooling among others. The model uses YGG-16 pre-trained on the ImageNet dataset and provides an accuracy of 88.10%. The sensitivity and specificity of the model are 97.62% and 78.57% respectively.

In this work, we demonstrate that a simple CNN model with minimum complexity can be trained to detect COVID-19 with 99% training and validation accuracy and 0.001% training and validation loss. We present different architectures of the CNN model for COVID-19 diagnosis using X-Ray images. The images have been retrieved from the GitHub platform with 1811 images in the training dataset and 484 images in the validation dataset. The model with the highest accuracy has been further trained using multiple epochs and different filter sizes. It has been shown that architecture 3 has the highest accuracy with the smallest number of trainable parameters.

The rest of the chapter has been designed as follows. Section 2 describes the basics of the CNN model and the data utilized. Section 3 describes the proposed CNN models and their use in COVID-19 diagnosis. Section 4 describes the results and discussion and the conclusion is presented in Sect. 5.

2 Method

2.1 Convolution Neural Network

The CNN is a sequential model used in Deep learning for image classification and segmentation [19, 20]. The model takes raw images as input that are convolved with various filters to generate feature maps. The convolution operation is used to extract features from the images that are used to identify the objects to be classified [21, 22]. The architecture of CNN often consists of multiple layers of convolution and pooling operations followed by the fully connected layers. The convolution layer consists of linear convolution operation and nonlinear operation i.e., application of activation function. The convolution operation involves the multiplication of the image array with the kernel leading to feature extraction. The output value called the feature map is generated by the element-wise multiplication of the input image and the kernel [23]. The output is subsequently passed through an activation function like SoftMax or sigmoid function to get the final feature map from the images. The rectified linear unit (ReLU) and sigmoid functions are the most common activation functions utilized in the CNN and are represented by Eqs. (6.1) and (6.2) respectively.

$$f(x) = \max(0, x) \tag{6.1}$$

$$S(x) = \frac{1}{(1 + e^{-x})} \tag{6.2}$$

Leaky ReLU is represented in Eq. (6.3).

$$\mathrm{F(x)} = \begin{cases} 0.01\mathrm{x}, & \mathrm{x} < 0 \\ \mathrm{x}, & \mathrm{x} \geq 0 \end{cases} \tag{6.3}$$

In the pooling operation, the output is taken as the mean or maximum value of any predefined input array. The data is processed subsequently in the layers and an error between the predicted output and ground truth is calculated in the forward propagation. The error is utilized to update the weight values which leads to updated prediction values from the model. The model observes the dataset several times and generates an optimal error value and a predicted output that most corresponds with the ground truth. The feature map f'_j is calculated as shown in Eq. (6.4).

$$\mathrm{F(x)} = \begin{cases} 0.01\mathrm{x}, & \mathrm{x} < 0 \\ \mathrm{x}, & \mathrm{x} \geq 0 \end{cases} \tag{6.4}$$

Where, f'_j and f_k^{l-1} is the jth *and* k^{th} feature map in the lth layer and $(l - 1)^{th}$ layer respectively. The $'\sigma'$ is the activation function, W_{jk}^l is the filter, and b^l represents the bias term.

2.2 Data

The dataset utilized in this work has been retrieved from the GitHub website using the link mentioned as https://github.com/education454/datasets.git. This dataset contains a total of 2295 images of size 64 × 64 × 3 wherein 545 are of COVID-19 class and 1266 of normal X-Rays used as training dataset, 167 COVID-19 class and 317 normal images of validation dataset. Therefore, there is a total of 1811 images in the training dataset and 484 images in the validation dataset. We further

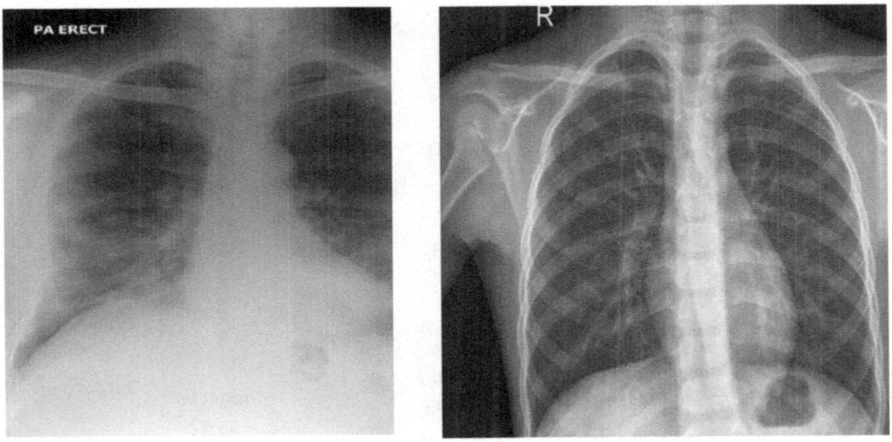

(a) (b)

Fig. 6.1 (**a**) Chest X-Ray sample image of a patient having COVID-19 (**b**) Chest X-Ray of a healthy individual [12]

perform data augmentation and pre-processing like horizontal flip, contrast enhancement, and normalization. The sample images from the dataset have been shown in Fig. 6.1.

3 Proposed Method

In this work, we develop six different CNN architectures using Convolution, Pooling, Drop-out, and fully-connected layers. The different CNN architectures are used to test the accuracy of the COVID-19 classification task. There are many complex architectures like AlexNet, VGG-19, and ResNet however the different models we have built are much simpler and can be deployed in any low-end medical center as well. The learning rate has been set at 0.001 and activation function 'ReLU' has been utilized for the convolution layer and the last layer makes use of the 'sigmoid' function. We employ the 'Adam' optimizer and loss function as binary cross-entropy. The filter size in the convolution layer for all architectures is 3×3 and for the pooling layer is 2×2. Furthermore, the number of filters in the convolution layer and pooling layers is 32 each. The block diagram for all the architectures is shown in Fig. 6.2 and the summary of architecture 3 has been shown in Fig. 6.3 that has the minimum number of trainable parameters.

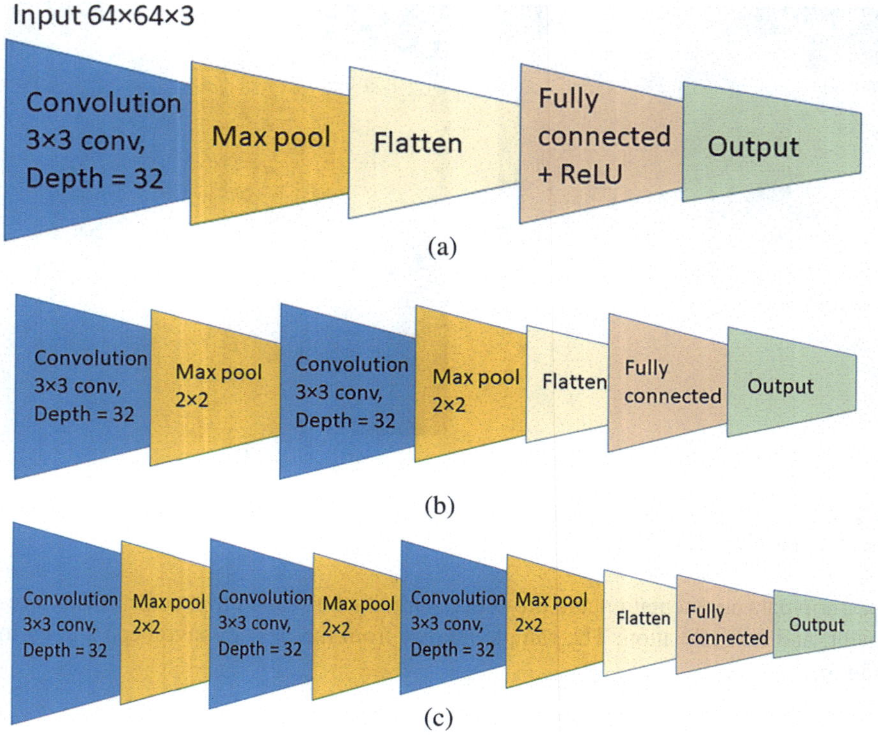

Fig. 6.2 (**a**) Architecture 1, (**b**) Architecture 2, (**c**) Architecture 3, (**d**) Architecture 4, (**e**) Architecture 5, (**f**) Architecture 6

4 Results and Discussions

To evaluate the proposed method, we perform many experiments wherein we use six different architectures and train the model on Tesla K80 GPU using a Google-Colaboratory notebook. The model is built using the tensor flow and Keras library in the Python programming language. All the models have been trained on the Chest X-Ray dataset in 20 epochs. The filter size for the convolution layer is 3×3 and the pooling layer is 2×2. The number of filters in the convolution layer and pooling layers is 32 each. The plots for the accuracy and loss for architecture 1, 3, and 6 have been shown in Fig. 6.4 for illustration.

The test accuracy and loss of the six architectures for 20 epochs have been shown in Table 6.1.

Architecture 3 is most efficient when trained on 20 epochs as the accuracy and loss values are 97.52% and 0.07% respectively with minimum trainable parameters equal to 93,249. The different training and validation accuracy and loss values are plotted for Architecture 3 with multiple epochs as shown in Fig. 6.5.

Architecture 3 has been further trained on multiple epoch values 50, 100, 200, 300, 400, and 500. The accuracy for multiple epochs for architecture 3 is shown in Table 6.2. The filter size is varied to 1×1, 3×3, 5×5, and 7×7. The trainable parameters for different filter sizes in architecture 3 are shown in Table 6.3.

The confusion matrix represents the performance of the system with the help of quantitative measures like True Positive (TP), False Positive (FP), True Negative (TN), and False Negative (FN). The confusion matrix for architecture 3 is shown in Fig. 6.6 and the accuracy in Eq. (6.5).

$$\text{Accuracy } (\%) = \frac{\text{TP} + \text{TN}}{\text{TP} + \text{FP} + \text{FN} + \text{TN}} \tag{6.5}$$

A comparison of different network accuracies for the dataset provided in [12] is shown in Table 6.4. The comparison of different techniques for COVID-19 classification using X-Ray images is shown in Table 6.5.

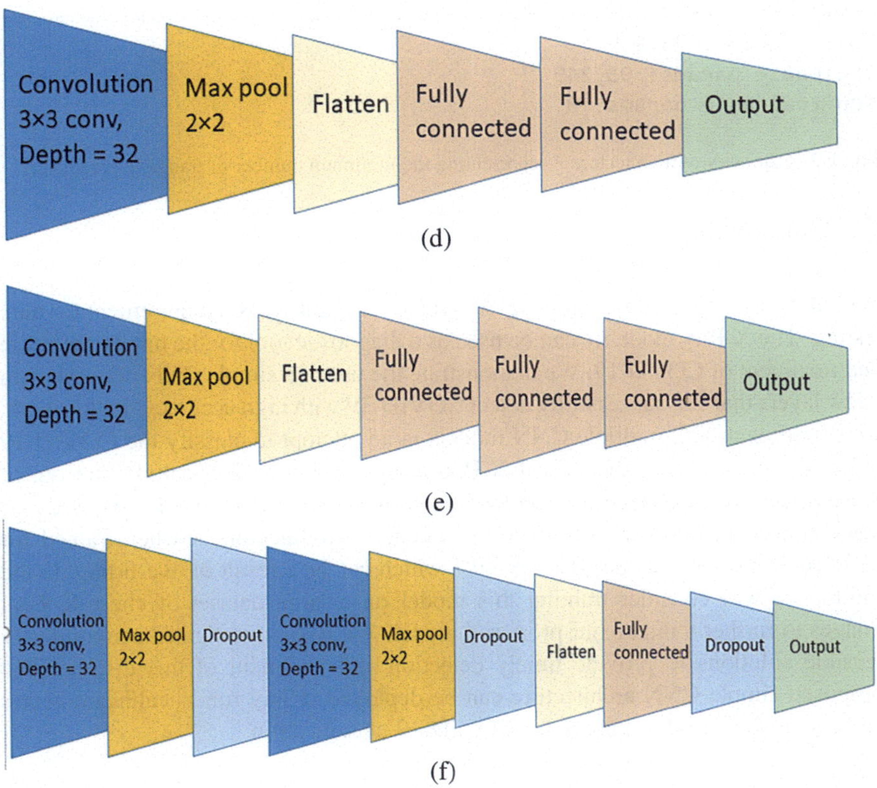

Fig. 6.2 (continued)

```
Layer (type)                 Output Shape              Param #
=================================================================
conv2d_53 (Conv2D)           (None, 62, 62, 32)        896
_________________________________________________________________
max_pooling2d_50 (MaxPooling (None, 31, 31, 32)        0
_________________________________________________________________
conv2d_54 (Conv2D)           (None, 29, 29, 32)        9248
_________________________________________________________________
max_pooling2d_51 (MaxPooling (None, 14, 14, 32)        0
_________________________________________________________________
conv2d_55 (Conv2D)           (None, 12, 12, 32)        9248
_________________________________________________________________
max_pooling2d_52 (MaxPooling (None, 6, 6, 32)          0
_________________________________________________________________
flatten_16 (Flatten)         (None, 1152)              0
_________________________________________________________________
dense_32 (Dense)             (None, 64)                73792
_________________________________________________________________
dense_33 (Dense)             (None, 1)                 65
=================================================================
Total params: 93,249
Trainable params: 93,249
Non-trainable params: 0
```

Fig. 6.3 Summary of architecture 3 representing the minimum number of trainable parameters

5 Conclusion

With the ever-increasing number of COVID-19 cases, there is a requirement for bulk testing. The X-Ray modality can be used as a diagnostic tool for the timely detection and treatment of COVD-19. We demonstrate the use of a simple CNN network with a few layers that can successfully detect COVID-19 with high accuracy. In this work, we experiment with multiple CNN models in an attempt to classify the COVID-19 affected patients using their chest X-Ray scans. Further, we conclude that out of these six models, architecture 3 has the best performance and is suited to be used as it has a minimum number of trainable parameters. Architecture 3 when trained for 500 epochs provides an accuracy of 99% which can be a result of overfitting. In the future, we will consider training this model on a large dataset of chest X-Rays images to further validate our proposed model. We have investigated economically feasible solutions to provide timely detection and treatment of this disease. The proposed simple CNN architecture can be deployed in any rural healthcare center and can achieve high accuracy for COVID-19 classification.

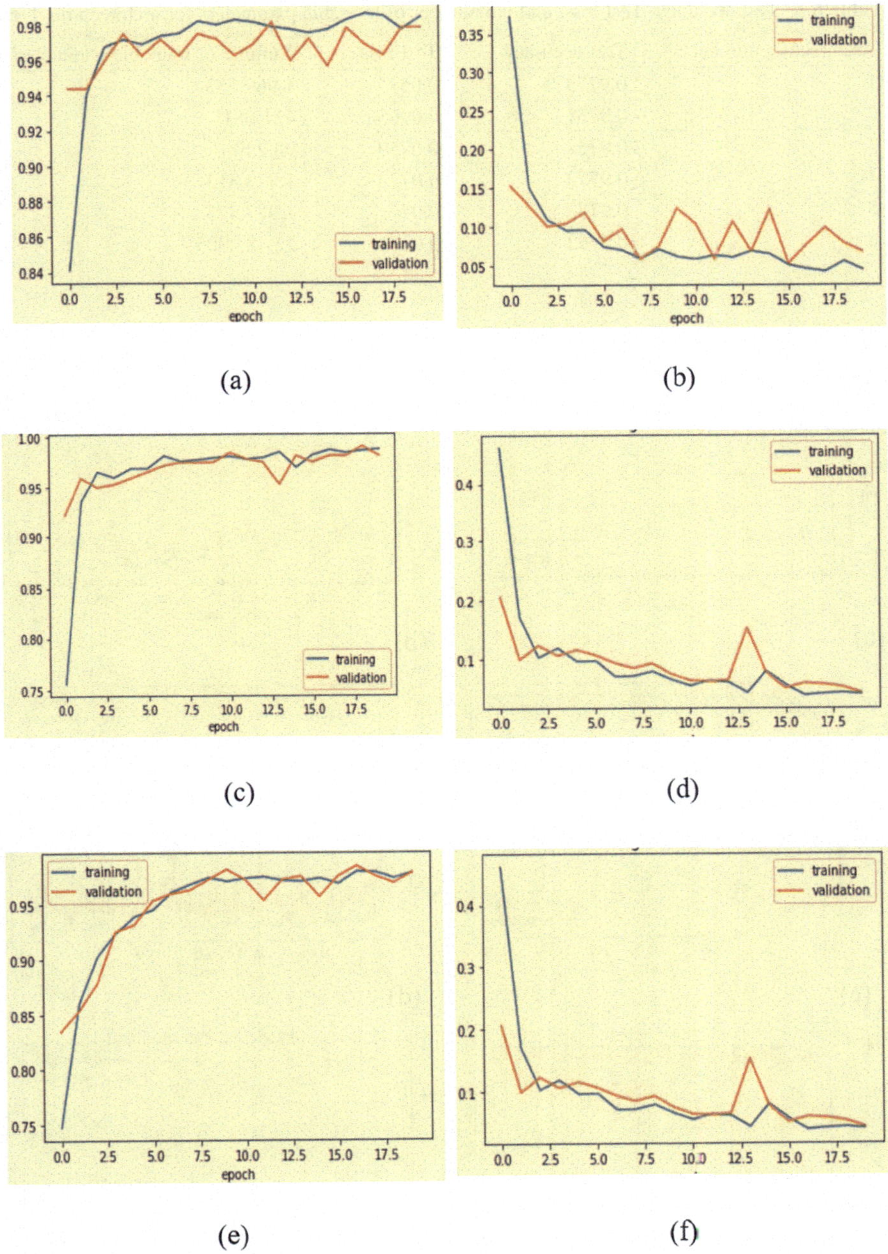

Fig. 6.4 (**a**), (**c**), and (**e**) Training and validation Accuracy of architecture 1, 3, and 6 respectively. (**b**), (**d**), and (**f**) Training and validation Loss of architecture 1, 3, and 6 respectively

Table 6.1 Test accuracy, Test loss, and the number of trainable parameters for architectures 1–6

Architecture number	Test accuracy	Test loss	Number of trainable parameters
1	0.9773	0.054	1,969,153
2	0.9731	0.0905	411,681
3	0.9752	0.0759	93,249
4	0.9772	0.0723	1,973,313
5	0.9772	0.07	1,977,473
6	0.9752	0.0771	22,483,905

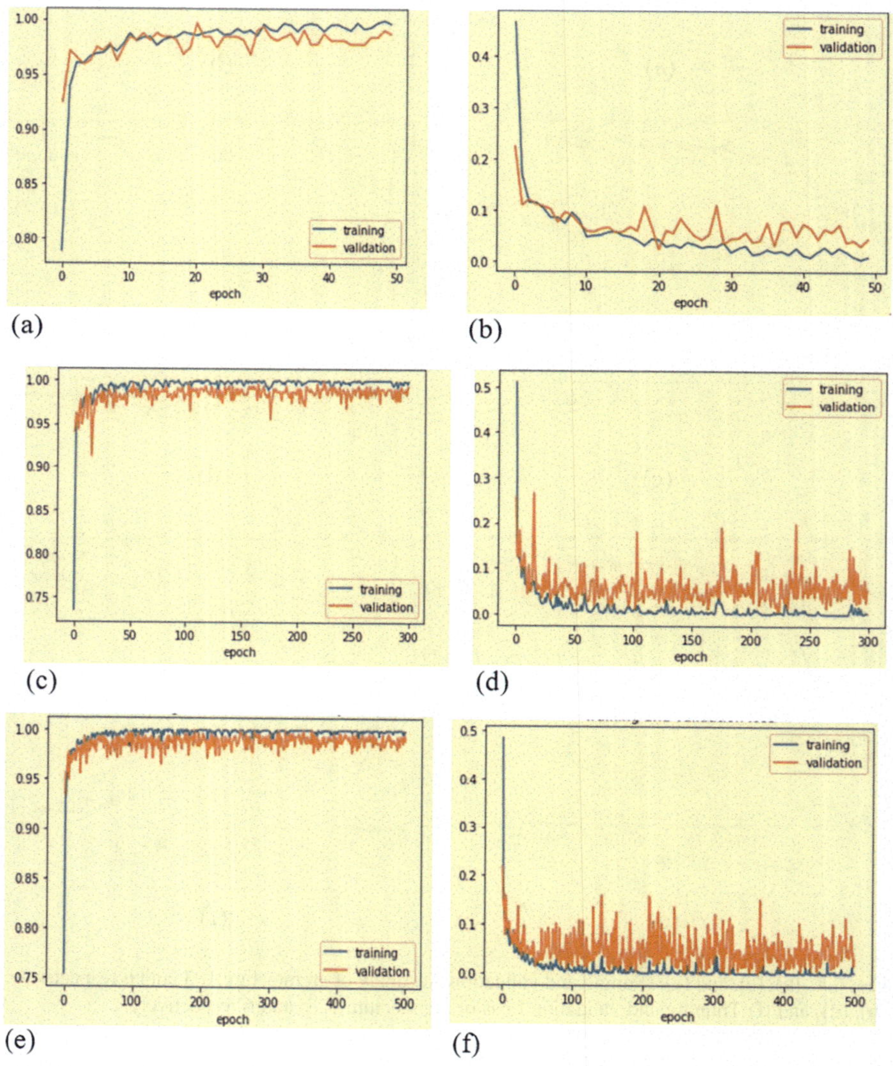

Fig. 6.5 Plots of accuracy and loss obtained for architecture 3 for different epochs. (**a**) Accuracy of architecture 3 for 50 epochs. (**b**) Loss of architecture 3 for 50 epochs. (**c**) Accuracy of architecture 3 for 300 epochs. (**d**) Loss of architecture 3 for 300 epochs. (**e**) Accuracy of architecture 3 for 500 epochs. (**f**) Loss of architecture 3 for 500 epochs

Table 6.2 The accuracy of architecture 3 when trained for a variable number of epochs

Number of epochs	Accuracy
20	97.52
50	98.9
100	98.9
200	98.9
300	98.9
400	99.4
500	99.4

Table 6.3 Number of trainable parameters in architecture 3 with different filter sizes

Filter size	Number of parameters
1 × 1	133,441
3 × 3	93,249
5 × 5	86,593
7 × 7	113,473

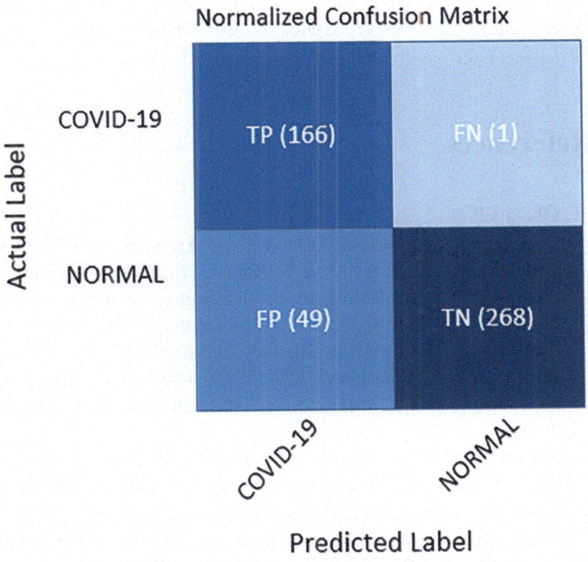

Fig. 6.6 Confusion matrix for architecture 3

Table 6.4 Accuracy values obtained for different well-known models

Network	Accuracy 2-class (%)
InceptionResNetV2 [24]	97.40
Inception [24]	86.13
Xception [25]	85.57

Table 6.5 Comparison of different proposed models

Scheme	Model	Dataset (chest X-ray)	Accuracy (%)
Proposed Scheme	CNN (Architecture 3)	The training dataset contains a total of 1811 images of size 64 × 64 × 3 (545 of COVID-19 class and 1266 of normal)	99.4 (500 epochs)
Ioannis D. Apostolopoulos et al. [12]	VGG19, MobileNet	1427 X-Ray images (700 for pneumonia, 504 for normal, 224 for COVID-19)	97.8
Asif Iqbal Khan et al. [17]	CoroNet	1251 images (330 for Bacterial pneumonia, 310 for normal, 284 for COVID-19, and 327 for viral pneumonia)	90
Tulin Ozturk et al. [26]	DarkNet-19	Chest X-Ray database of images developed by J. P. Cohen	98.08

Acknowledgments The authors would like to thank the Department of Science and Technology (DST) New Delhi, Government of India for providing financial support under the DST Inspire Fellowship Scheme with reference number DST/INSPIRE/03/2018/000093.

References

1. Ohata EF et al (2021) Automatic detection of COVID-19 infection using chest X-ray images through transfer learning. IEEE/CAA J Automat Sin 8(1):239–248
2. Parah SA, Sheikh JA, Ahad F, Bhat GM (2018) High capacity and secure electronic patient record (EPR) embedding in color images for IoT driven healthcare systems. In: Dey N, Hassanien A, Bhatt C, Ashour A, Satapathy S (eds) Internet of Things and Big Data analytics toward next-generation intelligence, Studies in Big Data. Springer, New York, p 30
3. Musleh AAWA, Maghari AY (2020) COVID-19 detection in X-ray images using CNN algorithm. In: 2020 International conference on promising electronic technologies (ICPET), pp 5–9
4. Rehman A, Saba T, Tariq U, Ayesha N (2021) Deep learning-based COVID-19 detection using CT and X-ray images: current analytics and comparisons. IT Professional 23(3):63–68
5. Parah SA et al (2021) Efficient security and authentication for edge-based Internet of medical things. IEEE Internet Things J. https://doi.org/10.1109/JIOT.2020.3038009
6. Haque KF, Haque FF, Gandy L, Abdelgawad A (2020) Automatic detection of COVID-19 from chest X-ray images with convolutional neural networks. In: 2020 International conference on computing, electronics & communications engineering (iCCECE), pp 125–130
7. Mporas I, Naronglerdrit P (2020) COVID-19 identification from chest X-Rays. In: 2020 International conference on biomedical innovations and applications (BIA), pp 69–72
8. Gull S, Loan NA, Parah SA, Sheikh JA, Bhat GM (2018) An efficient watermarking technique for tamper detection and localization of medical images. J Ambient Intell Human Comput 11: 1799–1808
9. Kaw JA, Loan NA, Parah SA, Muhammad K, Sheikh JA, Bhat GM (2019) A reversible and secure patient information hiding system for IoT driven e-health. Int J Inf Manag 45:262–275
10. Gull S, Parah SA, Muhammad K (2020) Reversible data hiding exploiting Huffman encoding with dual images for IoMT based healthcare. Comput Commun 163:134–149
11. Sarosh P, Parah SA, Bhat GM, Muhammad K (2021) A security management framework for Big Data in smart healthcare. Big Data Res 25:100225

12. Apostolopoulos ID, Mpesiana TA (2020) Covid-19: automatic detection from X-Ray images utilizing transfer learning with a convolutional neural network. Phys Eng Sci Med 43:635–640
13. Shibly KH, Dey SK, Islam MT, Rahman MM (2020) COVID Faster R-CNN: a novel framework to diagnose novel coronavirus disease (COVID-19) in X-ray images. Informatics Med Unlocked 20:100405
14. Sethi R, Mehrotra M, Sethi D (2020) Deep learning-based diagnosis recommendation for COVID-19 using chest X-ray images. In: 2020 Second international conference on inventive research in computing applications (ICIRCA), pp 1–4
15. Taresh MM, Zhu N, Ali TAA, Hameed AS, Mutar ML (2021) Transfer learning to detect COVID-19 automatically from X-ray images using convolutional neural networks. Int J Biomed Imaging 2021:8828404
16. Das AK, Ghosh S, Thunder S et al (2021) Automatic COVID-19 detection from X-ray images using ensemble learning with a convolutional neural network. Pattern Anal Applic 24:1111–1124
17. Khan AI, Shah JL, Bhat MM (2020) CoroNet: a deep neural network for detection and diagnosis of COVID-19 from chest x-ray images. Comput Methods Prog Biomed 196:10558
18. Panwar H, Gupta PK, Siddiqui MK, Menendez RM, Singh V (2020) Application of Deep learning for fast detection of COVID-19 in X-Ray using nCOVnet. Chaos, Solitons Fractals 138:109944
19. More SS, Mange MA, Sankhe MS, Sahu SS (2021) Convolutional neural network-based brain tumor detection. In: 2021 5th International conference on intelligent computing and control systems (ICICCS), pp 1532–1538
20. Jha N, Prashar D, Rashid M, Shafiq M, Khan R, Pruncu CI, Tabrez Siddiqui S, Saravana Kumar M (2021) Deep learning approach for discovery of in silico drugs for combating COVID-19. J Healthc Engineering 2021:6668985
21. Dautov E, Astafeva N (2021) Convolutional neural network in the classification of architectural styles of buildings. In: 2021 IEEE conference of Russian young researchers in electrical and electronic engineering (ElConRus), pp 274–277
22. Mondal S, Agarwal K, Rashid M (2019) Deep learning approach for automatic classification of x-ray images using convolutional neural network. In: In 2019 Fifth international conference on image information processing (ICIIP). IEEE, New York, pp 326–331
23. Li Z, Liu F, Yang W, Peng S, Zhou J (2020) A survey of convolutional neural networks: analysis, applications, and prospects. In: IEEE transactions on neural networks and learning systems. https://doi.org/10.1109/TNNLS.2021.3084827
24. Szegedy C, Ioffe S, Vanhoucke V, Alemi AA (2017) Inception-v4, inception-resnet and the impact of residual connections on learning. In: Thirty-first AAAI conference on artificial intelligence
25. Collet F (2017) Xception: deep learning with depthwise separable convolutions. ArXiv preprint. ArXiv:161002357
26. Ozturk T, Talo M, Yildirim EA, Baloglu UB, Yildirim O, Acharya UR (2020) Automated detection of COVID-19 cases using deep neural networks with X-Ray images. Comput Biol Med 121:103792

Chapter 7
AI-Based Deep Random Forest Ensemble Model for Prediction of COVID-19 and Pneumonia from Chest X-Ray Images

A. Jothi Prabha, N. Venkateswaran, and Prabaharan Sengodan

Contents

1 Introduction

The coronavirus (COVID-19) disease started with the detection of new viral pneumonia in Wuhan, China, in December 2019, which eventually blew out like a pandemic worldwide. Patients of COVID-19 have signs that are similar to other viral conditions. The correlations between other disorders and reactions create challenging problems about the clinical diagnosis. The standard methodology for distinguishing patients with COVID-19 is currently the Reverse Transcription-Polymerase Chain Reaction (RT-PCR) [1]. Although the RT-PCR specificity is pretty reasonable for the detection of COVID-19, its sensitivity was comparatively poor for COVID-19 detection. Computed tomography of the Chest is also used for

A. Jothi Prabha (✉)
Department of Computer Science & Engineering, Kakatiya Institute of Technology and Science, Warangal, Telangana State, India

N. Venkateswaran · P. Sengodan
Department of Computer Science & Engineering, Jyothishmathi Institute of Technology & Science, Karimnagar, India

S. A. Parah et al. (eds.), *Artificial Intelligence for Innovative Healthcare Informatics*,
https://doi.org/10.1007/978-3-030-96569-3_7

diagnosing abnormal COVID-19 pneumonia findings. It was distinguished primarily by the findings of ground-glass opacity widely spread on lung peripherals. The CT impression of COVID-19 Pneumonia is observed to be different from that of bacterial and viral pneumonia. The main concern of using CT for diagnosis is it has a high risk of facility contamination hence not preferable for COVID-19 detection [2, 37–39]. Chest X-Ray (CXR) is economical and widely used for diagnostic uses. Major medical associations advocate the use of chest radiography for individuals having chances of developing COVID-19 because of its wide range of availability. Most of the emergency service centers, hospitals, including both urban and rural areas have radiography facilities. Moreover, it is less prone to contamination and can be easily disinfected [3, 40–42].

Machine learning models, especially deep learning have the major advantage of learning a huge amount of data quickly. It has proven to perform well in diagnosing several diseases including COVID-19 pneumonia [4]. In this research work, the main aim is to develop a deep random forest ensemble model for the diagnosis/detection of COVID-19 pneumonia from other kinds of pneumonia using CXR. The proposed AI-Based Ensemble model combines the advantages of deep learning and Random Forest. Although deep learning is powerful in the diagnosis of diseases, they have some limitations when it comes to real-world detection tasks. They cause high computational overhead and also require hyper-parameter optimization [5, 49–52]. The computational overhead is mainly due to backpropagation.

Major Contributions of this investigation are as below:

- In the proposed ensemble model, tree learners are used instead of backpropagation. Considering the above advantages, this work proposes a deep random forest ensemble algorithm for the detection/diagnosis of COVID-19 Pneumonia and other kinds of pneumonia.
- The proposed deep forest ensemble model shows improved predictive accuracy with less computational overhead and works well on a small-sized dataset where deep learning usually underperforms [6–8].
- The deep forest model uses random-sized grains at each level of the sliding window. Hence it does not suffer from overfitting. The ensemble deep forest uses cross-validation to generate class vectors.

The structure of the remaining chapter is as follows. Section 2 gives an introduction to work done on COVID-19 classification/detection methods. Section 3 explains the proposed deep forest ensemble model. Section 4 describes the datasets, experimental setup, and results. Section 5 shows the comparison with existing works and Sect. 6 depicts the conclusion of the work.

2 Related Work

This segment highlights the research conducted or tasks done by researchers associated with the COVID-19 research. Recent mechanisms and technologies have made diagnosis and treatment significantly more accessible and better than existing. The accessibility of large datasets and invincible achievement of utilized learning techniques have attained diagnosis task efficient and optimal results. The researchers Pranav Rajpurkar et al. [9] proposed the cheXNet technique, a CNN of 121 model layers (DenseNet). It takes to consider the sample chest X-ray pictures and generate the probability of pneumonia, including a heat-map that locates pneumonia's most likely location. They adjust the last layer that has just a single output and then includes a sigmoid nonlinearity. They arbitrarily split the data set into practice as 98,637 sample images and patients strength 28,744, validation considered as 6351 sample images, total patients involves is 1672, and testing image samples are 420, patients are 389 to train the model. Before feeding the images as input into the network, they will be resized to 224 × 224 and applied to normalize it, and training data augmented with random horizontal flipping. Finally, it compared their framework model with various radiologists on the F1 metric. It gains a score of 0.435, more decadent than the average of 0.387 for the radiologist. In this article AsifIqbal Khan et al. [10], researchers proceed with a deep CNN model (CoroNet) that made the system detect coronavirus infection automatically with the support of digitally scanned X-ray image samples. The proposed techniques employed Xception structure and pertained to the image database. Finally, the model familiarised and validated well with the fine-tuned dataset, and desired results confirmed that the framework model reached a remarkable high accuracy rate of 89.6%. In this study Sekeroglu Boran and Ozsahin Ilker [11], researchers have performed several experiments to acquire the remarkable level-accuracy of coronavirus detection rate in digitally scanned X-ray samples using ConvNets model. During the investigation process, various categories like COVID-19-Normal (i.e. healthy), COVID-19-Pneumonia state (i.e. infected), and COVID-19 Pneumonia state healthy (i.e. Normal) were measured for classification. The various network structures and the machine-learning (ML) model were built and assessed using numerical data. The sum of digital scanned X-ray image samples in the datasets and the mean testing & detection time of COVID-19 will be 0.03 s/image computed with the remarkable ConvNets technique. The results projected that the ConvNets approach with fully connected layers and reduced convolutional is proficient in diagnosis COVID-19 images with two classes. Finally, the proposed model secured accuracy as ROC AUC's mean values as 0.965 and 0.963, respectively.

In this novel Hussain et al. [12], researchers focused on and developed an Artificial Intelligence (AI) based mega technique to diagnose coronavirus pneumonia and lung disease under portable chest X-rays. Utilized the open benchmark datasets with different categories of X-rays images such as COVID-19 with 130 patients, 145 bacterial pneumonia patients, viral pneumonia with 145 patients, and 138 regular patients were analyzed. The proposed work employs machine learning techniques to classify COVID-19 with various conditions. They used texture and morphological methods for feature extraction. The performance is made with two-class and multi-class classification. Finally, we secured 97.56% for the two-class category. In this work Farukh Hashmi Mohammad et al. [13], the researchers focused on an optimal framework model that used digitally scanned chest X-ray samples to detect pneumonia efficiently. The article introduced a highly impacted classifier that includes impacted predictions from DL (Deep Learning) techniques such as DenseNet121, ResNet-18, and InceptionV3 in the most favorable way. It used a quality dataset to predict the result with high accuracy. The transfer learning method is employed to reach an advanced training dataset, validate accuracy, and bias-based data augmentation methods to further increase the training dataset to fine-tune the proposed DL models. Finally, the model is evaluated and achieved a high performed accuracy rate of 98.43% and an AUC rate of 99.76%.

In this article Rahimzadeh Mohammad et al. [14], authors developed a combined Neural Network depending on ResNet50V2 and Xception networks to classify the scanned X-ray digital image samples into three classical clusters of the normal state, pneumonia state, and coronavirus state. There are two sets of benchmark datasets, which contained around 6054 and 180 digitally scanned X-ray samples from pneumonia and infected coronavirus patients. They have proposed techniques for educating the neural network to balance the dataset. They achieved 99.50% as a high-level accuracy and 80.53% sensitivity for the coronavirus [15]. Habib Nahida et al. [15] has proposed ensemble-based techniques which help for pneumonia diagnosis from scanned sample chest X-ray pictures. A model trained representatives with deep CNN and VGG-19 and extracted features from the image dataset. Techniques Random Under and Over Sampler (RUS and ROS) are used on the focused ensemble feature vector to avoid data abnormality issues. Finally, the model classifies the framework proposed and diagnosis pneumonia 98.93% optimal accurately than other existing models for pneumonia detection.

The researchers Rachna Jain Gupta et al. [16] came up with ideas for deep learning with CNN framework models. The proposed techniques compared their performance and accuracy with ResNet, Inception V3, and Xception models. They analyzed sample scanned chest X-ray from the benchmark repository to detect pneumonia cases, in which 84.99% were used for training the model and 15% for validation. Finally, In the analysis and performance part, the Xception model framework produced better performance accuracy as 97.9% for detecting scanned X-ray pictures compared with other existing models. This article Rafid Mostafiz et al. [17] has proposed a novel approach to discovering coronavirus from the digital chest sample pictures using hybridization of the DWF (Discrete Wavelet Transform) features and deep CNN. The best possible components are extracted along with recursive feature removal through less redundancy and high relevance methodologies. Then, they adapted the random forest-based approach to action the determination task. Finally, a proposed model has a better accuracy of 98.5% with satisfactory performance matched to the existing techniques.

This article Rahul Kumar et al. [18] author has presented work and focused utilization of ResNet152 and effective machine learning classifiers of diseases COVID-19. The proposed model has used benchmark datasets and outperformed all the necessary classes. They tailored the SMOTE algorithm to handle unbalanced class variation from the datasets. Finally, the Random Forest classifier using XGBoost obtained the best accuracy of 0.998 compared to existing methodologies. This article [19] proposed a competent DL model which trained with scanned X-ray samples to diagnose COVID-19 patients quickly. Researchers suggested Artificial Intelligence-based models for coronavirus and other chronic contagious diseases. AI-based models are fine-tuned and trained thoroughly with a transfer learning model and effectively classified with the scanned X-ray sample images demonstrating noticed conditions. Further, in the article Saleh Albahli et al. [20, 30, 31], researchers developed a model using transfer learning methodology for mechanical diagnose of coronavirus infection using digitally scanned CHX [Chest X-ray] image samples. The novel article engaged three models, likely NASNetLarge, InceptionNetV3, and Inception ResNetV2, to fine-tune to automate the process to detect coronavirus disease using scanned digital X-ray 2235 images out of that 850 samples are positive COVID-19 patients, 500 as non-COVID-19 patients and 915 as normal healthy lungs. Finally, InceptionNetv3 achieved high performance with the best accuracy of 98.63% without any data augmentation.

The proposed Sima Sarv Ahrabi et al. [27, 28] deep learning model established a well-structured design and randomly fine-tuned quality images shuffled in the benchmark dataset. The proposed model access and detects most of the coronavirus digitally scanned X-ray samples accurately, with an exceptionally high volume accuracy of 99.8% [21]. Tanvir Mahmud et al. [20] presented CovXNet as the architecture of a deep neural network model capable of investigating the coronavirus and the rest of infected pneumonia from digitally scanned X-ray samples. The proposed model made the system understand with a considerable volume of X-ray scanned samples and refined the dataset. The CovXNet model employed stacking and optimization techniques to design various forms of image resolution. Finally, the article achieved incredible detection performance with high accuracy of 0.97 for ordinary patients, with a rate of 0.97 for COVID-19 or viral infected patients, and at a rate of 0.95 for bacterial or COVID-19 patients. In this novel article Tawsifur Rahman et al. [21], researchers mainly focused on automatically detecting infection, either viral or bacterial using digitally scanned X-ray image samples. The authors employed four Deep Convolutional Neural networks such as AlexNet, SqueezeNet, ResNet18, and DenseNet201 mainly utilized for transfer learning. Almost 5247 digital chest X-ray samples, which consist of regular, infected, bacterial, and viral, were fine-tuned and trained for classification. In this proposed work, the authors performed various schemes. Finally, the model achieved a classification accuracy of 98% for regular and pneumonia patient schemes, 95% for bacterial and viral pneumonia patient's systems, and 93.3% as usual, respectively. The novel work Abdullahi Umar Ibrahim et al. [22] proposes the AlexNet model using a Deep Learning based model to diagnose coronavirus infection pneumonia state, bacterial pneumonia state, viral pneumonia state, and digital chest scanned samples acquired from the benchmark dataset. The proposed model performed two-way, three-way, and four classifications like viral state, bacterial state, COVID-19 infected state, and healthy state (i.e. non-COVID-19) use of X-rays scans. Finally, the novel approach achieved 0.95 accuracies, and ultimately COVID-19 infected viral and healthful (i.e. normal) with digital X-rays samples and secured 99.16% accuracy, 98% of sensitivity, and 100% specificity. This novel article D. Haritha et al. [23] proposed a VGG model using the CNN approach to predict the COVID-19 disease. The novel approach employed AI with significant support in transfer learning in the prediction of COVID-19. Transfer learning techniques are used to minimize the training time for a neural network proposed model [34–36]. Finally, the article scored a high accuracy of 99.49% as the detected rate of COVID-19 patients from chest scanned samples.

In the research article Muhammad Umer et al. [24, 25], the authors proposed the CNN [Convolutional Neural Network] model to extract all the weighted features from digital CX-ray (scanned X-ray) pictures for the prediction of classes. The selected model used three variations of filters that help to get the boundaries of X-ray images with the infected region. KerasImageDataGenerator [KIDG] is used to generate a thousand hundred augmented images [43, 44]. Classification techniques used with 2, 3, and 4 classes were normal cases, virus pneumonia cases, and bacterial pneumonia cases. Finally, the proposed model predicts coronavirus COVID-19 infected patients with high accuracy of 98.8%, and results indicated as 97% for 2-classes, 90% for 3-classes, and 85% for 4-classes, respectively. Research article [26, 28, 29] describes coronavirus as one of the most infected and deadly viruses that influence the body. The authors have adopted an automated technique to detect coronavirus using digitally scanned images. The proposed model CNN and HOG [Histogram Oriented gradient] are used for feature extraction to enhance classification. To fine-tune the edge of the pictures used diffusion filtering and watershed segmentation techniques. Using the deep learning model proposed, the feature fusion techniques ensure a better performance in detecting coronavirus and achieved a testing accuracy of 99.49% compared to existing methods such as KNN, ANN, and SVM, respectively. The research Parnian Afshar et al. [26] presents the COVID-Caps method, referred to as capsule networks, to handle nominal datasets with chest scanned digital pictures [45–48]. The novel approach secured better result investigation, than existing techniques. COVID-CAPS methods unanimously reached an accuracy of 95.7%, 95.8% of Specificity, 90% as Sensitivity, and 97% of AUC [Area under the Curve] with limited numbers of trainable parameters.

3 Proposed Deep Random Forest Ensemble Model

3.1 Architecture

Figure 7.1 depicts the architecture of the proposed deep random forest ensemble model for detection and classification of COVID-19 Pneumonia and other kinds of pneumonia.

Raw CXR images are resized, converted to grayscale, and fed as input to the next stage of the model for classification. The proposed model employs the deep forest ensemble for the identification and classification of COVID-19 and other kinds of pneumonia. The proposed deep random forest model has two stages such as sliding window scanning (SWS) and Cascade forest layering (CFL) [32–35].

The initial stage is the sliding window scanning which adopts the characteristics of Convolution Neural Networks (CNN). In this stage, the input image is processed parallel in two different sliding windows. Small instances of images are extracted from every sliding window, which is further trained by Random Forest and

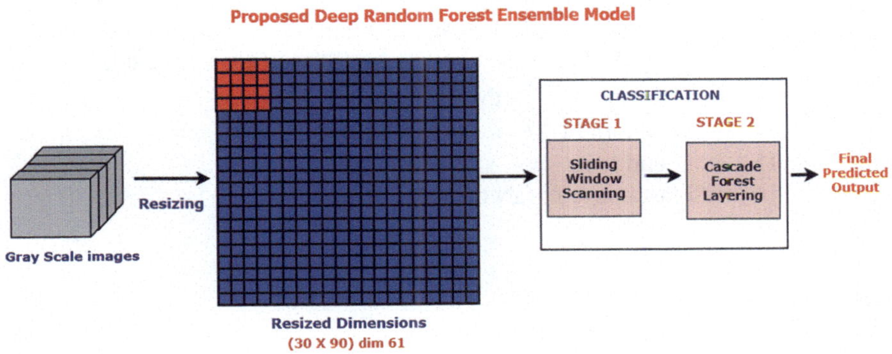

Fig. 7.1 Proposed deep random forest ensemble model

Completely Random Forest ensembles. In each sliding window, both the output of the ensemble generates a class vector. These class vectors are joined to form a multi-dimensional feature vector which aids in improving the performance of the classifier.

The multi-dimensional feature vector from SWS is then passed as input to the CFL stage. CFL stage has multiple layers that follow a sequential manner. Each of these layers has four ensemble forests. Two out of the four are Random Forests and the remaining two are Completely Random Forest. The number of layers to be learned is adaptively chosen by the deep random forest ensemble model. This feature of the deep forest helps in reducing the complexity of the model. The model also does not suffer from overfitting as the class vectors are generated using fivefold cross-validation technique. Feature representation is done by averaging the class vector probability of each forest. The layering stops when there is no increase in accuracy. The outputs of the ensembles are observed and the image is assigned to a class based on the maximum average probability value of a class. The algorithm of the proposed COVID-19 Pneumonia Classification Model is depicted below.

Algorithm 7.1 Proposed COVID-19 Pneumonia Classification Model

Input: $T=\{(a_n, b_n)\}_{n=1}^{N}$: Training data
Output: Final Predicted class bn

repeat
loop each image in T
Convert to grayscale image r=f(i,j)
Resize the image g: i × j
Set Sliding window size SW €{SW1,SW2 of size K× L)
repeat
    loop SW
        Call Slide_scan()
    end loop
    until SW

```
        Call Cascade_Forest_Layering()
        Calculate mean class probabilities of each ensemble
        avn= 1/Ex ∑_{e=1}^{Ex} av_f, e
        return bf
    end loop
until last image f=(aN,bN)
```

$$avn = \frac{1}{Ex}\sum_{e=1}^{Ex} av_{f,e}$$

3.2 *Image Processing Phase*

The chest X-ray images are resized as square images with an aspect ratio of 1:3 is inputted to the deep forest ensemble. Various sizes such as 10:30, 20:60, and 30:90 have been experimented with. Images with small dimensions may lead to information loss, hence image dimensions of 30:90 were used in this work for all experiments.

3.3 *Sliding Window Scanning Phase*

Figure 7.2 depicts the workflow of the sliding-window-scanning phase. The images are scanned with the aid of two sliding windows of dimensions (10 × 10) and (30 × 30). The size of the sliding window, the number of smaller image instances, and its stride value are decided based on the input dimensions.

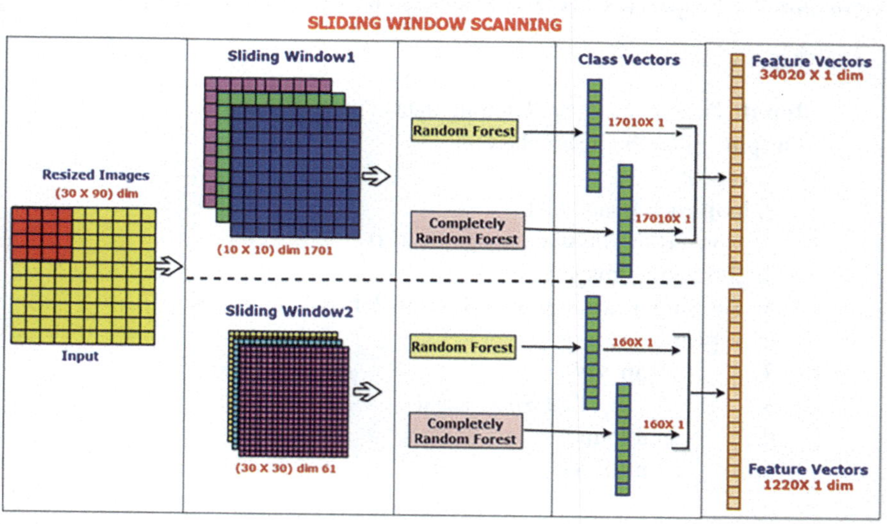

Fig. 7.2 The workflow of the Sliding Window Scanning phase

The reduced image instances are further processed using random forest and completely random forest ensembles. Each forest makes its own decisions by training decision trees. The ensemble generates feature vectors based on class probabilities. The leaf node of the tree is used to decide the class of the image. The final feature vectors are computed by concatenating the feature vectors outputted from both the sliding windows. The pseudo-code of the sliding-window-scanning phase is shown below.

Algorithm 7.2 Sliding_Window_Scanning_Stage

Input: g- Images resized and grayscale.
Output: k_f^{odd}, k_f^{even}: feature vectors.
1: gs : a × b; P ∈ {p1,p2 : M × N; s:stride; M ∈ {M1.....Ms}:
Set of compressed images: X ∈ {x1.x2: group of ensembles.
2. Output smaller images S= k1 × k2
Where, k1← a – m + s; k2 ← b – n + s.
3. **while** (element in X)
4. **loop** (each x1, x2 ∈X)
5. Train M
6. Obtain class probability vectors kC
Where, kC ∈ {kC1, kC2 : group of class probability
Vectors; kC1 =(kM1,1,,,,kMs,C) and kC2 =(kM1,1,,,,kMs,C)
7. **end loop**
8. Compute feature vectors k_f^{odd} ← kC1 & kC2, k_f^{even} ← kC1 & kC2
Where kf1: 2S1 × 1 dim's, for p1 ∈ P;
kf2: 2S2 × 1 dim's, for p2 ∈ P;
S1 and S2 – number of compressed images from p1 and p2 respectively.

3.4 *Cascade Forest Layering Stage*

Figure 7.3 illustrates the workflow of the Cascade-Forest-Layering stage. The smaller instances of images processed by the sliding windows are given as input to this phase. This stage has multiple layers and a new feature vector is generated at each layer. The first and second layers process the feature vector got after the sliding window 1 and sliding window 2 respectively. The ensembles in each layer (Random Forest and Completely Random Forest) generate class vectors that are integrated into the feature vector generated by sliding window 2. Cross-validation with fivefolds is used to generate class vectors. The new feature set generated by layer 1 is given as input to layer 2. The layering process continues until there is no improvement in accuracy. The algorithm of cascading forest layering is shown below.

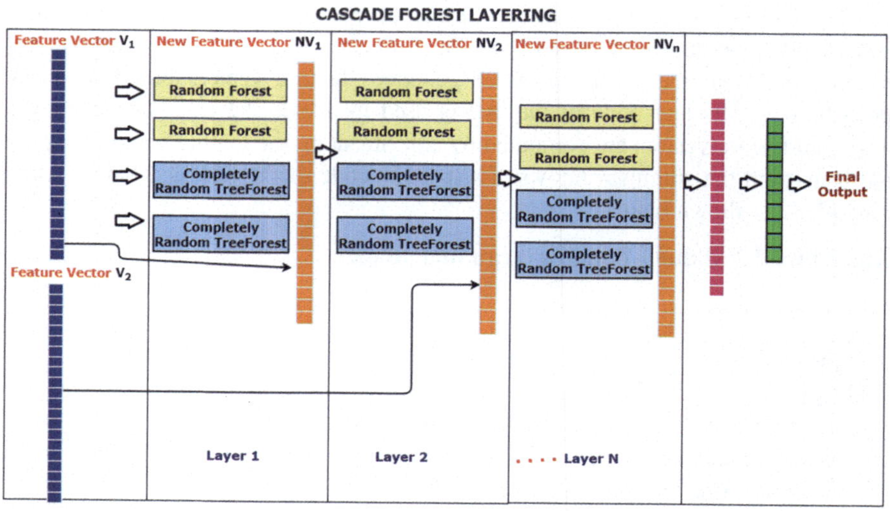

Fig. 7.3 Workflow of cascade forest layering

Algorithm 7.3 Cascade_Layering_Phase

Input: k_f^{odd}, k_f^{even}: feature vectors obtained from p_1 & p_2 ∈. **P**

Output: k_f^t**: new feature vector;** acy_t: accuracy of the current layer

1. **X** ∈ {x_1, x_2, x_3,x_4} : group of ensembles; t: layer_variable: acy_{t-1} initialize 0
2. **Repeat** t = 1
3. $acy_{t-1} = acy_t$
4. **if** t= 1
5. call C_Layering (k_f^{odd} , 0)
6. t = t + 1
7. **end if**
8. **if** t= even
9. call C_Layering (k_c^t, k_f^{even})
10. **else**
11. call C_Layering (k_c^t, k_f^{odd})
12. **end_if**
13. t = t + 1
14. **Until** $acyt_{-1} < acy_t$
15. **procedure** C_Layering(k_1,k_2 → k_f^n, acy_t);
16. **loop** each layer Lt (t = 1)
17. Train k^{t-1} with all necessary elements of X
18. **loop** each x_1, x_2, x_3, x_4 ∈ X and CL classes
19. output class probability vectors **X** → k_{cl}^t

Where, $k_{cl} \leftarrow k_{cl}^{x1}$ &k_{cl}^{x2} & k_{cl}^{x3} & k_{cl}^{x4} : CL-dimensional class vectors

k_{cl}^{x1}, k_{cl}^{x2}, k_{cl}^{x3} , k_{cl}^{x4} - class vectors obtained from x_1, x_2, x_3, x_4

respectively;
x- number of ensembles (x = 4).
20. **end loop**
21. **end loop**
22. Compute new feature vector $k^t_f \leftarrow k_1 \& k_2$, acy_t
23. **end procedure**

4 Experiments and Results

4.1 Datasets

Three public datasets were used to develop and evaluate the proposed deep random forest ensemble model for the detection of COVID 19 pneumonia and other types of pneumonia. CXR images of healthy, COVID-19 pneumonia and other kinds of pneumonia were taken from two public datasets in the COVID-19 data repository of GitHub (https://github.com/jurader/covid19_xp). The number of images for other types of pneumonia was less hence used images from the Pneumonia detection challenge dataset from Kaggle (https://www.kaggle.com/c/rsna-pneumonia-detection-challenge). Images were randomly selected from three different datasets and checked for class imbalance. The final data has 1248 chest X-ray images out of which 215 are of COVID-19 pneumonia, 533 images of other types of pneumonia, and 500 images of healthy individuals. Figure 7.4 shows sample chest X-ray (CXR) images of COVID-19 pneumonia, other kinds of pneumonia, and healthy individuals.

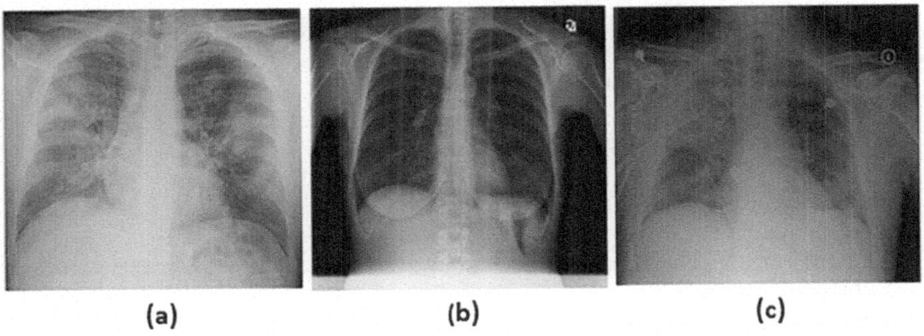

Fig. 7.4 Sample images of three classes COVID-19, other kinds of pneumonia, and healthy individuals. (**a**) CXR image of COVID-19 Pneumonia. (**b**) CXR image of Healthy individual without Pneumonia. (**c**) CXR image of other Pneumonias

4.2 Experimental Setup

The experiments in this work are performed on Windows 10 64 bit operating system having 16 GB-RAM and 1 TB hard disk drive. Python framework with required packages was installed. The experimental setting included two random forests and two completely random forests at each level. Fivefold cross-validation was performed to obtain the class vectors. The algorithm selects the number of layers centered on the data. The few hyperparameters used in this setting are the number of forests(2), the number of sliding windows(2), and the number of trees for each forest (4). The train test ratio for validation is 80:20.

4.3 Results and Discussion

The experimental results of the proposed deep random forest ensemble model and other existing models are tabulated in Table 7.1. The model gave a high performance with 96% accuracy while using two sliding windows and four trees in a forest with the default settings.

The confusion matrix of the validation set is shown in Fig. 7.5. From the confusion matrix, it can be observed that it was able to correctly predict all the COVID-19 images. The misclassification rate is too less for both healthy and other pneumonia individuals. The precision and recall of the proposed model are 0.96 and 0.97 respectively indicating that the proposed model exhibits high precision and recall. Hence the proposed deep random forest ensemble model is highly promising for the prediction of COVID-19 pneumonia and other kinds of pneumonia.

Performance measures used in this research work are computed as in Eqs. (7.1–7.5).

Table 7.1 Performance measures of the proposed deep random forest ensemble model

Author	Methods	Accuracy (%)	Precision	Recall	F1-Score
Nishio M. et al. (2020) [1]	Deep Learning Model	83.6	0.84	0.82	0.83
Ran Zhang et al. (2021) [2]	Pre-trained Deep Learning Model	92.0	0.88	0.79	0.91
Arun Sharma et al. (2020) [3]	Transfer Learning model	93.8	0.92	0.90	0.93
Harsh Panwar et al. (2020) [8]	Deep Learning model	88.1	0.97	78.5	0.89
Tanvir Mahamud et al. (2020) [20]	Deep Learning model CovXNet	90.2	0.89	0.87	0.89
	Proposed Deep Random Forest Ensemble Model	**96.63**	**0.97**	**0.96**	**0.96**

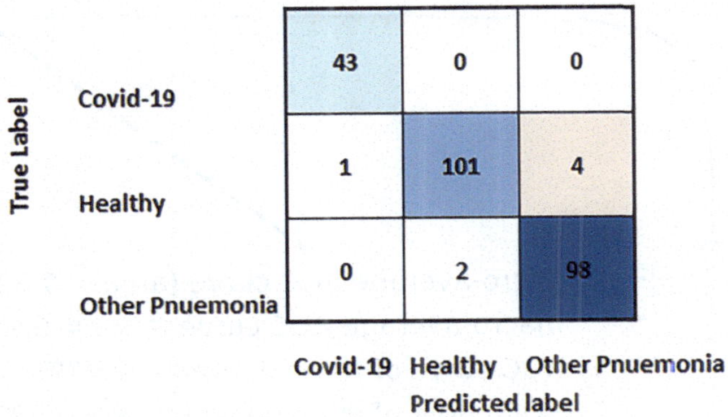

Fig. 7.5 Confusion Matrix

$$Accuracy = \frac{\sum Correctlyclassifiedinstances}{\sum Allinstances} \tag{7.1}$$

$$Specificity = \frac{TrueNegative}{FalsePositive + TrueNegative} \tag{7.2}$$

$$Recall = \frac{TruePositive}{TruePositive + FalseNegative} \tag{7.3}$$

$$Precision = \frac{TruePositive}{TruePositive + FalsePositive} \tag{7.4}$$

$$F1\ Score = 2 * \frac{precision * recall}{precision + recall} \tag{7.5}$$

Figure 7.6 shows the ROC curves of three classes COVID-19 Pneumonia, other kinds of pneumonia, and healthy individuals. Another important metric to evaluate classifier performance is Receiver Operating Characteristic (ROC). The ROC curve has a True Positive. Rate (TPR) on the y axis and False Positive Rate (FPR) on the x-axis. It has been observed that there is a large area under ROC which shows that the proposed model performs well in the classification of COVID-19 and other types of pneumonia.

5 Comparative Analysis

Table 7.1 shows the results of the proposed deep random forest ensemble model along with the other existing models for the detection and classification of COVID-19 and other types of pneumonia from CXR datasets. Evaluation metrics used to measure the performance of the model include Accuracy, precision, recall, and F1-score. From Table 7.1, it can be seen that deep learning models are widely used for the detection and classification of COVID-19 and other types of pneumonia.

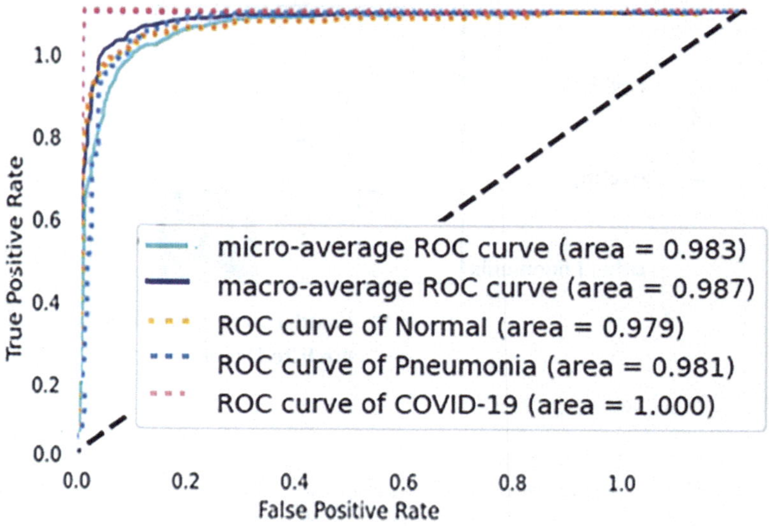

Fig. 7.6 ROC curve of three classes COVID-19, other types of pneumonia, and healthy individuals

The deep learning models show good accuracy levels but the proposed deep random forest ensemble model has outperformed the performance of these models. Moreover, the number of hyperparameters used in the proposed model is very less when compared to deep learning models. Hence, the comparative results show that the proposed deep random forest ensemble model is effective than that of other existing deep learning models for the classification of COVID-19 and other types of pneumonia.

6 Conclusion

This research work proposes a simple and efficient deep random forest ensemble model for the prediction of COVID-19 and other types of pneumonia. The proposed model does not require hyperparameter tuning and backpropagation reducing the complexity. The model uses a deep forest model that is based on three main aspects, image processing, sliding window scanning, and cascade forest which is similar to deep neural networks but does not have backpropagation which aids in reducing the complexity of the model. The proposed model shows a high accuracy of 96% and low complexity when compared to the state-of-the-art models used in literature for detection and classification of COVID-19 Pneumonia and other types of pneumonia. The precision and recall of the proposed model are 0.96 and 0.97 respectively indicating that the proposed model exhibits high precision and recall. The ensemble deep forest uses cross-validation to generate class vectors and does not suffer from overfitting.

Acknowledgments The authors would like to thank the management of the Jyothishmathi Institute of Technology & Science for their encouragement and support in doing this research work.

References

1. Nishio M, Noguchi S, Matsuo H, Murakami T (2020) Automatic classification between COVID-19 pneumonia, non-COVID-19 pneumonia, and the healthy on chest X-ray image: combination of data augmentation methods. Sci Rep 10(1):1–6
2. Zhang R, Tie X, Qi Z, Bevins NB, Zhang C, Griner D, Chen GH (2021) Diagnosis of coronavirus disease 2019 pneumonia by using chest radiography: value of artificial intelligence. Radiology 298(2):E88
3. Sharma A, Rani S, Gupta D (2020) Artificial intelligence-based classification of chest X-ray images into COVID-19 and other infectious diseases. Int J Biomed Imaging 2020:8889023
4. Rajaraman S, Siegelman J, Alderson PO, Folio LS, Folio LR, Antani SK (2020) Iteratively pruned deep learning ensembles for covid-19 detection in chest x-rays. IEEE Access 8:115041–115050
5. Zhang J, Xie Y, Pang G, Liao Z, Verjans J, Li W, Xia Y (2020) Viral pneumonia screening on chest X-rays using confidence-aware anomaly detection. In: IEEE transactions on medical imaging
6. Kong Y, Yu T (2018) A deep neural network model using random forest to extract feature representation for gene expression data classification. Sci Rep 8(1):1–9
7. Mahmud T, Rahman MA, Fattah SA (2020) CovXNet: a multi-dilation convolutional neural network for automatic COVID-19 and other pneumonia detection from chest X-ray images with transferable multi-receptive feature optimization. Comput Biol Med 122:103869
8. Panwar H, Gupta PK, Siddiqui MK, Morales-Menendez R, Singh V (2020) Application of deep learning for fast detection of COVID-19 in X-rays using nCOVnet. Chaos Solitons Fractals 138:109944
9. Rajpurkar P et al (2017) CheXNet: radiologist-level pneumonia detection on chest X-rays with deep learning. Bibcode:2017arXiv171105225R
10. AsifIqbal K et al (2020) CoroNet: a deep neural network for detection and diagnosis of COVID-19 from chest x-ray images. Comput Methods Prog Biomed 196. https://doi.org/10.1016/j.cmpb.2020.105581
11. Boran S, Ilker O (2020) Detection of COVID-19 from chest X-ray images using convolutional neural networks. Slas Technol Transl Life Sci Innov 25(6):553–565. https://doi.org/10.1177/2472630320958376
12. Hussain et al (2020) Machine-learning classification of texture features of portable chest X-ray accurately classifies COVID-19 lung infection. BioMedEngOnLine 19:88. https://doi.org/10.1186/s12938-020-00831-x
13. Mohammad FH et al (2020) Efficient pneumonia detection in chest Xray images using deep transfer. Learning 10(6):417. https://doi.org/10.3390/diagnostics10060417
14. Mohammad R et al (2020) A modified deep convolutional neural network for detecting COVID-19 and pneumonia from chest X-ray images based on the concatenation of Xception and ResNet50V2. Informatics Med Unlocked. https://doi.org/10.1016/j.imu.2020.100360
15. Nahida H et al (2020) Ensemble of CheXNet and VGG-19 feature extractor with random forest classifier for pediatric pneumonia detection. SN Comput Sci 1:359. https://doi.org/10.1007/s42979-020-00373-y
16. Gupta RJ et al (2020) Deep learning based detection and analysis of COVID-19 on chest X-ray images. Appl Intell 51:1690–1700. https://doi.org/10.1007/s10489-020-01902-1

17. Mostafiz R et al (2020) Covid-19 detection in chest X-ray through random forest classifier using a hybridization of deep CNN and DWT optimized features. SN Comput Sci. https://doi.org/10.1016/j.jksuci.2020.12.010
18. Kumar R et al (2020) Accurate prediction of COVID-19 using chest X-ray images through deep feature learning model with SMOTE and machine learning classifiers. BMJ. https://doi.org/10.1101/2020.04.13.20063461
19. Albahli S et al (2020) Detection of coronavirus disease from X-ray images using deep learning and transfer learning algorithms. J Xray Sci Technol 28(5):841–850. https://doi.org/10.3233/XST-200720
20. Mahmud T et al (2020) CovXNet: a multi-dilation convolutional neural network for automatic COVID-19 and other pneumonia detection from chest X-ray images with transferable multi-receptive feature optimization. Comput Biol Med 122:103869. https://doi.org/10.1016/j.compbiomed.2020.103869
21. Rahman T et al (2020) Transfer learning with deep convolutional neural network (CNN) for pneumonia detection using chest X-ray. Appl Sci 10(9):3233. https://doi.org/10.3390/app10093233
22. Ibrahim AU et al (2021) Pneumonia classification using deep learning from chest X-ray images during COVID-19. Cogn Comput. https://doi.org/10.1007/s12559-020-09787-5
23. Haritha D et al (2021) Covid prediction from X-ray images. In: 5th International conference on computing, communication and security (ICCCS), Patna, India, pp 1–5. https://doi.org/10.1109/ICCCS49678.2020.9276795
24. Umer K et al (2021) COVINet: a convolutional neural network approach for predicting COVID-19 from chest X-ray images. J Ambient Intell Human Comput. https://doi.org/10.1007/s12652-021-02917-3
25. Nur-A-Alam et al (2021) COVID-19 detection from chest X-ray images using feature fusion and deep learning. Sensors 21(4):1480. https://doi.org/10.3390/s21041480
26. Afshar P et al (2021) COVID-CAPS: a capsule network-based framework for identification of COVID-19 cases from X-ray images. Pattern Recogn Lett 138:638–643. https://doi.org/10.1016/j.patrec.2020.09.010
27. Ahrabi S et al (2021) An accuracy vs. complexity comparison of deep learning architectures for the detection of COVID-19 disease. Computation 9(1):3. https://doi.org/10.3390/computation9010003
28. Bassi PR, Attux R (2020) A deep convolutional neural network for covid-19 detection using chest x-rays. arXiv Preprint arXiv:2005.01578
29. Rao V, Priyanka MS, Lakshmi A, Faheema AGJ, Thomas A, Medappa K, Masood S (2020) Predicting COVID-19 pneumonia severity on chest X-ray with convolutional neural network: a retrospective study. Indian J Med Sci 72(3):132–140
30. Wang Z, Xiao Y, Li Y, Zhang J, Lu F, Hou M, Liu X (2021) Automatically discriminating and localizing COVID-19 from community-acquired pneumonia on chest X-rays. Pattern Recogn 110:107613
31. Roseline SA, Geetha S, Kadry S, Nam Y (2020) Intelligent vision-based malware detection and classification using deep random forest paradigm. IEEE Access 8:206303–206324
32. Zhou ZH, Feng J (2017) Deep forest. arXiv:1702.08835. http://arxiv.org/abs/1702.08835
33. Hemdan EED, Shouman MA, Karar ME (2020) COVIDX-Net: a framework of deep learning classifiers to diagnose COVID-19 in X-Ray images. arXiv 2020, arXiv:2003.11055. https://arxiv.org/abs/2003.11055. Accessed 5 Aug 2020
34. Cohen JP, Dao L, Morrison P, Roth K, Bengio Y, Shen B, Abbasi A, Hoshmand-Kochi M, Ghassemi M, Li H et al (2020) Predicting COVID-19 pneumonia severity on chest X-ray with deep learning. arXiv 2020, arXiv:2005.11856. https://arxiv.org/abs/2005.11856. Accessed 5 Aug 2020
35. Pasa F, Golkov V, Pfeiffer F, Cremers D, Pfeiffer D (2019) Efficient deep network architectures for fast chest X-Ray tuberculosis screening and visualization. Sci Rep 9:6268

36. Kermany D, Zhang K Goldbaum M (2019) Labeled optical coherence tomography (OCT) and chest X-ray images for classification. https://data.mendeley.com/datasets/rscbjbr9sj/2. Accessed 7 Oct 2019
37. Rathour N, Alshamrani SS, Singh R, Gehlot A, Rashid M, Akram SV, AlGhamdi AS (2021) IoMT based facial emotion recognition system using deep convolution neural networks. Electronics 10(11):1289
38. World Health Organization (2020) Coronavirus disease (COVID-2019) Situation Report—32.2020. https://www.who.int/docs/default-source/coronaviruse/situationreports/20200221-sitrep-32-covid-19.pdf. Accessed 11 Dec 2020
39. Huang C, Wang Y, Li X et al (2019) Clinical features of patients infected with 2019 novel coronavirus in Wuhan, China. Lancet 395(10223):497–506. [Published correction appears in Lancet 2020;395(10223):496]
40. Kumar I, Alshamrani SS, Kumar A, Rawat J, Singh KU, Rashid M, AlGhamdi AS (2021) Deep learning approach for analysis and characterization of COVID-19. Comput Mater Continua 70: 451–468
41. Jha N, Prashar D, Rashid M, Shafiq M, Khan R, Pruncu CI, Tabrez SS, Saravana KM (2021) Deep learning approach for discovery of in silico drugs for combating COVID-19. J Healthc Engineering 2021:6668985
42. Kim HW, Capaccione KM, Li G et al (2020) The role of initial chest X-ray in triaging patients with suspected COVID-19 during the pandemic. Emerg Radiol. https://doi.org/10.1007/s10140-020-01808-y
43. Murphy K, Smits H, Knoops AJG et al (2020) COVID-19 on chest radiographs: a multi-reader evaluation of an artificial intelligence system. Radiology 296(3):E166–E172
44. Shah AA, Parah SA, Rashid M, Elhoseny M (2020) Efficient image encryption scheme based on generalized logistic map for real time image processing. J Real-Time Image Proc 17(6): 2139–2151
45. Shi H, Han X, Zheng C (2020) Evolution of CT manifestations in a patient recovered from 2019 novel coronavirus (2019-nCoV) pneumonia in Wuhan, China. Radiology 295(1):20
46. Mondal S, Agarwal K, Rashid M (2019) Deep learning approach for automatic classification of x-ray images using convolutional neural network. In: 2019 Fifth international conference on image information processing (ICIIP). IEEE, New York, pp 326–331
47. Showkat S, Parah SA, Gull S (2021) Embedding in medical images with contrast enhancement and tamper detection capability. Multimed Tools Appl 80(2):2009–2030
48. Kamili A, Fatima I, Hassan M, Parah SA, Vijaya Kumar V, Ambati LS (2020) Embedding information reversibly in medical images for e-health. J Intell Fuzzy Syst 39:8389–8398
49. Gull S, Parah SA, Muhammad K (2020) Reversible data hiding exploiting Huffman encoding with dual images for IoMT based healthcare. Comput Commun 163:134–149
50. Rashid M, Singh H, Goyal V, Parah SA, Wani AR (2021) Big data based hybrid machine learning model for improving performance of medical Internet of Things data in healthcare systems. In: Healthcare paradigms in the Internet of Things ecosystem. Academic, Cambridge, MA, pp 47–62
51. Hurrah NN, Parah SA, Sheikh JA (2020) Embedding in medical images: an efficient scheme for authentication and tamper localization. Multimed Tools Appl 79(29):21441–21470
52. Gull S, Loan NA et al (2020) An efficient watermarking technique for tamper detection and localization of medical images. J Ambient Intell Humaniz Comput 11(5):1799–1808

Part III
Use of AI-Enabled IoT in Healthcare

Chapter 8
Internet of Things and Artificial Intelligence in Biomedical Systems

S. V. K. R. Rajeswari and Vijayakumar Ponnusamy

Contents

1 Introduction

With the emergence of the twenty-first century, the world stepped into a new era. The modifications are much witnessed by generations from the millennium year 2001 in the era of technology. The method of communication has always been evolving. The technical and non-technical audience from the world has always appreciated the upliftment of possibilities that technology can bring in. This chapter binds the two thriving technologies internet of things and artificial intelligence, for making a decision in smart biomedical applications without or with negligible human interference.

The biomedical field has been progressing remarkably over the past few years. With the amalgamation of AI and IoT in biomedical empiric, health can be monitored remotely and the user and clinicians can access medical data for further diagnosis, which helps in near detection of diseases and selecting a treatment plan. AI with IoT will create powerful biomedical applications that would help maintain

S. V. K. R. Rajeswari · V. Ponnusamy (✉)
ECE Department, SRMIST, Kattankulathur, Tamilnadu, India

S. A. Parah et al. (eds.), *Artificial Intelligence for Innovative Healthcare Informatics*,
https://doi.org/10.1007/978-3-030-96569-3_8

transparency between the user and clinicians. The outcome can be easily predicted using AI techniques. Any error predicted can also be solved without interruption, thus in many cases, increasing life expectancy. In the following section, IoT, AI, and motivation behind both are discussed with a daily life application.

1.1 Internet of Things

Internet of Things (IoT) is the new communication paradigm that deploys things that can be wearable devices, machines, the human body with technologies, software, and network. The things are connected through the internet and share data where decisions are taken using artificial intelligence techniques in real-time and decisions are made based on real-time observations. IoT finds its application in consumer, organizational, vehicular communications, industrial, infrastructural, military digitalization, and product digitization fields. One of the most promising and potential-filled applications of IoT in healthcare. The Healthcare industry is the most expensive care service that cannot be avoided under any circumstances by a common person. The introduction of IoT in the healthcare industry has already touched milestones in creating wearable devices to monitor basic vitals, such as smartwatches that detect blood pressure in real-time and provide accurate observations. This has led to uplift the research in wearable devices, embedded systems using IoT in healthcare machines. Chronic diseases are increasing every day. The need to monitor vitals at home and other health conditions continuously has become essential.

Monitoring glucose before and after surgical procedures at home after being discharged from the hospital is very crucial. Hence IoT finds its potential in biomedical applications [1]. The IoT for medical things is known as the Internet of Medical Things.

1.1.1 Working of IoMT Architecture

Figure 8.1 depicts the architecture of IoMT. A biomedical application that works with IoT devices is known as IoMT. IoMT consists of various sensors, i.e., temperature, pulse rate, and motion sensor, which are responsible for sensing the physiological, psychological, and environmental parameters. The data collected through the sensors are sent to the IoMT gateway, where the data pre-processing takes place. The filtered data is sent to the cloud where the AI helps in making decisions and the assistance is then carried out towards an application in a smartphone, which may receive alerts depending on the biomedical application and to the healthcare provider for prediction of diseases. Much light will be thrown on AI in the next section.

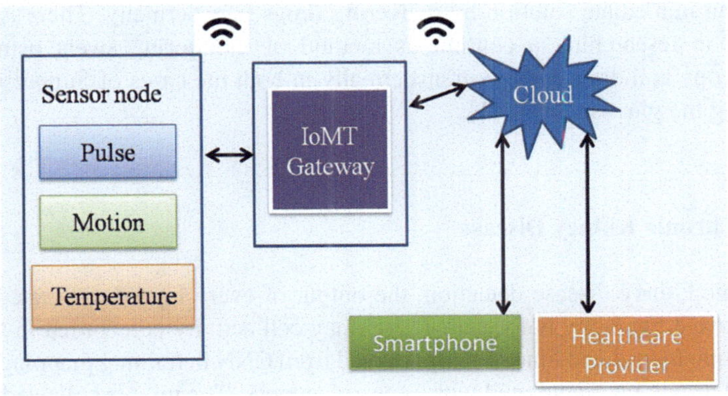

Fig. 8.1 Internet of Medical Things architecture

1.2 IoMT Application Frameworks

In this section, use cases in the current state of the art are discussed. These can be implemented either commercially or as working prototypes. IoMT applications are classified into the following broad categories:

1.2.1 Non-invasive Glucose Monitoring

A non-Invasive method of measuring Glucose in IoMT using sweat as a biomedical application is discussed. Further, pH, Temperature, and Humidity measurements are also considered. The drug is released transdermally when the glucose level goes up. The research considers a Nafion layer and sensors where the wearable patch consisting of a waterproof band and a non-porous material is placed. Humidity sensor, glucose sensor, pH sensor, temperature sensor is integrated for efficient sweat-based glucose sensing.

The detection accuracy is improved at the multipoint sensing for glucose and pH sensors. To make the system minimal, reference and counter electrodes are packed closely. The impedance changes of Poly (3,4-ethylene dioxythiophene) (PEDOT) and inter digitized electrodes were monitored by a humidity sensor to estimate the appropriate starting point of sweat analysis.

Glucose concentration range between 10 and 1 mM is calibrated by the Prussian blue-deposited porous gold electrode based on a glucose sensor using a galvanostatic method. On 8-to-12 week old diabetic mice, experiments were conducted by transdermal drug delivery using fabricated microneedles and integrated heaters (performing in vivo method). Blood glucose levels were suppressed more when metformin was delivered to the mice. It can be inferred that monitoring Glucose levels in sweat is possible with accurate results. Data aggregation can be done using a Deep Learning algorithm for minimum errors and accuracy. Microneedles can be used as an immediate solution by delivering drugs transdermally. There is a lot of potential in researching a continuous method of monitoring sweat using Light spectroscopy and drug delivery transdermally in both the cases of Suppressing and increasing the glucose levels [1].

1.2.2 Chronic Kidney Disease

In Chronic kidney disease detection, the output of every layer is extracted and its feature image hierarchy is formed. The kidney cell activity is recorded in CNN by representing hybridized functionality derived from CNN in training mapping of MRI signals. The patient is equipped with a sensor network. The images collected are sent for data pre-processing at the Local Processing Unit. Adaptive Hybridized Deep Convolution Network is applied at this stage. The Neural feed-forward network process signal without loops and cycles directly while considering the CECT image. Tumor cells are analyzed and algorithms are drawn. Doctors detect abnormalities by remotely tracking physical body state in IoMT. Two SVM classifiers derived from the CNN model are the local binary patterns with robust speed-up features and raw images wing deep features with generating probability scores. By establishing the right classification of the number of true positive TP, negative TN, false-positive FP, false-negative FN, probability analysis is observed. In the early treatment stages of certain diseases, the forecast results show the potential for integrating a classification model into the suggested system. In the IoMT cloud, the data is stored. The classification of renal cell subtypes has shown promising results by radiologists for deeper learning methods in the proposed approach. It can be inferred from [2], that Deep learning can be applied to image processing in Chronic disease detections. There is a lot of potential in this field of research [1].

1.3 Artificial Intelligence

Artificial Intelligence is the ability of computers to perform actions that require human intelligence.AI has gained popularity due to its critical advances in many fields. General applications of AI include speech recognition, visual perception, translations, and decision making [3].

Artificial Intelligence is the intelligent technology that enables machines to perform actions without or with negligible human interference. IBM's Watson to autonomous weapons, Google's search algorithms, SIRI, and self-driving cars are few examples of AI implemented technologies [3]. AI is implemented in areas where there are data and no theory. As discussed in the above paragraphs about IoT and its implementation in various fields, AI comes into the picture while performing actionable results for the data collected by IoT devices.AI algorithms produce possible solutions, decisions and predictions and create new propositions, business models, revenue streams, and models [4].

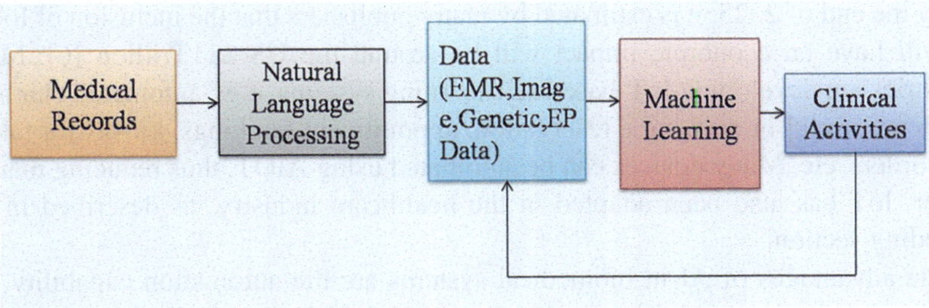

Fig. 8.2 Artificial Intelligence architecture for biomedical application

Healthcare is one of the most promising fields of AI. It has brought an enormous paradigm shift in the areas of availability of healthcare data and analytical techniques.AI finds its application both in structured and unstructured healthcare data. Cancer, Neurology, and Cardiology are the three aspects of healthcare that find solutions in AI machine learning methods. Support vector machine, neural network, and modern deep learning for structured data and natural language processing for unstructured data are the most used algorithms [3].

1.3.1 Working of AI Architecture

Figure 8.2 depicts the block diagram of Artificial Intelligence architecture in a biomedical application [5]. Human written medical records are converted into structured digital text by Natural Language Processing (NLP) for data enrichment and clinical decision making is taken place in Machine Learning data analysis. The decision making can be the process of screening a disease, diagnosis, or treatment, which can be drawn in any form of data. Artificial Intelligence has many algorithms that extract the features from this data and predict a disease that helps diagnose the disease and its treatment. Prediction of output and prognosis evaluation is the outcome of an efficient Artificial Intelligence algorithm [5]. The motivation behind stressing AI in a biomedical application is presented in the following section.

1.4 Motivation for the Use of Artificial Intelligence in Biomedical Systems

In the preceding section, IoT and how IoT can impact various fields, especially in the healthcare industry, have been discussed. In this section, blending Artificial Intelligence with BioMedical systems will be taken up.AI itself, being a very powerful technology when amalgamated with IoT will result as Artificial Intelligence of Things (AIoT) in much efficient and smarter devices, thus making human life easier.

By the end of 2025, it is estimated by many publishers that the inclusion of IoT in AI will have an economic impact will be around the US $11Trillion [6]. Many industries are developing IoT-based self-learning systems, e.g., automated chatbots, which are useful in booking a reservation, appointment bookings, kiosks for taking food orders, etc. Many devices can be automated using AIOT, thus reducing manual power. IoT has also been adapted in the healthcare industry, as described in the preceding section.

The advantages of AI in biomedical systems are the automation capability and decision-making process. The implementation of AI in the medical system saves time while providing healthcare. Lack of medical expertise to a large community of people is an issue where automation helps in managing healthcare. Villages lack proper healthcare service where the on-time diagnosis is not possible. As a point of care service (POC), amalgamating AI with automation helps in providing timely care and diagnosis. Often, the accuracy of treatment is based on doctors' perspectives, which may change if they are under stress. When implementing AI in biomedical systems, human errors are not possible, which is an added advantage. Another advantage of implementing AI in the biomedical system is encouraging the treatment. Many treatments currently are based on trial-and-error methods. Thus, if these methods are replaced by a well-trained intelligent AI system with knowledge on the effective medical process, the AI system can learn the effect of medical procedures. Thus, this experience of already handling the diagnosis can be modeled and can be used for large communities. Nowadays, smart application-based surgery using robots has emerged. The robotic surgery equipment is capable of performing surgery with more accuracy when compared to humans. "Prevention is better than cure"-AI justifies this statement and it can be concluded that it does more than the statement because AI can accurately predict, diagnose and also treat diseases in real-time.

Continuing with the same example of the CPAP machine, the data collected can be utilized to gain insights and make necessary decisions. IoT powered by AI may optimize operations by reducing the use of energy consumption. There are many AI techniques depending on the requirement, which help in processing complex amounts of data and make multitasking more efficient. Data communication can be much transparent with remote monitoring as well. Decision-making after implementing network learning algorithms in AI help in reducing human error from 0 to no error [7].

1.5 Internet of Things and Artificial Intelligence Application in Daily Life

Traditional health care processes in the past included the filing of medical reports and following up with doctors. Apart from reducing accuracy, the prediction of disease was not possible.AI and IoT together in Biomedical applications address this issue. IoT devices work with sensors and collect data from the sensing environments that can be things, animals, the human body. The data generated by IoT devices are further processed in AI using machine learning techniques. This amalgamation of two technologies helps in addressing the assistance issues. The assistance can be decision making, examining the healthcare sectors, patient assistance, and patient care, continuous health monitoring, etc.

There are many biomedical applications where patient assistance is essential. Patient assisting biomedical application will be discussed. CPAP (Continuous Positive Airway Pressure) is a biomedical application that provides pressure therapy for Sleep Apnea [8]. Sleep Apnea is a condition where a person suffers from abnormal snoring. The machine has a breathing tube that allows continuous airflow while sleeping, thus reducing snoring. The status of the patient is analyzed by the machine that works on IoT. By collecting and analyzing the sleep patterns' real-time data, the doctor prescribes changes and adjustments if needed. A large amount of data is collected with respect to sleep patterns. AI and Machine Learning come into the picture here.

The AI can deep dive into the accurate diagnosis by characterizing disease sub types. AI also helps in the prognosis of disease and treatment prediction. Different algorithms can be applied to receive accuracy and better performance. Support Vector Machine (SVM), Logistic Regression (LR), K-Nearest Neighbor (K-NN), Linear Discriminant Analysis, Gaussian Processes, Artificial Neural Network (ANN) are a few algorithms that can be applied.

The block diagram of the LSTM model for diagnosing sleep apnea is presented in Fig. 8.3. The noise-filtered version of respiratory signals is considered rather than extracting features. First, the respiratory data is collected through PSG signals as an input. To obtain the respiratory information, pre-processing of breathing signals is done. Epoch is created for each signal using American Academy of Sleep Medicine (AASM) annotations. Using AASM, the incoming signal is annotated with respect to Obstructive Sleep Apnea (OSA), Central Sleep Apnea (CSA), and Hyopnea (obstructive or central). These epochs are then sent to bootstrap. Bootstrapping helps in making estimations by transforming unbalanced datasets into multiple

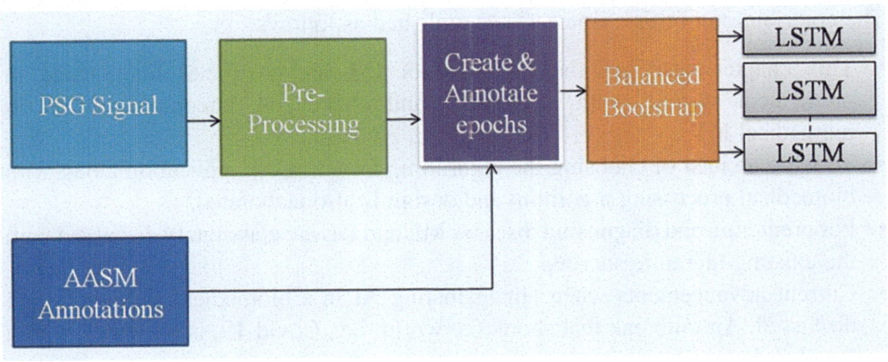

Fig. 8.3 Sleep Apnea model for LSTM algorithm

balanced datasets. Here epochs are separated into datasets. A balanced bootstrapping scheme is applied for a long stream of respiratory signals and to attain robustness and accuracy. These epochs are then trained into LSTM models. Each LSTM carries out the probability of having apnea events depending on the sigmoid activation function. All the LSTM outputs are averaged to a single epoch model. Readings at each sec are classified depending upon the condition of normal apnea, mild apnea, moderate apnea, severe apnea using AHI (Apnea-Hypopnea Index) where normal breathing: AHI ≤ 5, mild sleep apnea: $5 \leq$ AHI ≤ 15, moderate sleep apnea:$15 \leq$ AHI ≤ 30, severe sleep apnea: AHI ≥ 30 [8].

This method has the advantage of detecting OSA, CSA, and Hypopnea. Using sleep apnea metrics and specialized metrics for imbalanced data, the analysis is performed. Two thousand patients were considered using five sets of data. LSTM has provided much accuracy and improvement compared to the current state-of-the-art. AI analyzes and optimizes the data and provides personalized care for the patient. Current studies are going on teeth grinding while sleeping, providing an advanced research possible in the field of biomedical application and AI [8].

CPAP is one of the best examples of a remote health monitoring system. The implementation of IoT in healthcare has a lot of potential in resolving many deadly health conditions like Sleep apnea and has a huge potential in serving humankind. Another method of attaining reliability, accuracy for OSA is presented [9]. As the OSA severity increases, sleep staging decreases. For automatic classification of sleep stages, raw EEG and EOG signals are considered. The deep learning method is used to classify the sleep stages and the variability in sleep stage readings has been reduced.

1.6 Contribution of the Chapter

The application of AI in the biomedical system is discussed on different platforms. For a successful AI to be implemented in various applications of IoT in biomedical systems, it is important to learn and investigate the new methods and applications. The contribution of this chapter is accomplished as follows:

- This chapter describes the overview of IoT and Artificial Intelligence in biomedical systems with advantages and challenges, integration of AI in biomedical IoT.
- To have an idea of choosing the algorithm, designing an application along with biomedical processing algorithm and design is also elaborated.
- For predicting and diagnosing diseases ML and DL are elaborately discussed with the existing literature survey.
- Current advancements when amalgamating AI in a biomedical application are discussed. An outbreak that shook the world, i.e., Covid-19, is presented with a detailed discussion.

- Open research challenges are also thrown light on which hold the potential in the field of research.

This chapter is organized into six sections. The introduction of IoT and AI are discussed together in Sect. 1. Section 2 describes Artificial Intelligence in Biomedical Systems. Section 3 focuses on Integrating AI and IoT in biomedical systems (AIoT). Biomedical advances are explored in Sect. 4. The chapter is concluded with Sect. 5.

2 Artificial Intelligence in Biomedical Systems

2.1 IoT and Artificial Intelligence Architecture

With the emerging technological advances and the endless possibilities, combining IoT with AI has created enormous progress, especially in biomedical applications. An enormous amount of data sensed through IoT and its communication by implementing AI will be discussed in detail.

2.1.1 Working of an Artificial Intelligence Architecture

The block diagram of IoT and Artificial Intelligence Architecture is pictured in Fig. 8.4. The architecture is inspired by the wireless communication network [10]. The structure of AI consists of four bodies. The first body is data generators, i.e., user layer AI. It consists of IoT (Internet of Things) devices. IoT devices are a network of devices interconnected through the internet. Computer devices, actuators, sensors, and software embedded in a device altogether form an IoT device. It is responsible for generating data by using sensors directly or in wearable devices to sense the human body's physiological or ecological parameters. Inputs of data are recorded in this layer, e.g., smartwatches, security cameras, smart home/industrial devices, etc.

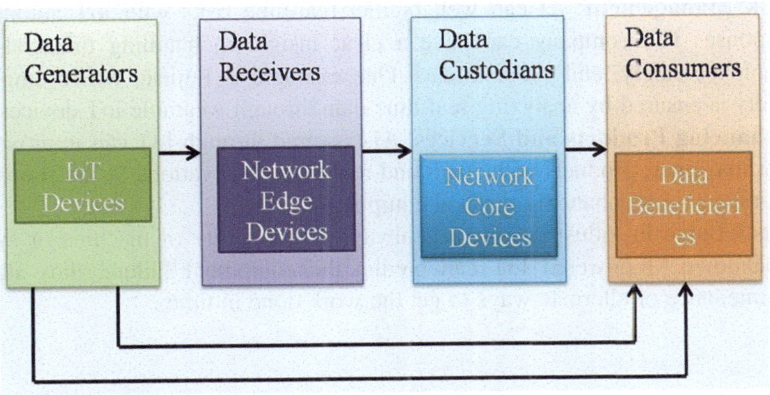

Fig. 8.4 IoT and Artificial Intelligence architecture block diagram

Data receivers are the second body where data from the generators are received wirelessly. This is where network device AI comes into the picture. The network edge devices can be 4G/5G networks, Wi-Fi, Lora, etc. The third body of AI architecture is the data custodians, where data is stored and organized. The data is received wirelessly through cloud services like Google Cloud, Microsoft Azure, etc. In this body, the data is privately and securely transmitted to the data consumers. Data Consumers are the beneficiaries of the whole process. They can be individuals for remote monitoring, government services, analysts, or industries depending upon the application. There are few applications where data receivers can be skipped entirely, for e.g., counting people application, human activity detection or monitoring, etc. Data receivers are able to see the physical world. This wireless framework works using a radio frequency spectrum. In a few applications like data surveying, report generation, cross-organizational data sharing, both data generators and data receivers can be skipped. The framework works from the physical world directly to data custodians, for e.g., authorized medical record sharing, tax return lodging, population census, etc. Edge computing is also one of the modules where AI is present in the edge devices at the data receivers performing edge computing tasks. The need to push AI near the network devices close to the data generators and receivers is because there are security challenges at the data custodians. To overcome the challenge of data theft, security issues, reducing latency, saving power and cost with increasing reliability by less communication, edge computing is performed at the Data Receiver body itself.

2.1.2 Advantages of AI-Enabled IoT Techniques

There are many advantages of amending AI with IoT. Proactive intervention, automating a system with respect to the requirement, AI helps automate IoT with decision making without human intervention [11–13].

1. **Optimal Efficiency**: AI, when amended with IoT, increases optimal efficiency. AI has the ability to predict the current status of an operating system and suggest any modifications required for a perfect outcome. One of the examples is Google, where AI in IoT reduces the cooling cost of the data center.
2. **Risk Management**: AI can well predict real-time risks with IoT automation response. The company can have a clear insight in handling financial loss, employee safety, and cyber threats. One example is Fujitsu, where employee safety is ensured by analyzing real-time data through wearable IoT devices.
3. **Enhancing Products and Services**: AI-powered through IoT can improve current machines, products with smart and real-time observations. A lot of research is going on for enhancing medical equipment.
4. **Predictions**: In industries, there is always a probability of machine or system breakdown.AI powered IoT can predict the equipment failure, thus alerting maintenance or alternate ways to get the work done in time.

5. **Privacy and Security**: AI with IoT provides extra security and privacy thus avoiding any cyber thefts, threats and enabling workplace security.
6. **Lightweight models**: There are many learning models in AI, such as *Machine* learning (ML), enabling a lightweight model for IoT enabling accurate detection and analytics with low complexity.
7. **Object Detection**: Without the need for physical measurements, I can locate objects or nodes of an IoT system. In a dynamic network, I can estimate the location of an object/node without mathematical formulation.

There are many advantages of integrating AI with IoT, which will be discussed elaborately in the next sections. Though this composition comes with many advantages, there are challenges that have a strong research potential to be taken off.

2.1.3 Challenges of AI-Enabled IoT Techniques

1. **Obtaining Feature**: AI can facilitate feature selection to obtain data from signals. Amplitude, phase, and frequency are the data from a signal when working with signal features. IoT has its advantages of large data streaming, heterogeneity of data, time and space correlation. ML implements big data in AI can help in human activity recognition, object detection, etc. Obtaining hidden information and knowledge from IoT becomes a challenge [11–13].
2. **Self explainability**: AI models are self-explainable without human intervention. The IoT system is comprised of many devices where communication in between the devices can become complex. Accuracy can be achieved if other AI models can collaborate with the existing system. AI being self-explanatory, doesn't allow other AI models to work with. This field has a large potential for research.
3. **Computational costs**: AI model has many techniques were few techniques like Explainable AI(XAI), when implemented for the self-explainability challenge, increases computational cost based on the operation of model-agnostic assumption. This remains an open area of research.
4. **Security Issues**: As IoT devices are exposed to the outer environment for sensing real-time parameters, they are vulnerable to security. There is a need for a solution regarding the security of data maliciousness.
5. **Energy Efficiency**: IoT devices are operated through batteries. In a few applications, tiny batteries are needed. To be able to connect to all the devices using a battery with less complexity is a challenge. The additional challenge includes the implementation of AI on IoT devices.

3 Amalgamation of IoT and AI as AIOTBS

AIoTBS (Artificial Internet of Things Biomedical System) finds its healthcare application for biomedical devices and systems. The IoT network consists of things that can be humans or devices. Healthcare IoT has many categories: IoT for patients,

IoT for physicians, IoT for hospitals, and IoT for healthcare insurance companies. Biomedical applications integrated with IoT enable remote monitoring of health, thus reducing hospital visits. While monitoring health remotely, health status can be accessed by the patient and also a doctor with absolute transparency, which helps in future diagnosis. There is a possibility of detection of diseases at an early stage. IoT in biomedical devices helps in decision-making by reducing error, system waste, and costs.

For designing biomedical hardware, processors considered are low power consumption and low complexity, and low cost of design. When combining AI in IoT devices, computational complexity with AI is not available in IoT nodes. There is a special design of processors that could be low cost, low power consumption for IoT applications, and it should support computational complexity requirements for implementing AI algorithms. Microcontroller, FPGA, and ASIC are the hardware platforms for developing biomedical systems.

SVM and KNN algorithm can be implemented for low complex/ low latency implementation when compared to other AI algorithms. FPGA provides better performance for higher complexity algorithms, e.g., Neural network computation algorithm. ASIC provides higher computational speed and ultra-lower power consumption which FPGA cannot provide. Hence depending on the requirement and needs of the system, AI-based algorithms are implemented. Though algorithms are different, they have noise filtering pre-processing module and segmentation, extraction of features, dimensionality reduction, and a module for classification and diagnosis.

To design AI-based biomedical processors for a wearable device, optimizing power and area consumption becomes a requirement without compromising accuracy. Power consumption reduction, classifying weak-strong hybrid structure, computing architecture for sparse matrix, serial processing architecture help architecture-level techniques. Near-threshold circuit design, switchable clocking circuit, analog computing device are circuit-level designs that is the third architecture.

3.1 Integrating AIoT in Biomedical Systems

In the preceding section, the importance of AI and IoT in the biomedical system is discussed. The biomedical algorithm based on AI and processor design with application and solution will be discussed in this section. Two approaches need to be achieved when integrating AI and IoT in Biomedical systems (a) AI-based biomedical processing algorithm design and (b) AI-based biomedical processor design.

3.1.1 AI-Based Biomedical Processing Algorithm

Among many algorithms present in an AI, choosing a perfect algorithm is based on many factors and also requirements. According to studies and extensive research, it is found that when two or more algorithms are combined, the performance of the system increases with accuracy. AI is classified into supervised and unsupervised learning. Mostly used methods of unsupervised learning include fuzzy clustering, k-proximity algorithm: linear decision analysis, SVM, Neural networks, Gaussian Bayesian networks.

1. **SVM**—Under supervised learning algorithm, Support Vector Machine is the machine learning algorithm. It has been observed that SVM categorizes data. Looking at the example of sleep apnea, using the ECG recordings, SVM identifies OSAS (obstructive sleep apnea syndrome) types from nighttime recordings. To train the SVM and to achieve the OSAS recognition with an accuracy of 92%, feature selection, classification, ROC (Receiver Operation Curve) analysis, and SVM classifiers are implemented. In another study of detecting ventricular fibrillation (VF) and rapid ventricular tachycardia (VT), it was observed that combining two or more techniques results in better performance in SVM. Hence, Least Square-SVM, Feedforward NN are combined to classify ECH beats and achieve high performance. When the same target was compared with single techniques, the accuracy is proved to be more in combined techniques, i.e., in LS-SVM and NN. In a study of detecting EEG, when SVM was combined with KNN and MLP (multi-layer perceptron), the accuracy reached 95–99%. In another study of epilepsy detection, LS-SVM (least square support vector machine) is shown to be 97.17% [7].
2. **ANN**—Artificial Neural Network (ANN) is another popular approach to supervised learning algorithm design. There are different applications of ANN that include CNN (Convolution neural network), PNN (Probabilistic neural network), RNN (Recurrent neural network), and BPNN (Backpropagation neural network). CNN is widely used in learning and recognizing human images. While considering ECG monitoring, individual CNN was trained. It was observed that it had greater performance in detecting ventricular ectopic beats and supraventricular ectopic beats. CNN is used as layers forming a structure. Eleven layered deep CNN structure is implemented to detect five main classes of non-life-threatening arrhythmias' classifiers are generally used in ECG applications. In another application, the PNN model is implemented to distinguish normal sinus rhythm and seven types of arrhythmias. For feature reduction, Fuzzy C-Mean (FCM) is used, which proved to show good classification accuracy. Hence, when PNN combined other algorithms, i.e., Principal component analysis (PCA), Linear discriminant analysis (LDA) proved to be the best solution. For processing time series in an ECG, RNN is found to be good. While the traditional RNN can have a long-term dependency, it was observed that subsequent RNN variants and LSTM (Long short-term memory) could be used together and solve the problem, thus becoming the best choice for ECG signal processing. In another study, BPNN was used in

ECG applications to automate ECG arrhythmia classification. To extract feature sets, DTCWT (dual-tree complex wavelet transform) was used [7].

3. **Fuzzy Clustering**: Fuzzy clustering is an unsupervised learning method. Fuzzy clustering is widely used in monitoring emotion recognition. In various studies, it was observed that fuzzy clustering itself could result in 97–99% recognition accuracy for four emotions (happy, disgust, surprise, fear) and 98% accuracy for blood pressure and hypertension risk diagnosis [7].
4. **DNN**—Deep Neural Network can be supervised or unsupervised. It can be run on mobile phones for image classification and human activity recognition applications. It finds its extensive application in the nonlinear relationship between artificial eigenvectors between the oscilloscope and reference blood pressure. Deep Belief Network (DBN)-DNN produces low error standard deviation, average error, average absolute error, and supine blood pressure [7].
5. **AI**-*based Biomedical Applications*—There are several AI applications that have been proved to be successful in the area of healthcare and the biomedical field. A lot of research is being carried out in the biomedical field. Covid-19 had a huge effect on the world and this pandemic also opened many areas of observations and research. In a recent study, the contribution of AI in scrutinizing CT scans was carried out. The radiologists can only see the affected part of the lung by looking at the CT scans. It was proposed that quantitative and objective minute details of the CT image may provide much more information. Deep learning was adopted and was proved to spot the abnormalities in the images. The abnormalities include the percentage of the lunch affected, Ground Glass Opacity (GPO), and other types of lung issues. These parameters altogether give the presence and severity of COVID-19. Currently, this work is waiting for Food and Drug Administration (FDA)approval. There is much-proven research and works that when combining different networks, the highest accuracy and best performance can be achieved. AI when applied in the healthcare and biomedical field, would change the way that humankind is receiving care from the hospitals by also enabling remote health monitoring [7].

3.1.2 AI-Based Biomedical Processor Design

When designing a processor, there are a few factors to consider. The factors vary for each application. In the seizure detection process, latency and power consumption are the two factors to consider while designing a processor. A two-stage processing engine is constructed for extracting the feature of an ECG signal. While designing a processor, a dynamic standby controller is used to minimize the consumption of power leakage [7].

However, these factors do depend a lot on the type of AI algorithm to work with and the processor, by continuing with a study of ECG monitoring, different work models and their outcomes will be discussed [7].

Primarily, AI processors work with sensors. Large power consumption and delay in data transmission are the two drawbacks of sensors. In a study of ECG detection and monitoring, smart ECG sensors are developed for diagnosis and avoiding any transmission of raw data. To make the sensor smart, integration of an ECG classification processor is required. The classification processor handles and works with AI-based algorithms, thus resulting in higher accuracy and performance. It has computational complexity and memory requirement. Hardware overhead and power consumption are important factors to be considered while implementing a classification processor [7].

Let us consider a study of a mobile health application for ECG monitoring [7]. A low-power machine learning is proposed. To extract the features of an ECG signal, 2-stage processing is designed. For heartbeat segmentation, DWT is implemented with QRS/P/T, and to analyze the characteristic of the heartbeat, MAR(Multivariate Auto-Regressive) estimator is used. The next segment for computation hardware reuse is designed for switching between SVM and maximum likelihood classification (MLC). Switching helps in working with different applications. The near-threshold circuit design is adopted where a standard cell library is characterized that filters cells with failure and reduces power consumption. Crystal less clock generator (kHz) is used for data sampling and critical path replica is used for MHz range. To minimize the leakage current in sleep mode and enable faster wake up, a dynamic standby controller is used. Finally, with SVM, 95.8% accuracy is achieved. In another study with the same application of ECG, by implementing SVM and WLC, 98.2% accuracy is reached [14]. Similarly, in addition to ECG, other studies with EEG and speech recognition are also verified. For Epilepsy seizure detection in the FPGA platform, 100% accuracy is met using a neural network [13]. Implementing the same application with KNN, LR, NB, and SVM in the ASIC platform gives an accuracy of 91%. EMG-based gesture recognition gives an accuracy of 98% with SVM [7].

3.1.3 Machine Learning in IoMT

A large number of health monitoring devices, wearable, assistive devices for health care are largely powered with AI. AI is intelligence that powers up a system and can function in any system. ML is the subset of AI that deals with computational statistics and makes predictions using computers. ML is a study of mathematical optimization delivering methods, theory, and application domains to the field of ML. Depending on the nature of the "signal" and "feedback", ML is divided into three categories are Supervised, Unsupervised, Reinforcement Learning [15] (Fig. 8.5 and Table 8.1).

Among the three categories of Machine Learning, Supervised Learning methods can recognize action-based discrimination between the environmental response and body movements. In the intelligent feature of DL (supervised learning), time efficiency and time sensitivity algorithms can be improved. As DL can handle a colossal amount of information when data is extracted, supervised learning helps in improving big data analytics. One of the most important advantages of DL is that it mimics the instruction of the human brain. It consists of multiple layers with higher

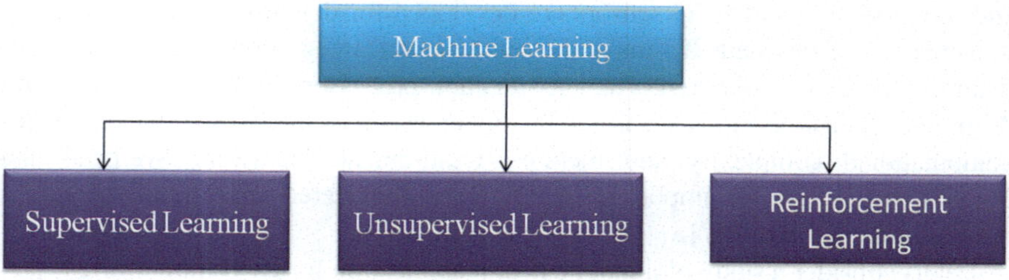

Fig. 8.5 Taxonomy of Machine Learning

Table 8.1 Difference between Supervised, Unsupervised, Reinforcement Learning

S. No	Supervised Learning	Unsupervised Learning	Reinforcement Learning
1.	Dependent and Independent are available.	No Dependent and Independent variables are available.	No need of Dependent or Independent variables.
2.	The machine learns by labeled data.	The machine is learned by unlabeled data.	By leading errors or rewards, an agent interacts with its environment.
3.	Maps the labeled inputs to the known outputs.	Understands pattern and discusses the output.	Follows the trial-and-error method.

efficiency. The standard algorithms of DL are CNN, DBN, RNN, LSTM. When RL and DL are combined together, Deep O-Network (DQN) is formed, which is much yielding and high-performance algorithm [15].

Applications of IoMT

ML finds its applications in MIoT in the following:

- Diseases and Diagnosis identification.
- Manufacturing of drugs and drug discovery.
  - Diagnosing medical images.
  - Personalized Medicine.
  - Behavioral modification using ML.
  - Saving and recording health parameters/information.
  - Research on clinical trials.
  - Data collection by crowdsourcing.
  - In Radiotherapy.
  - Predicting outbreak.Specific use cases in ML applications provide solutions for healthcare challenges like remote monitoring of health before and after surgeries, ICU care etc. It is also helpful for daily monitoring of physiological

parameters. Daily health monitoring help in real-time health monitoring. Implementing ML architecture in healthcare would help detect risk scores, precise resource allocation, and make better decisions like alerts, etc.

Case Study of Deep Learning ML in IoMT

Machine Learning algorithm is used for predicting chronic disease [16]. By extracting structured and data that is unstructured from the hospital, the author has proposed a CNN-based multimodal disease risk prediction model. Cerebral Infraction is considered for risk prediction as it is a fatal disease. Structured data is the easily searchable quantitative predefined format. Unstructured data is stored in a native format which is qualitative data. CNN-based multimodal disease risk prediction algorithm is discussed using structured and unstructured data from the hospital [16]. EHR, medical image, gene data are obtained from the hospital by taking 3-year data from 2013 to 2015 securely. Patients' age, gender, life habits come under structured data, whereas patients' narration comes under unstructured data. Patients, sex ratio, major diseases are taken into consideration. It was observed that patients who were hospitalized due to chronic disease, i.e., cerebral infarction, hypertension, diabetes, were observed among 5.63% with chronic diseases of cerebral infarction, hypertension, and diabetes were observed among 5.63% of the whole population that was admitted. CNN-MDRP and CNN-UDRP are the disease risk prediction algorithms derived for replacing missing data, i.e., data imputation. Due to human error, a large number of missing data is possible, which has to be found as the first step of data imputation. Data is modified or deleted to improve the data quality when uncertain or incomplete, medical data is identified. The second step, i.e., data pre-processing, takes place here to explain the observable variables, latent factor model is presented. An equation is derived as *R*(*m*×*n*) *Pm*×*kQTnk;m=total no.of patients=patient feature attributes=assumed latent factors*. First, this parameter is transformed into an optimization problem. The stochastic gradient descent method is used to solve this parameter and missing values are found.

For processing the medical data which is in text, the prediction algorithm used is based on CNN unimodal for disease risk prediction. *Rd*—dimensional vector, where $d = 50$. Maximum pooling is to be calculated as the text role is not equal. Max pooling operating is done by taking o/p of the convolution layer and giving it as an input to the pooling layer. Through the different lengths of training set samples, text data is then converted into a fixed-length vector. After convolution and pooling, 100 features of the text are obtained. CNN network is fully connected after the pooling layer is connected to the neural network.

Softmax classifier is connected to the following CNN layer. CNN-MDRP algorithm based on CNN-UDRP is designed for both structured and unstructured data. One hundred features are extracted for the text data set. Seventy-nine features are extracted using S-data and hundred features are extracted using T data. Word segmentation tool is used for training the word vector whose dimension is 50. Specific training parameters, W1; W3-b1; b3n are obtained by stochastic gradient method in CNN-MDRP algorithm.

Thus, risk assessment if the patient suffers from cerebral infarction or not is defined. In CNN, UDRP and MDRP are the two algorithms where the run time, the sliding window, text feature, and iterations are a few aspects that can be compared. It is observed that the run time of 178.2 s in a data center and a personal computer is 1637.2 s, i.e., 9.18 times more in the data center than on the personal computer. The T-data (CNN-UDRP) and S&T data (CNN-MDRP) are the same. It is also observed that the accuracy and recall of T-data are 0.95 and 0.98, whereas S&T data are 0.95 and 1.00.

As the number of iterations increases, the training error rate of the T-data is decreased, thus increasing the accuracy. S&T data also shows a similar trend in terms of error rate and test accuracy. The training data of the S&T data algorithm is shorter that implies that the convergence speed of CNN-MDRP is faster.

This chapter also discusses unstructured data by CNN. Text feature effect with accuracy, recall of T-data, and S&T data is discussed. For S-data, traditional ML algorithm, NB, KNN, DT algorithms are used to predict the risk of cerebral infarction disease.

To estimate discrete feature attributes, the formula of conditional probability is used. Gaussian distribution is implemented to estimate continuous feature attributes. Training data set is given to KNN classification and k instance closest to KNN is found. Selection of k value, distance measurement is required. To measure the distance, Euclidean distance is used. It is also found that the accuracy of the three ML algorithms is 50%. S data has the best NB classification. It is inferred from the results that due to the simple, lightweight features; it is hard to predict whether a patient is at higher risk with cerebral infarction. The accuracy for the data that is structured and the T-data is 0.9420, where recall is 0.9898 in the T-data whereas 0.9480 and recall of 0.99923 for CNN-MDRP (S&T data). There is a small difference in the accuracy of T-data, i.e., CNN-URDP and S&T data, i.e., CNN-MDRP algorithm. With the faster convergence speed, CNN-MDRP (S&T data) recall is high. It can be concluded that MDRP (S&T data) is better than UDRP (T-data) in CNN. The accuracy can be reached to 94.80% in S&T data. On the diversity feature of hospital data, accuracy depends on disease risk prediction. The highest accuracy can be achieved by a better feature description of the disease. The higher the accuracy and faster convergence speed than CNN-UDRP disease risk prediction algorithm [16].

Summary of ML Applied in IoMT

See Table 8.2.

Table 8.2 Summary of ML in the field applied in IoMT

Reference	Proposed work and use case	Outcome
M. Panwar et al. [17]	The author proposed a single channel PPG data with LRCN based PP-Net DL framework to monitor HR and BP continuously.	It was observed that for a total population of 1557, accurate measurements of Average NMAE i.e., 0.09(DBP) and 0.04(SBP) mmHg for BP, and 0.046 bpm for HR estimation was achieved.
Z. Zhou et al. [18]	The author proposed a HAR based on IBCN network. EDL design is also considered for addressing security issues.	It was observed that the system consisted of Wearable sensors that were successful in sensing various sources of uncertainty and provided information about the variety of behaviors by detecting any suspicious activities using DL technology.
W. N. Ismail et al. [19]	The author used the Pearson correlation coefficient for the regular target detection and recognition model by overcoming the limitations of a CNN-model. Readings of high blood pressure, obesity, diabetes are derived.	It was observed that when three different techniques LSTM, SVM, TNN, were compared, the proposed model CNN had better accuracy and low computational load.
X. Qian et al. [20]	The author proposed the architecture of DHNN for fall detection. The work is based on a smartwatch, smart insole and smartphone.	It was observed that while preserving privacy, the DHNN had better accuracy, specificity, precision and sensitivity.
T. Zhang et al. [21]	The author proposed a framework for cardiac image processing for elderly patients using DL-IoMT. In a DL architecture, an Effective-Aware-Approach is proposed to reduce energy consumption and enhance battery lifetime and reliability.	It was observed in elderly healthcare, the proposed scheme (EEA) has performed better by enhancing energy efficiency, reliability, sustainability during data transmission.
G. Ascioglu et al. [22]	The performance of each neural network (CNN, LSTM, ConvLSTM) for each category type is compared and examined based on HAR (Acceleration and Gyroscope).	ConvLSTM outperforms CNN and LSTM concerning Human Activity Recognition.
V. Bianchi et al. [23]	The author presented a HAR system with wearable devices integrating deep learning techniques.	97% of Global accuracy is reached using CNN-based architecture.
M. Amin-Naji et al. [14]	Deep Learning automated method for Alzheimer's disease diagnosis is proposed implementing SCNN.	98.72% is the accuracy achieved.
M. Rashid et al. [24]	ResNet architecture (CNN Network) is used to detect Parkinson's disease sustained phonation and a dedicated originally to image classification.	The proposed technique has an accuracy of 90%.
W. Chang et al. [25]	An intelligent medicine recognition system is proposed based on ST-Med-Box Deep Learning Technique.	The overall accuracy of 96.6% is achieved.

3.2 Challenges in Integrating AI and IoT in Biomedical Systems

As discussed, there are many AI techniques to attain great accuracy and high performance. Before developing any biomedical system, it is important to consider the challenges that are already existing. The challenges that are needed to be addressed are:

1. **High performance**: In this chapter, we have discussed ECG and EEG applications. In future biomedical applications that would work on different signal features and processing approaches, e.g., in diabetic foot monitoring and endoscopy where the electrical signal is changed into sound, image, or pressure distribution, the system would demand a higher computation is required [4].
2. **Interoperability**: Systems should be able to communicate effectively without losing any data. Interoperability is limited in AI. It is important to consider which algorithm can be trusted in an application [4].
3. **Scalability**: With high-performance requirements, larger storage and high-power consumption are also other challenges. These factors depend on the selection of classifiers and thus are needed to be addressed [7].
4. **Computational Complexity**: When combining two or more algorithms, better accuracy is achieved but increases the computational complexity. This increases power consumption and processing time [7].
5. **Security**: Security issues such as tampering with the original data and modifying is the nightmare of any technology. When integrating IoT and AI, the security of data must be taken into account [4].
6. **Privacy**: The ease of access to AIoT system datasets and computational power (GPU's) has been considered as a serious threat for growing AIoT technology [4]. Hence privacy is an important concern when integrating AI and IoT.

3.3 Solutions that May Advance Biomedical-AIoT in Healthcare and Possible Areas of Research

1. **Solution for achieving High performance**: AI arrives as a solution in providing higher-performing algorithms. Machine learning is a nest under AI that has algorithms used to build based on the data available. There are methods of ML (Machine learning) classified depending on the availability of data. Each method has a specific variety of algorithms. To choose a specific algorithm, the size, characteristics, behavior, type of data should be considered. The speed and accuracy, which are proportional, depending on the objective of the problem. For, a time-sensitive, simple algorithm must be chosen and for accuracy, a complex algorithm will address it [4].

2. **Solution for Interoperability**: The diversity in IoT devices that include different devices, protocols, technologies, networks, middleware etc., makes the system heterogeneous. By assigning global reference standards, IoT can provide homogeneity to the devices, thus reducing interoperability [4].
3. **Solution for scalability**: When two technologies are combined, i.e., IoT and AI, where IoT becomes the center for sensing and collecting massive amounts of data through sensors, the AI is responsible for stimulating the data and making decisions. This makes the system hectic with all the data traffic. Edge computing comes into the picture as a solution. With edge computing, many computational tasks can be handled at the edge of the devices. Another advantage other than achieving scalability is reducing the latency and increasing response time [7].
4. **Solution for complexity**: Considering low power complexity algorithms and low power hardware architecture while designing an AI-based biomedical application will provide the solution for complexity [7]. Implementing Edge Computing in AI is a solution for reducing complexity [26].
5. **Solution for security**: solution such as defense techniques and attack detection in Deep Learning (ML) may help in handling security issues in AIoT [4].
6. **Solution for privacy**: Nature of data collected by AIoT device, data that the device should not collect, data used, access to the storage, and expiration of the data are to be considered for differential privacy mechanisms [4].

While the mentioned challenges are not limited to, but by taking into consideration these challenges and possible solutions, a new algorithm that can achieve higher accuracy with great response time has research potential in an AIoT biomedical application.

4 Current Advances in Biomedical Application

As the year 2020 hit, all chaos and uncertainties were happening in the world. It was declared by World Health Organization (WHO) on March 11th, 2020, COVID-19 a pandemic. The WHO director-general, Dr. Tedros Adhanom Ghebreyesus, is addressing the media, said that, "This is not just a public health crisis, it is a crisis that will touch every sector". There were already 111,800 cases of coronavirus illness among 110 countries, and it was predicted that the risk of spread would grow further [27].

During this pandemic situation, along with the people attacked by the virus, a lot of frontliners working in healthcare were also affected by a coronavirus. Healthcare front-liners were deprived of sleep, family visits and were constantly at risk for their lives. Let us appreciate the frontliners who have served and a few who lost their lives while serving humanity selflessly with dedication and bravery. Along with healthcare professionals, there were scientists who worked to help hospitals to find a smarter solution that would ease the way how COVID-19 was being handled.

4.1 An Advanced AI Biomedical Application that Is Currently Serving Hospitals in the COVID-19 Pandemic

In this section, one of the applications developed by Dirk Smeets, Ph.D., Preetham Sreenivas, AI scientist, and Maryellen L. Giger will be discussed. AI as it has always been used to make a qualitative interpretation; in radiology, qualitative analysis is broadly gauged. To monitor and diagnose void-19, a lot of research was conducted in parallel by reading and analyzing through X-rays and computer tomography (CT). Clinicians and radiologists recognized the abnormalities in the lung CT images in Wuhan, Hubei Province of China. All around the world started to notice the abnormalities in CT scans and X-rays. The images helped to understand how much of the lung was infected and to monitor the patients' health condition in treatment. Though this process surprised many health organizations, it was still doubtful [28].

4.1.1 AI for X-Ray Images

The abnormalities in COVID-19 affected lung is the presence of localization of lesions in the lower part of the lungs, Ground Glass Opacities (GGO), and consolidations (lungs filled with fluid). Other abnormalities noted are cavities, nodules, pleural effusions. Using these, the X-Ray model was created, which displayed the risk report at the right side of the report, enabling the radiologists to quickly analyze. The sensitivity and specificity are found out to be 91% and 78% with respect to identifying the disease and those without the disease (COVID-19). The risk assessment was provided by qXR (name of the X-Ray developed by the scientists) [28]. It was implemented in around 60 clinics to benefit the triage purpose of patients and the simultaneous monitoring of health. The minute detail of lung function, e.g., If there is a 5% decrease of lung involvement, it will show up. It has then become a traditional way to detect if a patient is improving by taking a chest scan. The monitored results were also shared in a mobile app, 'qScout' [28]. AI was implemented in the app for secured and private Electronic Medical Records (EMR) storage. The EMR includes patients' health status and tracking for personalized care by clinicians.

4.1.2 AI for CT Scans

For a detailed investigation of the CT images, AI was implemented to quantify the CT images. The already existing X-Ray AI (qXR) developed by Qure.ai helped find 20 abnormalities in lungs that also could predict Tuberculosis and other respiratory illness, came for rescue. Solution for detecting, monitoring, and diagnosing coronavirus started by training qXR with deep learning.

To monitor COVID-19, 'Icolung' was developed by Icometrix using AI algorithms. With collaborative efforts from all over the world, the COVID-19 detecting framework was developed, which received CE marking (European Conformity marking). AI helped in detecting the percentage of lungs affected and where to diagnose. Hence the quantification method of using AI is useful in mass requirement of diagnosis in rural areas and economically deprived/lagging countries. Isometrics has also received the U.S. Food and Drug Administration to quantify CT chest scans in lung pathology for COVID-19 patients.

4.2 Future Biomedical AIoT Applications

Some of the future applications of Biomedical AI are developing augmented reality glasses where it would be possible to detect a person's activity and location. Smartwatches and Fitness Bands are another application of biomedical AI. Existing smartwatches and fitness bands are responsible for displaying the heart rate, whereas further advances include detecting blood pressure, blood glucose parameters and providing accurate real-time readings. By overcoming the challenges in the preceding section, the development of an adaptive AI is the key to empowering advances in biomedical applications. Edge/fog computing is another approach that reduces latency and reduces computational complexity with limited resources. IoT devices benefit by implementing edge/fog computing resulting in a powerful application [29].

5 Future Directions

From the projection of growth stated as, "AI in the IoT market is expected to grow at a CAGR of 27.3% during the forecast period (2021–2026)", it is quite evident that AIoT together can bring tangible benefits in healthcare with accessibility and quality in humanity [30]. The amalgamation of AI and IoT resulting in AIoT has made the possibility from disease classification to disease diagnosis and prediction. Real-time health monitoring, Virtual consultations, RFID Wristbands for the elderly with smart wheelchairs, GPS positioning applications for patients with heart diseases open wide areas of research potential fields. New devices and medical equipment are manufactured with intelligent systems. The old medical devices, for example, MRI scanners, X-Ray machines, etc., have an open challenge of enhancing the machines smarter with AI. Hindrance of security in AIoT is another open challenge which is a field of research that has to be explored more. The integration of AI in biomedical systems with different devices while interconnecting has an open challenge of complexity and unification issues. Smart glass-based applications are emerging [31] which could be used effectively for biomedical systems.

6 Conclusion

Healthcare can benefit from the amalgamation of IoT and AI, i.e., AIoT. Reduction of human errors, continuous monitoring of vitals, emergency assisting systems, automatic detection of complicated patterns makes healthcare advanced. In this chapter, the motivation behind AIoT and its anatomy and the architecture, working model with advantages and challenges is presented. Advanced and enhanced biomedical application is possible with the integration of IoT and AI, which has been discussed with processor algorithm and design. An advanced biomedical application that is being served in hospitals is also detailed. Future directions with research potential fields have also been discussed.

References

1. Lee H et al (2017) Wearable/disposable sweat-based glucose monitoring device with multistage transdermal drug delivery module. Sci Adv 3(3):e1601314
2. Chen G et al (2020) Prediction of chronic kidney disease using adaptive hybridized deep convolutional neural network on the Internet of Medical Things platform. IEEE Access 8: 100497–100508
3. Sarosh P et al (2021) Secret sharing-based personal health records management for the Internet of Health Things. Sustain Cities Soc 74:103129
4. Cai Q et al (2019) A survey on multimodal data-driven smart healthcare systems: approaches and applications. IEEE Access 7:133583–133599
5. Rashid M, Hamid A, Parah SA (2019) Analysis of streaming data using big data and hybrid machine learning approach. In: Handbook of multimedia information security: techniques and applications. Springer, Cham, pp 629–643
6. Parah SA et al (2020) Efficient security and authentication for edge-based internet of medical things. IEEE Internet Things J 8:15652–15662
7. Wei Y et al (2020) A review of algorithm & hardware design for AI-based biomedical applications. IEEE Trans Biomed Circuits Syst 14(2):145–163
8. Steenkiste TV et al (2019) Automated sleep apnea detection in raw respiratory signals using long short-term memory neural networks. IEEE J Biomed Health Inform 23(6):2354–2364
9. Korkalainen H et al (2020) Accurate deep learning-based sleep staging in a clinical population with suspected obstructive sleep apnea. IEEE J Biomed Health Inform 24(7):2073–2081
10. Paranjape K et al (2020) Short keynote paper: Mainstreaming personalized healthcare–transforming healthcare through new era of artificial intelligence. IEEE J Biomed Health Inform 24(7):1860–1863
11. Gull S et al (2020) A self-embedding technique for tamper detection and localization of medical images for smart-health. Multimed Tools Appl 80(19):29939–29964
12. Chen Z et al (2018) An energy-efficient ECG processor with weak-strong hybrid classifier for arrhythmia detection. IEEE Trans Circuits Syst II Express Briefs 65(7):948–952
13. Mondal S, Agarwal K, Rashid M (2019) Deep learning approach for automatic classification of x-ray images using convolutional neural network. In: 2019 Fifth international conference on image information processing (ICIIP). IEEE, New York
14. Amin-Naji M et al (2019) Alzheimer's disease diagnosis from structural MRI using Siamese convolutional neural network. In: 2019 4th International conference on pattern recognition and image analysis (IPRIA), Tehran, Iran, pp 75–79. https://doi.org/10.1109/PRIA.2019.8786031

15. Qadri YA et al (2020) The future of healthcare Internet of Things: a survey of emerging technologies. IEEE Commun Surv Tutorials 22(2):1121–1167
16. Shah AA et al (2020) Efficient image encryption scheme based on generalized logistic map for real time image processing. J Real-Time Image Process 17(6):2139–2151
17. Panwar M et al (2020) PP-Net: a deep learning framework for PPG-based blood pressure and heart rate estimation. IEEE Sensors J 20(17):10000–10011
18. Zhou Z et al (2020) Human activity recognition based on improved Bayesian convolution network to analyze health care data using wearable IoT device. IEEE Access 8:86411–86418
19. Ismail WN et al (2020) CNN-based health model for regular health factors analysis in Internet-of-Medical Things environment. IEEE Access 8:52541–52549
20. Qian X et al (2020) Wearable computing with distributed deep learning hierarchy: a study of fall detection. IEEE Sensors J 20(16):9408–9416
21. Zhang T et al (2020) A joint deep learning and Internet of Medical Things driven framework for elderly patients. IEEE Access 8:75822–75832
22. Ascioglu G et al (2020) Design of a wearable wireless multi-sensor monitoring system and application for activity recognition using deep learning. IEEE Access 8:169183–169195
23. Bianchi V et al (2019) IoT wearable sensor and deep learning: an integrated approach for personalized human activity recognition in a smart home environment. IEEE Internet Things J 6(5):8553–8562
24. Rashid M, Singh H, Goyal V (2020) The use of machine learning and deep learning algorithms in functional magnetic resonance imaging—a systematic review. Expert Syst 37(6):e12644
25. Chang W et al (2019) A deep learning-based intelligent medicine recognition system for chronic patients. IEEE Access 7:44441–44458
26. Gong C et al (2020) Intelligent cooperative edge computing in Internet of Things. IEEE Internet Things J 7(10):9372–9382
27. WHO Director-General says be prepared as coronavirus declared a pandemic. Riverine Herald, 12 Mar 2020. www.riverineherald.com.au/news/2020/03/12/1079364/who-director-general-says-be-prepared. Accessed 21 Feb 2021
28. Mertz L (2020) AI-driven COVID-19 tools to interpret, quantify lung images. IEEE Pulse 11(4):2–7
29. Gong C, Lin F et al (2020) Intelligent cooperative edge computing in Internet of Things. IEEE Internet Things J 7(10):9372–9382
30. AI in IoT Market | Growth, trends and forecasts (2021–2026). www.mordorintelligence.com, www.mordorintelligence.com/industry-reports/ai-in-iot-market
31. Rashid M et al (2019) Novel big data approach for drug prediction in health care systems. In: 2019 International conference on automation, computational and technology management (ICACTM). IEEE, New York

Chapter 9
Role of IoT in Healthcare Sector for Monitoring Diabetic Patients

Kumar Gourav and Amanpreet Kaur

Contents

1 Introduction

Technology has become an indispensable part of our day-to-day life since the last few decades and someway we all are depending on it to obtain extreme benefit and comfort. We are living in an era of Information Technology i.e., the era of smart technologies where every person is associated with this technology either intentionally or unintentionally. According to the survey conducted by Cisco Internet Business Solutions Group (IBSG) in 2003, that there were more than 500 million devices connected to the Internet and approximately 6.3 billion people were living [1]. There was tremendous growth of smartphones and tablet PCs through which the number of devices connected to the Internet to 12.5 billion in 2010, while the world's human

K. Gourav (✉)
University Institute of Computing, Chandigarh University, Chandigarh, India

A. Kaur
Chitkara University Institute of Engineering & Technology, Chitkara University, Punjab, India

S. A. Parah et al. (eds.), *Artificial Intelligence for Innovative Healthcare Informatics*,
https://doi.org/10.1007/978-3-030-96569-3_9

population increased to 6.8 billion. It also predicts that there will be more than 50 billion devices connected to the Internet by 2020 [2]. To enhance our modern-day to day lifestyle, Wireless Sensor Network (WSN) technologies enable the Global Sensing Technology that offers the ability to measure, infer and understand the various environmental indicators from delicate ecologies and natural resources to urban environments. This changing scenario of these advents in technology enlightens the world in the form of the Internet of Things (IoT). Internet of things is a dignified domain that leads us to real-world scenarios where each object can perform some tasks while communicating with some other objects. The world with full of devices, sensors, and other objects that will communicate and make human life far better and easier than ever. The propagation of these devices in a collaborating and actuating network creates the Internet of Things whereas, sensors and actuators blend seamlessly with the environment around us and the information is shared across platforms to improve a common operating picture (COP).

Changing the way that we live today by making keen gadgets around us, performing day-by-day activities and tasks is the center of the motivation behind IoT. It is the platform where everyday devices become smarter, everyday processing becomes intelligent, and everyday communication becomes revealing. It has the potential to add a new dimension to this process by enabling communications with and among smart objects, thus leading to the vision of any time, anywhere, any media, anything communications [3]. Internet of Things is the new paradigm that provides a set of new services for the next wave of technological innovations. It is considered an immensely important global infrastructure that enables connectivity between both virtual and physical objects and can change the way people work, learn, and live. In other words, IoT is an interconnected ecosystem of uniquely addressable physical objects with varying degrees of sensing, processing, and actuation capabilities, sharing the ability to communicate and interoperate through the Internet as their common denominator. In IoT the sensor-equipped devices can provide fine-grained information about the physical world, allowing cloud-based resources to extract value from such information and possibly make decisions to be implemented by actuator-equipped devices. Thus it is the next big revolution of the world on digitalization of commercializing various modules that are associated with the internet, some involve controlling and some involve monitoring the parameters from anywhere which is the most trending technology in the present scenario that stands alongside wearables and robotics. The Internet of Things (IoT) makes smart objects that are known as ultimate building blocks in the development of cyber-physical smart pervasive frameworks. IoT is gaining momentum due to its potential and capacity that is to be integrated into any complex system. As a result of the rapid development of sensing technologies such as radio frequency identification sensors and the conversions of information technologies such as wireless communication and the internet, IoT is emerging as an important technology for monitoring systems. The rapid expansion of IoT and wireless technology leads to find new opportunities for growth in various fields such as education, transportation, agriculture, and most importantly in the healthcare sector. There is no doubt that IoT will change people's quality of life. The creation of integrated tools will bring about many positive changes to integrated information systems services, systems processing, and communications with a wide range of control. This Embedded technology has entered almost all aspects of our day-to-day life and the healthcare field is no exception for that. Researchers [4–6] have stated in their study that the healthcare and modern technology industries enlarged crucial intentions in present day's life. According to the researchers [7–11], the main objective in incorporating the technology with the healthcare systems is to felicitate the improved interface among patients and health service providers to enhance the efficacy and convenience of medical devices and services. According to Kumar [12], this new technology will act as a vital part in the monitoring of patients in hospitals and at their homes conveniently. The fully-equipped hospitals and diagnostic centers are gaining momentum, as most people are unaware of their health problems because health is an essential part of life. In this context, the wide diffusion of powerful embedded hardware together with the development of smart medical sensors and devices for ubiquitous healthcare has made the Internet of Medical Things (IoMT) drastically change the way healthcare is approached worldwide, so that the number of healthcare devices using IoT and wearable technologies is expected to reach 162 million by the end of 2020 [13]. Mistry [14] highlights in his study that monitoring patients globally offers various opportunities to improve the quality of healthcare as well as lessens the expenses in the field of healthcare by recognizing and preventing chronic diseases and is side effects. As we all know these days our healthcare is very expensive than ever mostly patients require hospitalization through their treatment. The usage of devices that can monitor patients remotely can somehow overwhelm these issues. By gathering patient health-related information through IoT devices and then moving that information to health service providers may decrease the healthcare expense and make it conceivable to deal with health problems earlier they become serious [15]. There is no disbelief that this technology will change the lifestyle of people globally but also establish the set of gears that will enhance system performance in terms of services, processing, and communication. Due to these different technologies based on the Internet of Things for the healthcare sector were developed [16].

Inappropriately, the progressively aging of the population and rapid increase in chronic illness is placing substantial worry on modern healthcare systems and the demand for resources from hospital beds to doctors and nurses is enormously high [17]. A solution is required to reduce the pressure on healthcare systems whilst continuing to provide high-quality care to critical patients. There is resourceful use of IoT technology in healthcare not only to bring the benefits to doctors and managers to access wide ranges of data sources but also allows to meet the challenges in accessing data, especially in a mobile environment of real-time IoT application systems. For the majority of the population who are living in remote places, healthcare is the predominant issue to this nation as they are not availing the benefits of the modern healthcare system. IoT technology plays an important monitoring tool at all levels in the larger interest of the global as a whole. The health monitoring system is beneficial to the patients as well as to the society where the implementation of such systems will save hospital bills, waiting time, and also reduce the long queues in the hospitals. Thus, this technology provides a solution to healthcare issues and connects the patients across the country and also doctors to monitor, track and record patients' vital data and medical information on a real-time basis so that timely and effective solutions to the patients on regular basis can be met. IoT allows heterogeneous devices and technologies to smoothly interact with each other in a common intellectual framework with connected networks and centralized data. The IoT revolution is redesigning modern health care with promising technological, economic, and social prospects. This technology has attracted much attention in recent years for its potential to alleviate the strain on healthcare systems. The power of IoT for health and medical services is harnessed by smart sensors (sensors and a microcontroller) that accurately measures, monitor, and analyze a variety of health status indicators. These include basic vital health signs such as pulse rate and blood pressure, oxygen and glucose level in the blood, and heart rate. Smart sensors can be incorporated into medicines and pill bottles that are connected to a network and can generate alerts about whether the patient has taken a scheduled dose of medication. With the help of IoT potential, doctors are now able to collect real-time raw data from numerous patients for a continual period through smart devices connected to an interconnected network, which ensure them not only with trustable and reliable results but also time-saving which will be of maximum benefits. Internet of Things is going to revolutionize healthcare by significantly lowering costs and improving quality. Health monitoring systems based on Internet-of-things have been recently introduced to improve the quality of health care services. The IoT technology helps to manage or monitor remote health services, personal fitness care at home, chronic diseases [18] like bone disease, disease related to breathing, cancer, diabetes [19] attention for old people like Heart-related issues [20].

Diabetes is a major health concern in today's lifestyle. According to the report given by WHO in 2016, the number of people with diabetes has exceeded 422 million in 2012 and as a result over 1.5 million people died because of diabetes. The WHO has classified diabetes as a top ten cause of death due to its dangerous effects on the well-being of a person and the society as a whole and unfortunately, there is still no permanent cure for diabetes till now [21]. Diabetes is one of the major health threats in many parts of countries, according to recent statistics from the ministry of health in Saudi Arabia, around one-third of the population is diabetic. These terrifying numbers are threatening the young nation where more than 70% of the population under 30 years of age group are suffering from diabetics. The number of diabetic patients in the United Kingdom has also jumped from one in ten to one-third according to The Economist. The main reasons are unhealthy eating habits and inadequate exercise. More than 30 million population till now have been suffering from diabetes in India. This growing prevalence of diabetes has earned India a tag of the world's diabetes capital [22]. According to the survey conducted by International Diabetics Federation in 2014, in India, there were 387 million individuals with diabetes, and this number is estimated to become 592 million by 2035 [23]. Worldwide, the total number of people with diabetes is projected to rise from 171 million in 2000 to 366 million in 2030 [24]. Diabetes mellitus has become a worldwide epidemic and also a long-term metabolic disorder in which the blood glucose (BG) level varies and is caused by either insufficient insulin production in the body Type 1 diabetes (T1D) or by the body's inability to utilize its produced insulin

Type 2 diabetes (T2D) [25]. The diagnosis of both T1D and T2D has increased, but the rise has been greater for T2D, which accounts for 90–95% of all cases of diabetes especially in developing countries.

Most diabetic patients can manage their disease by complying with self-management guidelines at home. Poor monitoring is the main issue in managing effective glycemic control. Enhanced results are related to better monitoring of medications, blood sugar self-monitoring, diet and lifestyle changes, and routine doctor checkups. Barriers include time constraints, knowledge deficits, denial, limited social support, inadequate resources, declining cognitive abilities, and low self-efficacy. To evaluate the effectiveness of diabetes health guidance by using devices like Glucometer, Continuous Glucose Monitoring System (CGMS), Ambulatory Blood Pressure Monitoring System (AMBP), Hypoglycemia Alarm, Activity Tracking Wearable Technologies (ATWT), Target Heart Rate Monitoring Devices (TMD) and Diet & Nutrition Apps have advanced sensors and actuators that are the type of intelligent devices. These devices can communicate with cloud-based applications, which use IoT Backend to help in managing diabetes management efficiently. IoT uses sensors to assist diabetes management by monitoring blood pressure, glucose level, calorie intake, and physical activity. To facilitate the process of patient diagnosis and personal monitoring Internet of Things (IoT) system is used. IoT in medical devices (IoMT) can help improve the health of patients who need special care and constant supervision from specialized doctors. IoMT refers to a collection of medical devices connected to the internet of things. Glucose checking is a fundamental piece of diabetes administration and the support of physiological blood glucose fixation is the main route for a diabetic to evade perilous diabetic confusions.

This study aims to explore how the Internet of Things assists and benefit the life of diabetes suffering patients by improving their quality of life. The main contribution of this chapter is in studying the role of IoT in healthcare for diabetic patients by reviewing the following aspects: Study of architecture for IoT-based healthcare applications, benefits, and challenges with its solutions for monitoring diabetic patients. The remainder of this chapter is organized as follows. Section 2 discusses the related work and literature review Sect. 3 explores a comparison of existing architectures used for IoT healthcare applications with proposed architecture based on edge computing. Section 4 depicts the benefits of IoT for diabetes patients. Section 5 highlights the challenges with its solutions related to IoT for diabetes patients. Section 6 depicts the latest security trends and its solutions to deal with healthcare data in IoT. At last Sect. 7 concludes the chapter.

2 Related Work

Internet of Things (IoT) has become the most developed and prominent technology in recent years that associates our working devices and day-to-day sensors with internet-based architecture which also links our virtual and physical objects that have proficiencies like data communication and data storage [26, 27]. This new technology has many innovative features that provide services in various fields and the healthcare sector is one of them [28]. It facilitates the patients by providing care, improving the diagnosis quality, enabling the various medical services, and centralizing the patient records in the form of repositories at very nominal cost by using devices that are embedded with sensors and other wearable devices [29]. There is rapid growth in the number of patients suffering from various chronic diseases in the present scenario. The IoT-based healthcare system is the improved way to deal with issues related to elderly patients suffering from these chronic diseases and also deal with the problem of health experts. Internet of Things is also beneficial in the situation of COVID-19 pandemic [30] because devices that are associated with IoT have the proficiency of monitoring the patient remotely that making the patient safe and healthy. These days according to the lifestyle of people, diabetes is one of the major chronic diseases widespread that have social as well as economic influence on the population. Various studies have been carried out in this recent field of the Internet of Things in the healthcare sector concerning diabetes. This section represents the various research views related to IoT specific to healthcare applications.

Internet of Things is the set of intelligently associated systems and gadgets that are used to collect information from implanted wearable sensors, actuators as well as physical items linked with it [31]. Many researchers highlighted in their study that the Internet of Things is an innovation and has completely transformed ourselves by contributing its benefits like progress the access to care, enhancing the value of care, and decreasing the expenses for care. The study highlighted by [18, 32] reveals that the IoT has been associated with several application fields like smart homes, smart cities, logistics, waste management, retails, vehicles, industrial control, traffic congestion, public surveillance, weather forecasting, and healthcare. According to [33–35] IoT is supposed to be benefited for various industries healthcare sector is one of them and these days almost all the healthcare associations globally are capitalizing and implementing this newly embedded digital technology to make new worth in the industry. Omar [36] projected in his study that, within this field are continuously considering novel and improved methods to help patients' requirements in a secure, reliable, and cost-effective way. According to Bhatt [37] by incorporating this latest technology with healthcare equipment advances the eminence and efficacy of service that will bring more worth particularly for the old aged peoples and patients suffering from chronic diseases. Gomeza [38] highlighted that this technology improves the quality of life for the patients by applying personal care and routine monitoring.

Selvaraj [39] highlighted in their study related to the applications, advantages, and future difficulties in the field of healthcare. They addressed the incredible role of IoT applications that will provide and recognize the most projecting challenges in the field of healthcare. A study accompanied by Rodrigues [40] on the utilization of the Internet of Things in the field of healthcare. His study reveals several approaches and conducts to utilize IoT in the field of medicine and also debated on the procedure for using IoT in healthcare that will benefit and ease the process of decision making. Jain [41] proposed a novel procedure for moving the patient's medical data into the medical cover picture by encapsulating the data by using the concept of the decision tree. The study conducted by Maksimivic [42] shows the impact of IoT in the building of E-health applications. Their study will also have analyzed that the successful positioning of IoT-based e-health applications has been beneficial for healthcare organizations. Suhardi [43] discussed the latest trends and concerns associated with E-health applications and also briefs to handle these issues. The issue related to security is a major concern and quickly developed for the IoT E-health framework. This IoT-based monitoring system guarantees the arrangement of benefits like remote real-time health monitoring with rarer faults, reduced medical administration expenses, and improves patient gratification. In the study of Islam [18], there is a review of various technologies related to healthcare based on IoT. They examine the separate IoT privacy and security aspects for healthcare that includes security specifications, threat models, and attack classifications. According to Natarajan [44], there is a well-organized machine-to-machine correspondence is to be achieved by using IoT in the field of healthcare.

Researcher [45] suggested a framework for monitoring and following the day-to-day activities by using smartphones to gather information of the elderly or disabled patients. Shi [46] also proposed another framework for old and chronically ill patients. The framework was actualized on smartphones and allows the patients to manage and supervise their condition independently from their homes that avoid hospitalization for a while. Ahmed [47] has examined the Remote healthcare system for senior citizens. In his study health checking, recovery, and aided living for the old and medically challenged patients. An adaptable IoT-based framework was proposed that can be used to gather the information required to ease the free living of senior citizens to improve their quality of life. Yehia [48] suggested different healthcare applications applied in an IoT environment that is based on a wireless medical sensor network (WMSN). Priyan [49] presented the mobile health application to forecast the type of disease by using IoT sensors. Mobile application-based gathered unique client identifier (UCI) repository dataset was utilized to diagnose the disease in the human body efficiently. Abdulhamit [50] established a mobile health application with the help of IoT sensors to foresee human activities. In this system patients were trained to do 12 physical activities as well as appropriate health information was collected through the mobile health application. This system was more reliable, effective, and robust though forecasting numerous human activities.

Researchers [51, 52] designed an IoT-based Smart Health Care Monitoring System that studies the rural and urban areas people's health-associated problems like diabetics, Pulse rate and kidney functioning, body temperature, heart health, etc. A study conducted by the World Health Organization in 2014 reveals about 422 million people globally suffer from diabetes that has a frequency of 8.5% of the adult population [53]. According to the study highlighted by researchers [54–56] that from the last few years numerous healthcare applications that were based on the Internet of Things have been projected for the management of diabetes. Rodriguez [57] proposed an architecture that is made up of sensors, a smartphone (a local gateway), and a cloud-based system to deal with diabetes suffering patients. A glucose monitoring system gathers the sensor information by using sensors attached to the body. Menon [58] recommend a blood glucose monitoring system by using near-infrared (NIR). In this framework level of glucose in the blood is projected by analyzing the variations in the signal intensity attained from a NIR sensor. Lucisano [59] also presents glucose monitoring in persons by using a long-term embedded sensor system. Glucose data is transferred every 2 min to peripheral the receivers and this system stores data for approximately 180 days for further reference. Chen [60] suggested a mobile health system by using 5G for continuous valuation and monitoring of diabetes patients. In their study, the authors present the 5G-Smart Diabetes framework by joining the current technologies like Wearable 2.0, Artificial Intelligence, and big data for making complete observing and investigation for diabetic patients. Chang [61] suggested the patient monitoring by the mhealth. It is the self-assessment system for diabetic patients that is monitored by the patient as well as by the doctor too. The connectivity is done by the GSM networks, sensors are linked with an n node of mobile devices and the patient data will be transferred to the cloud storage.

Ahmed [62] presents a framework for forecasting the absorption of glucose for a diabetic patient. GlucoSim software was used to examine the information from the diabetic patient that is produced by a continuous glucose monitoring system (CGS). Bruen [63] stated in his study that it is essential to screen the level of glucose in the body of diabetic patients to control and monitor the condition of patients are necessary. Glucose levels can be improved by changing the lifestyle and adopting habits like medications, exercise, and diet. Rasyid [64] proposed a framework used to monitor the level of glucose in the blood by using a wireless body area network for diagnosing diabetes. The framework worked by using a glucometer sensor, Arduino Uno, and a Zigbee module. A case study was proposed by Rodrigues [40] on the assessment of constant checking of a diabetes patient and factors monitoring by using biomedical sensors for type 1 diabetes mellitus. Breton [65] considered Type 1 diabetes and continuous glucose monitoring for different age groups of women that depicts that the system of insulin educated warning and proved safe and sound. Joubert [66] presented in his study that Type 1 and type 2 diabetes, insulin treatment, and distant checking for diabetes patients are considered for a cloud system. Researcher [67] suggested a monitoring system for type 2 diabetes mellitus. This system is intelligent to make decisions on the figures of diabetes control and forecast future glucose for an individual. A distant patient checking architecture is proposed by Ahmad [68] that uses E-health records for a decision support system. A conversation on the development of inpatient diabetes management is covered by Rushakoff [69] that makes a model for remote patient checking and management from the proper consultations.

3 The Architecture of IoT in Healthcare

In the Internet of Things (IoT) healthcare becomes the fastest growing sector that requires attention instantly, many healthcare applications are mending that serve the patients with the various services. Healthcare Management System provides consistent and secure services to medical staff, doctors, and patients. Each framework that is designed gives reliable communication and low latency. Cloud computing is used as an information service to complete a huge number of health-related applications. The layout of the layered architecture for the global network comprises other different networks for the recognition and combination of components of various networks having the same functions as an individual layer. In the architecture of IoT in healthcare new technology Fog computing is used instead of Cloud computing in the architecture of healthcare because cloud computing has issues like latency, low bandwidth, etc. that do not fulfill the specifications for the IoT devices. In fog computing devices works at the edge of the network that reduces the effect of issues that occurs in the cloud. To do this task many researchers propose layered architectures.

Cerina [70] proposed four-layered multi-level architectures in his study for context awareness and fog computing that includes interaction layer, mesh layer, fog layer, and cloud layer. Nandyala [71] proposed a four-tier architecture for monitoring real-time healthcare data globally that was determined by CISCO fog architecture and consists of smart devices tier, fog tier, core tier, and cloud tier. Verma [72] proposed five-layered architectures applied by the smart gateway at the fog layer for monitoring patient health remotely that includes data acquisition layer, event classification layer, information mining layer, decision making layer, and cloud storage layer. Azimi [73] proposed a hierarchical fog-assisted computing architecture in his study for observing health systems based on IoT consisting of sensor layer, fog layer, and cloud layer. Debauche [74] projected a system for healthcare based on IoT that includes three layers: sensors layer, fog layer, and cloud layer. In their proposed architecture data visualization and acquisition of data was done at the fog layer by using a smart gateway. Paul [75] proposed three-layered architectures to keep track of patients' health who are going through chronic diseases involves sensors, fog computing, and cloud computing. Analysis of data as well as data aggregation is performed at the fog computing tier performs. Awaisi [76] projected an architecture for medical applications based on fog comprised of IoT devices network layer, fog layer, and cloud layer. Abdelmoneem [77] suggested architecture for various applications related to healthcare based on cloud-fog pattern includes four layers: things layer, sink layer, fog layer, and cloud layer. The corresponding study of these IoT architectures for monitoring the health conditions of patients is subjected to several layers. These architectures are responsible for serious issues that need immediate attention, ambulance as well as for the issues that are not serious like doctor appointments. Ghoneim [78] proposed a smart healthcare framework that comprises three modules client and doctor module, edge computing module, and cloud computing module. The study proposed a novel system for image forgery recognition for the medical structure to authenticate the images related to the medical and can't be transformed or changed. Hossain [79] also proposed smart healthcare architecture that consists of four constituent's smart sensors, edge computing, cloud computing, and stakeholders i.e. patients and doctors. This framework is developed by using the concept of deep and projected to perceive Electroencephalogram (EEG) pathology and transfer the data from the edge to the cloud for its

Table 9.1 Comparison of existing architectures with proposed architecture

Reference	No. of layers	Fog/edge computing	Complication	Real-time support	Security
Cerina et al. [70]	4	Fog	Mild	Mild	High
Nandyala and Kim [71]	4	Fog	Mild	Mild	High
Verma and Sood [72]	5	Fog	High	Mild	Mild
Azimi et al. [73]	3	Fog	Low	Mild	High
Debauche et al. [74]	3	Fog	Low	Mild	Mild
Paul et al. [75]	3	Fog	Mild	Mild	Mild
Awaisi et al. [76]	3	Fog	Mild	Mild	Mild
Abdelmoneem et al. [77]	4	Fog	Mild	Mild	Mild
Ghoneim et al. [78]	3	Edge	Mild	Mild	High
Hossain and Muhammad [79]	4	Edge	Mild	Mild	High
Qadri et al. [80]	3	Fog and Edge	Mild	Mild	Mild
Proposed Architecture	3	Edge	Low	High	High

authentication check. Qadri [80] proposed a three-tier architecture that comprised of three layers things or sensor layer, communication layer that consists of fog/edge node, and processing layer or server layer that consists cloud.

Here an architecture in the Internet of Things for healthcare monitoring based on edge computing is proposed. After reviewing the study, conducted by the various authors as mentioned in Table 9.1 but the study revealed that most of the authors preferred fog computing in their architecture. Only a few of them preferred edge computing in their study. Edge computing is preferred over fog computing as fog computing works on the substructure side whereas edge computing stresses the effective side [81]. In the proposed architecture edge computing is associated with cloud computing that results in high-performance computing, low latency, and real-time output. This architecture comprises three layers as shown in Fig. 9.1, Device layer, Edge layer, and Cloud layer. This architecture effectively responds to emergency services like ambulance call, call to the doctor, etc. as well as to the non-emergency services. The device layer is the first layer in the architecture. It is also recognized as the bottom layer in the architecture. It is associated with various gadgets like body sensors, wearable devices, glucose monitoring sensors, etc. that are associated with wireless technology and to collect the information that is related to the vitals of the patient and required for monitoring patient health. The sensors that communicate the data with application devices or hardware platforms like mobiles, Arduino, Raspberry Pi, etc. These signals that are collected at this level are broadcasted to the next layer i.e. Edge layer through wired or wireless protocols. At this level of architecture, various edge computing servers are included. The virtual platform is created at different edge servers that deal with various functions like computation, storage, and computing services among end devices and cloud data centers. Data that is collected through various sensors become huge and unable to

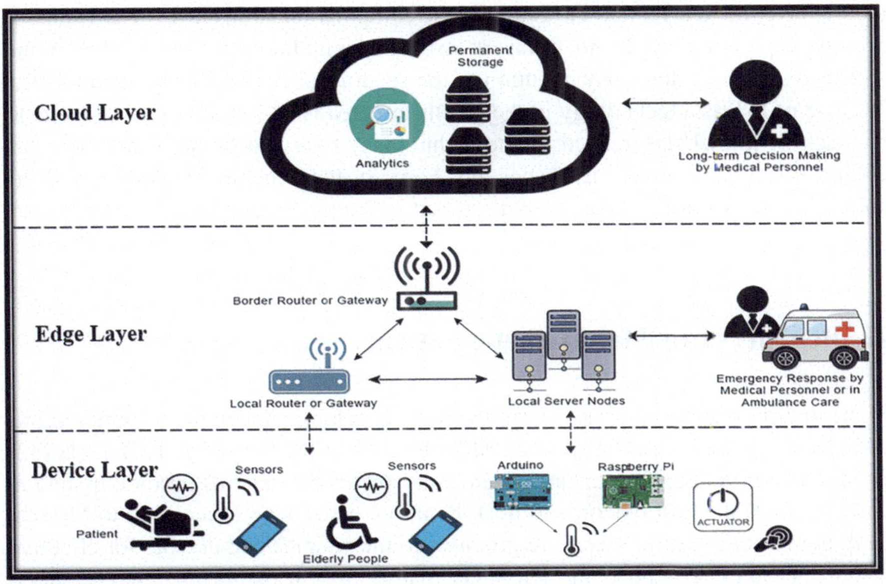

Fig. 9.1 Proposed Architecture in IoT for Healthcare based on Edge Computing

manage at the cloud computing level and generates latency, low-quality data, and low storage. To overcome these issues edge computing is used that improves the issues like system performance, speed, latency, bandwidth, etc. This layer also contains the local gateway that executes privacy and security strategies. Data is also filtered and analyzed at this level according to the requirement of the application. At the third level of architecture i.e. at the cloud layer also known as the core computing layer where the data is transferred into the bigger gateway that will send the data to the cloud, a firewall is also used for data security and privacy. This core network is liable for accommodating different services and also end-to-end communication. Here the data is permanently stored on servers for future use by the patients and hospitals that are categorized into public and private data, public data is accessed by the patient whereas private data is the trustworthy information that was not accessed by the patients.

Table 9.1 depicts the analysis of the association between existing architecture with the proposed architecture. The constraints that are taken into consideration for the association of various architectures are no. of layers, fog/edge computing, complication, real-time support, and security. Several layers represent the layers that are utilized for designing the architecture. Use of computing technology like fog computing or edge computing. The complication for the architecture is represented by parameters like low, mid, or high. The value for the complication or complexity of the architecture is considered based on the number of layers and its functionality segmented at each layer. Real-time support is also represented by parameters like low, mild, or high and security. The possible values for the chosen parameters can be any one of the following: low, moderate, or high and it is selected by the presence of the fog layer/edge layer and the extent of the computation at this level. The value for security is preferred on the no. of layers associated with the architecture. Most of the former researchers don't pay attention to the security of the healthcare architecture. The use of IoT as a technology in the healthcare area is still in its early stage due to the lack of knowledge related to the technology. Every technology has benefits, challenges as well as security issues too. Some of the benefits, challenges with its solutions, and security trends were discussed in the next sections.

4 Benefits of IoT for Diabetic Patients

In the present scenario Internet of Things is the developing technology for numerous industries as well as for the specialized sectors. With the help of IoT, Hanada [82] developed a combined healthcare system that benefits the patients for their treatment and also finds the best outcome to treat them in a better way. According to Mumtaj [83], numerous opportunities were provided to the patients and doctors for effective resources. Sun [84] reflects in their study that the use of platforms based on cloud analytics and wireless networks shows improvement in patients' health problems. These IoT-based healthcare resolutions can be used in different zones like monitoring and handling chronic diseases, remote health observing, treatment for elder patients, fitness plans, and pandemic conditions. Aniket [85] projected in his study that various persons were interacting with different technologies associated with the Internet of Things in many ways that were based on communication and usage. Following are the various benefits offered by IoT especially for diabetic patients.

1. **Benefit of IoT for Hospitals**—This technology helps the hospital to use various devices for monitoring patient health situations daily. Moreover, hospitals also can keep eye on the patient daily blood sugar levels by using the glucose sensors and recording those inputs on daily basis. By using the associated sensors, the hospital can track the current position of the various medical devices like nebulizers, wheelchairs, oxygen pumps, defibrillators, and other monitoring tools. Contamination of patients was also avoided by observing the hygiene-related issues. Technology also helps in managing inventory for pharmacies [85].
2. **Benefit of IoT for Doctors**—IoT benefits doctors to be more practical and more concentrating during their work. The data generated by various IoT devices will assist the doctors to diagnose the problem with its best outcome. By implanting remote home monitoring tools and wearable sensors, doctors can more precisely keep track of patient daily schedules, check glucose levels, manage diet plans and exercise for them [85].
3. **IoT for Patients**—To monitor the patient daily wearable health devices and sensors play an important role. Such devices like blood pressure monitoring, blood glucose monitoring, heart rate monitoring cuffs, and wearables like fitness

trackers can be connected or linked with the smart mobile device for additional investigation by doctors.

4. **Data Analysis**: Devices connected with IoT can able to collect, analyze, capture, and report the data extensively. That will reduce the necessity of storing the unanalyzed data. Here the data is directly stored on the cloud server in a very less period and easily accessible by the patients or by the healthcare providers.
5. **Uninterrupted Monitoring and Reporting**: At the time of medical emergency uninterrupted real-time monitoring of patients like stroke, heart attack, high diabetes attack, asthma attack, etc. can save the lives of many patients. Sloane [86] suggested in their study that various sensors linked to the patient body immediately transfer the data to the cloud form where the doctors and hospitals easily accessed the data and the treatment will be managed before it becomes more serious.
6. **Emergency Support**: By using this technology, patients can use mobile applications easily to interact with doctors and other medical staff globally in case of an emergency.
7. **Tracking and Connectivity**: At the time of emergency data collected by IoT devices is immediately transferred to the doctors as well as hospitals for real-time monitoring. It will also allow the machine to machine communication, sharing knowledge, movement of data, and interoperability that makes this healthcare service effective.
8. **Enhance Patient Care**: This latest technology provides better service to patients. IoT also provides accuracy for the diagnosis of disease, its improved treatment, and timely follow-up by the doctors benefit the patients in every manner.
9. **Better Diagnosis, Treatment, and Results**: Healthcare system when combined with other infrastructures benefit the medical practitioners to diagnose the disease, take better decisions to treat that disease, and follow with the patients on a routine basis. Daily monitoring of patients helps the doctors to detect indications at an initial phase or before the problem starts.
10. **Lower Cost**: Online monitoring will reduce avoidable doctor and hospital visits. Healthcare workers can assist the patients with their healthcare solutions that will help the patients, as well as the hospital, reduce their expenses [6].
11. **Managing Medicines and Equipment**: With the help of this technology, it is very easy to keep track of the medicines inventory and manage the medical equipment. According to [87] a system was developed that manages by the identification of important medicines, keeping stock of medicines, and placing an order for those medicines that are less in stock.
12. **Reduce Errors**: IoT in healthcare offers accuracy of data and automatic flow of data [88]. Moreover, data-based decisions were managed that will reduce bugs and also the cost of the system.

5 Challenges in IoT and Its Solutions for Diabetic Patients

Every technology has its positive as well as negative aspects. IoT is benefiting many fields especially the healthcare sector. Apart from these benefits in healthcare, there are some drawbacks of this technology that also exists. Researchers [89–91] in their study have discussed these drawbacks related to healthcare as part of their study. This section highlights some of the challenges and its state-of-the-art solutions.

1. **Latency**: Latency is defined as the amount of time taken by data to reach its destination. In healthcare applications latency at the communication and transport layer plays an important role in its effectiveness. The impact of latency also relies on the type of healthcare application used [92]. Applications that may be used become any emergency service like live surgeries latency causes a very radical impact. To deal with such a situation [93] proposed an IoT healthcare architecture based on fog computing that will decrease the communication latency by processing the data nearer to the sensors at the gateway instead of transferring data to the cloud that causes more latency.
2. **Consumption of Energy**: As technology increases, there is a rapid increase in the use of wearable sensors, and gadgets require higher consumption of energy and loss of power. The sensors associated with the perception layer are battery-operated. Battery exhaustion leads to the closure of these sensors that was dangerous for patients who are suffering from critical diseases in case of emergency [92]. To overcome this challenge various optimization algorithms were used to decrease the consumption of energy because of the intricacy of gadgets it becomes very difficult. Researcher [93] proposed an autonomous Wireless Body Area Network in his study that uses solar power instead of as an alternative to the battery. In this model, the energy consumed by the sensors through solar panels and framework worked throughout the day.
3. **Lack of Training and Education**: As such the technology has multiple benefits but it has hazards too. IoT devices gave accurate results only when they are properly used. To use these devices proper knowledge of these devices is required. Healthcare associations and hospitals need to appoint trained staff who have proper knowledge related to these devices. There are a lot of difficulties while using these gadgets. Consumers are aware of these devices and their proper usage because they are customary buyers [94].
4. **Availability of Service**: In IoT medical care applications like observing and emergency services, the information of a patient ought to be accessible all day, every day for proper measures to be taken by the doctors and specialists [95]. The lack of nodes accessibility or organization accessibility at the perception layer or the processing layer causes the non-accessibility of basic information, which may lead to a patient's demise. Further research is required to get the framework at the processing layer, which incorporates advances like big data, cloud computing, etc. Cloud computing incorporates numerous dangers and weaknesses, which ought to be alleviated for the high accessibility of an IoT healthcare framework [96].

5. **Lack of Interoperability**: IoT traverses various areas and includes an extensive variety of applications with clashing guidelines that raise the issue of interoperability. This issue is reduced in the medical services area as the current guidelines and norms request severe prerequisites to be fulfilled [93]. A real-time monitoring framework was proposed, which utilizes 6LoWPAN, an open standard based on top of IEEE 802.15.4, and addresses the interoperability issues among imparting devices [97]. Another solution recommended to address the interoperability issues is by abstracting the unpredictable details through various interfaces [98]. Researcher [99] proposed an IoT semantic interoperability model to deal with the problems between mixed gadgets in the framework of IoT. This model uses Resource Description Framework (RDF) and SPARQL for combining the things and querying them for extracting the data.
6. **Fault Tolerance**: The dependability of an IoT healthcare framework is influenced by the working of sensors and corresponding nodes that move the information to the cloud or processing layer. Their work is vital for the dependable and credible working of healthcare administrations during an emergency. Gia [100] proposed an IoT framework that was the solution to the fault tolerance and uses additional backup devices in case of communication failure. The gateway in this arrangement leads the analysis of sensors by noticing the information patterns occasionally and makes suitable actions.
7. **Huge Data**: IoT healthcare applications create an enormous volume of information because of the huge amount of data generated by gathering patient information. Moreover, as indicated by federal and state laws, healthcare organizations should be especially attentive in taking care of patient information from IoT applications. The flow of information made by the IoT gadgets utilized in the healthcare settings could likewise cause unexpected issues if mindful associations/partners do not have the information important to deal with it cautiously [90, 101].

6 Latest Security Trends in IoT for Healthcare Data and Its Solutions

There is a rapid increase in the concept of data hiding in the past few years. This technique deals with the challenges like data security and preservation of information while shifted over networks. To handle these issues researchers projected various studies related to the hiding of data globally. Various trends and techniques in the internet of things related to the security of data by hiding the information were used by different researchers as part of their study some of them are:

6.1 Digital Watermarking

Data that is collected through various sensors and other wearable devices securely exchanged that data in different situations with high network insecurity numerous techniques like steganography, digital signatures, encryption, and digital watermarking have been used [102–105]. To manage the concerns like data security, localization, and authentication of data digital watermarking techniques have been used. By using this technique data is embedded gradually in the form of multimedia contents like text, audio, image, or video [106]. It also deals with covering the data in the form of digital content that can be gathered only when there is proper knowledge of encoding the information by using secret keys. This technique is classified into two ways; the Robust watermarking technique and the Fragile watermarking technique. The robust technique is used for copyright protection whereas the fragile technique is used for content authentication [107]. This technique of watermarking can be used in various applications such as e-commerce defense, e-healthcare, etc. [108–110]. The use of digital watermarking techniques in the field of healthcare provides many benefits. It modifies the data in the form of an image that includes the patient's as well as the doctor's information [111]. Many researchers projected watermarking method as part of their study to deal with the security and other issues in the field of healthcare.

Parah [112] proposed dual watermarking schemes for the preservation of copyright and validation of digital content. In their study proposed schemes have been estimated the medical images that are in greyscale as well as color format. Kamili [113] presented a secure dual watermarking framework for content validation, preservation of copyright, and tamper localization for developed colored images generated by sensors are communicated over the insecure networks. In this study, a dual encrypted robust watermark has been created in the Y channel as well as a fragile watermark has been created in the Cb channel. Researcher [114] proposed a robust watermarking technique for copyright preservation and privacy of data that is based on a hybrid transform field. In this study, a block-based image watermarking algorithm along with a cryptographic algorithm was used to obtain the locations of the cover image where the watermark is to be embedded.

Gull [115] proposed a low computational and with less complexity an efficient fragile watermarking technique for the detection of tamper as well as localization of images related to medical. In this study, the cover image has been distributed into 4×4-pixel blocks with each block further sub-divided into two 4×2 blocks one is known as Upper Pixel Block (UHB) whereas another one is known as Lower Pixel Block (LPB). The information related to the watermark and features of each block has been used to develop two-bit streams; one used for tamper detection and the second one for tamper localization. Puvvadi [116] projected a well-organized watermarking technique for medical images in e-healthcare applications that are based on the hybridization of compression and cryptography algorithm. This study reveals that the security aspect has been enhanced by combining the images with patients' health information and also by compressing the information by using an arithmetic coding algorithm. Anand [117] developed a compression-then-encryption based on dual watermarking to assign the Electronic Patient Record (EPR) data for the healthcare system. The authors used the combination of redundant discrete wavelet transform (RDWT)-randomized Singular value decomposition (RSVD) and set partitioning in hierarchical trees (SPIHT)-stereo images using encryption (STE) to confirm the strength and safety of EPR.

6.2 *Pixel Repetition*

To hide data there are different schemes available, each scheme has its own use pixel repetition technique is one of it. In this technique, the input image is scaled up by utilizing the pixel repetition method in which that image is escalated by changing each pivot pixel into a small block by repeating that pixel that generates the cover image that has dimensions double than the input image. This technique doubles the original image size by repeating the number of pixels of that image which is why it is known as the pixel repetition technique. Kaw [118] proposed a high-capacity technique for hiding the information that is based on the pixel repetition method and special data shifting. This proposed technique generates the cover image by repeating the pixels of the original image that resulting in the decrease of computational complexity.

Parah [119] proposed reversible and high-capacity techniques for hiding data related to healthcare based on pixel repetition technique. This proposed technique is used for the recognition of tampered blocks by embedding the fragile watermark in the electronic records of patients. To embed the information Block-wise division of cover image and intermediate significant bit substitution have been used. Loan [120] proposed a high capacity and semi reversible scheme for hiding the information related to medical images based on pixel repetition method (PRM) and hybrid edge detection. In this proposed scheme PRM is used to enhance the size of small-sized images whereas hybrid edge detection that is based on Canny and Prewitt edge detection techniques confirms no important information is missed and maximum utilization of edge has been recorded.

6.3 *Reversible Data Hiding*

Data can be secured and embedded by using various techniques like steganography, cryptography, encryption, and watermarking. But these data embedding techniques cause damage to the cover image of data. There are some sensitive areas such as defense, healthcare, banking, military, and so on where the loss of information is not permissible. To deal with such a problem reversible data hiding technique came into existence. By using this technical information is retrieved in its primary form after the alleviation of the embedded data. Bhagat [121] highlighted the Encrypted domain, spatial domain, and compressed domain as the various types of domains that are used in reversible data hiding techniques. Ayyappan [122] designed a method that is the combination of encryption as well as reversible data hiding technique for data compression that will decrease the transmission time and also enhance the security of the system. The author also proposed a novel reversible crypto-watermarking system that utilized cryptographic algorithms for hiding and encrypting Electronic Patient Record (EPR) into an image related to that patient by using Rhombus Prediction Scheme.

Kaw [123] proposed a secured framework-based reversible data hiding technique. The proposed system is proficient in enclosing the Electronic Patient Records in the form of medical images securely for a cloud-based e-healthcare system where the cloud administrators restrict unauthorized access to the patient data. This system uses the Optical Pixel Repetition technique to change every pixel of the input image to simplify the process of reversibility. The proposed technique can retain the statistical attacks because it can present a histogram invariant among the stego image as well as the cover image. Gull [124] proposed a dual image reversible data hiding technique for IoMT based networks. In this study, data that is collected through sensors are transformed into a binary format than to the decimal format by taking four bits at a time. Huffman encoding schemes have been used to decrease the size of the data and also improve the embedding capacity.

6.4 Image Encryption

As we discussed earlier the various schemes for hiding information, among them image encryption technique becomes an adequate resolution to retain the security for all kinds of images [125]. It is the process in which the information is encoded into a secret image by using some encryption algorithms like blowfish, data encryption standard, advanced encryption standard, etc. to protect the data from unauthorized access. Manjula [126] proposed a framework that is secured for the encryption of medical images based on advanced encryption standards. This framework utilizes the hash function to design dynamic s-box generation and increase the system performance by decreasing the encryption processing time and increasing the stego image quality. Khashan [127] projected a selective encryption scheme based on edge detection to partially encrypt the digital images related to medicine. In this proposed scheme a large keyspace is presented where these different keys are used to detect the blocks that are created by using a chaotic map. A one-time pad algorithm is used to encrypt the substantial blocks. This scheme also attains high security as well as low computational complexity.

Khan [128] proposed a secure surveillance mechanism with probabilistic image encryption on smart healthcare IoT systems. The proposed system extracts the relevant images from the concise videos and then implements a well-organized probabilistic and lightweight encryption algorithm (TensorFlow, python, light-weight YOLOv3 algorithm) to the extracted image frames to protect the patient information keep safe. Researcher [129] projected a homomorphic encryption algorithm to encrypt as well as to decrypt the medical images. This homomorphic algorithm supports both additives as well as a multiplicative homomorphism. Ahmed [130] proposed a novel encryption mechanism for the privacy preservation of patient records based on controlled alternate quantum walks (CAQWs). CAQWs encrypt the colored as well as gray-scale images and based on two phases; permutation and substitution that have their parameters. Parah [119] proposed a secure and high-capacity image embedding scheme that is proficient to hide the patient information in colored image format. A fragile watermark is also embedded in the patient records to detect tamper of these records during transit.

7 Conclusion

The Internet has transformed significantly the way we live and lead us to the refined technical world. This technology allows communications among people virtually in various circumstances from our professional life to social life. Internet of Things allows everything to be connected to the internet. It allows the process of communication by using smart objects like sensors that work on the principle of any time, anything, any media, Anywhere communication. The role of the Internet of Things in the field of healthcare helps people globally in the diagnosis and monitoring of chronic diseases. This novel technology enhances the quality of service, individual's gratification and also supports elderly people, doctors, medical staff, etc. As IoT has benefited various segments of healthcare, diabetic patients are also monitored and get helped by this technology by using various sensors and wearable devices. Thus, this chapter provided the role of the Internet of Things in Healthcare for monitoring diabetic patients. Architecture based on edge computing in Internet of Things for healthcare monitoring. The proposed architecture is compared with the existing architecture for state of art parameters in terms of healthcare. Benefits for diabetes suffering patients and challenges with its solutions related to IoT for diabetic patients were also discussed. Lastly to deal with healthcare data in terms of its security with its remedial solutions was also highlighted as part of the study. In brief, the research also offers the role of IoT that is envisioned to be useful for diabetes patients. In the future, the proposed architecture in IoT for healthcare based on edge computing will be implemented and evaluated.

References

1. Internet of Things: science fiction or business fact?. Harv Bus Rev. Accessed 22 March 2021
2. Arampatzis T et al (2005) A survey of security issues in wireless sensors networks, in intelligent control. In: Proceeding of the IEEE international symposium on, Mediterrean conference on control and automation, pp 719–724

3. Tiwary A, Mahato M, Chidar A, Chandrol MK, Shrivastva M, Tripathi M (2018) Internet of Things (IoT) research, architecture, and applications. Int J Futur Revol Comput Sci Commun Eng 4(3):23–27
4. Chen ET (2020) Examining the influence of information technology on modern health care. In: Data analytics in medicine: concepts, methodologies, tools, and applications, pp 1943–1962
5. Gupta S et al (2020) Technologies in health care domain: a systematic review. Int J e-Collab 16(1):33–44
6. Izaddoost A, McGregor C (2016) Enhance network communications in a cloud-based real-time health analytics platform using SDN. In: 2016 IEEE international conference on healthcare informatics (ICHI), pp 388–391
7. Hassan H, Bashir AK, Ahmad M, Menon VG, Afridi IU, Nawaz R, Luo B (2021) Real-time image dehazing by superpixels segmentation and guidance filter. J Real-Time Image Proc 18(5):1555–1575
8. Hassan H, Bashir AK, Abbasi R, Ahmad W, Luo B (2019) Single image defocus estimation by modified Gaussian function. Trans Emerg Telecommun Technol 30(6):e3611
9. Jagadeeswari V et al (2018) A study on medical Internet of Things and Big Data in the personalized healthcare system. Health inf Sci Syst 6(1)
10. Navjot R et al (2021) IoMT based facial emotion recognition system using deep convolution neural networks. Electronics 10(11)
11. Tuli S et al (2020) Health fog: an ensemble deep learning-based smart healthcare system for automatic diagnosis of heart diseases in integrated IoT and fog computing environments. Futur Gener Comput Syst 104:187–200
12. Kumar P, Silambarasan K (2019) Enhancing the performance of healthcare service in IoT and cloud using optimized techniques. IETE J Res. https://doi.org/10.1080/03772063.2019.1654934
13. Akmandor AO, Jha NK (2017) Smart health care: an edge-side computing perspective. IEEE Consum Electron Mag 7(1):29–37
14. Mistry I et al (2019) Blockchain for 5G-enabled IoT for industrial automation: a systematic review, solutions, and challenges. Mech Syst Signal Process 135:106382
15. Rashid M et al (2020) Securing E-health IoT data on cloud systems using novel extended role-based access control model. In: Internet of Things (IoT). Springer, Cham, pp 473–489
16. Sarosh P, Parah SA, Bhat GM, Heidari AA, Muhammad K (2021) Secret sharing-based personal health records management for the Internet of Health Things. Sustain Cities Soc 74:103129
17. Perrier E (2015) Positive disruption: healthcare, ageing & participation in the age of technology. The McKell Institute, Australia, pp 43–51
18. Islam SMR, Kwak D, Kabir MH, Hossain M, Kwak KS (2015) The Internet of Things for health care: a comprehensive survey. IEEE Access 3:678–708
19. Bisio I, Delfino A, Lavagetto F, Sciarrone A (2017) Enabling IoT for in-home rehabilitation: accelerometer signals classification methods for activity and movement recognition. IEEE Internet Things J 4(1):135–146
20. Gourishankar S, Prachita MY, Prakash A (2017) IoT based heart attack detection, heart rate, and temperature monitor. Int J Comput Appl 170(5):26–30
21. WHO Global report on diabetes. http://apps.who.int/iris/bitstream/10665/204871/1/9789241565257eng.pdf. Accessed 22 Feb 2021
22. Reddy VR, Choudhury AD, Deshpande P, Jayaraman S, Thokala NK, Kaliaperumal V (2017) DM sense: a non-invasive diabetes mellitus classification system using Photoplethysmogram signal. In: Pervasive computing and communications workshops (per com workshops), 2017 IEEE international conference, pp 71–73
23. World Health Organization (1999) Definition, diagnosis, and classification of diabetes mellitus and its complications. Part 1: Diagnosis and classification of diabetes mellitus. World Health Organization, Geneva, Switzerland

24. Wild S, Roglic G, Green A, Sicree R, King H (2004) Global prevalence of diabetes: estimates for the year 2000 and projections for 2030. Diabetes Care 27:1047–1053
25. Acciaroli G, Vettoretti M, Facchinetti A, Sparacino G (2018) Calibration of minimally invasive continuous glucose monitoring sensors: state-of-the-art and current perspectives. Biosensors 13:24
26. Kamilaris A, Pitsillides A (2016) Mobile phone computing and the Internet of Things: a survey. IEEE Internet Things J 3(6):885–898
27. Jan A et al (2021) Secure data transmission in IoTs based on CLoG edge detection. Futur Gener Comput Syst 121:59–73
28. Kadhim KT, Alsahlany AM, Wadi SM, Kadhum TH (2020) An overview of patient's health status monitoring system based on Internet of Things (IoT). Wirel Persn Commun 114:2235–2262
29. Mishra V (2017) Uses of wireless devices and IoT in management of diabetes. In: Proceedings of national conference on emerging trends in science, technology & management, pp 14–21
30. Singh RP, Javaid M, Haleem A, Suman R (2020) Internet of things (IoT) applications to fight against COVID-19 pandemic. Diabetes Metab Syndr 14:521–524
31. Moharana SR, Jha VK, Satpathy A, Addya SK, Turuk AK, Majhi B (2017) Secure key-distribution in IoT cloud networks. In: 2017 Third international conference on sensing signal processing and security (ICSSS)
32. Rajput DS, Gour R (2016) An IoT framework for healthcare monitoring systems. Int J Comput Sci Inf Secur 14(5)
33. Sajid O, Haddara M (2016) NFC mobile payments: are we ready for them? In: SAI computing conference. Springer, London, UK, pp 960–976
34. Browser J, Saxena S, Fraser H, Marshall A (2017) A healthy outlook: digital reinvention in healthcare. IBM, Armonk, NY, p 10504
35. Haddara M, Helgesen T (2018) Wireless power transfer solutions for 'things' in the Internet of Things. Adv Intell Syst Comput 880(1):92–103
36. Omar H, Khoshnaw A, Monnet W (2016) Smart patient management, monitoring and tracking system using radio-frequency identification (RFID) technology. In: IEEE EMBS conference on biomedical engineering and sciences (IECBES), pp 40–45
37. Bhatt Y, Bhatt C (2017) Internet of Things in healthcare. In: Internet of Things and Big Data technologies for next generation healthcare, pp 13–33
38. Gomeza J, Oviedob B, Zhuma E (2016) Patient monitoring system based on Internet of Things. Proc Comput Sci 83:90–97
39. Selvaraj S, Sundaravaradhan S (2020) Challenges and opportunities in IoT healthcare systems: a systematic review. SN Appl Sci 2(1):139
40. Rodrigues JJ et al (2018) Enabling technologies for the Internet of health things. IEEE Access 6:13129–13141
41. Jain M, Choudhary RC, Kumar A (2016) Secure medical image steganography with RSA cryptography using decision tree. In: Contemporary computing and informatics (IC3I), 2016 2nd international conference, pp 291–295
42. Maksimovic M, Vujovic V (2017) Internet of Things based E-health systems: ideas, expectations, and concerns. In: Khan S, Zomaya A, Abbas A (eds) Handbook of large-scale distributed computing in smart healthcare. Scalable computing and communications. Springer, Cham
43. Suhardi, Ramadhan A (2016) A survey of security aspects for IoT in healthcare, Lecture notes in electrical engineering information science and applications (ICISA), pp 1237–1247
44. Natarajan K, Prasath B, Kokila P (2016) Smart healthcare system using Internet of Things. J Netw Commun Emerg Technol 6(3)
45. Ketabdar H, Lyra M (2010) System and methodology for using mobile phones in live remote monitoring of physical activities. In: Proceedings of the IEEE international symposium on technology and society, Wollongong, NSW, Australia
46. Shi L et al (2015) Integrated care delivery and health care seeking by chronically-ill patients–a case-control study of rural Henan province, China. Int J Equity Health 14:98

47. Ahmed A, Kumar Y, Ahmed K (2017) IoT-based health monitoring system for active and assisted living. In: International conference on smart objects & technologies for social good, pp 11–20
48. Yehia L, Khedr A, Darwish A (2015) Hybrid security techniques for Internet of Things healthcare applications. Adv Internet Things 5(3):21
49. Priyan MK et al (2018) Cloud and IoT based disease prediction and diagnosis system for healthcare using fuzzy neural classifier. Futur Gener Comput Syst 86:527–534
50. Abdulhamit S, Radhwan M, Kurdi R, Khateeb K (2018) IoT based mobile healthcare system for human activity recognition. In: 15th Learning and technology conference (L&T)
51. Dinesh K et al (2018) IoT based smart health care monitoring system. Int J Inst Ind Res 3(1): 22–24
52. Gupta N, Chahande M, Pandey S (2017) Study of IoT based health monitoring devices. Int J Eng Technol 9:451–456
53. World Health Organization (2016) Global report on diabetes. World Health Organization, Geneva, Switzerland. Accessed 20 Mar 2021
54. Catarinucci L et al (2015) An IoT-aware architecture for smart healthcare systems. IEEE Internet Things J 2(6):515–526
55. Corno F et al (2016) A healthcare support system for assisted living facilities: an IoT solution. In: Proceedings of the 2016 IEEE 40th annual computer software and applications conference (COMPSAC), Atlanta, GA, pp 344–352
56. Philip V, Suman VK, Menon VG, Dhanya KA (2017) A review on latest Internet of Things based healthcare applications. Int J Comput Sci Inf Secur 15(1)
57. Rodriguez I, Rodriguez J, Zamora M (2018) Variables to be monitored via biomedical sensors for complete type 1 diabetes mellitus management: an extension of the "on-board" concept. J Diabetes Res:1–14
58. Menon KAU et al (2013) A survey on non-invasive blood glucose monitoring using NIR. ICCSP 2013:1069–1072
59. Lucisano J et al (2016) Glucose monitoring in individuals with diabetes using a long-term implanted sensor/telemetry system and model. IEEE Trans Biomed Eng 64(9):1982–1993
60. Chen M, Yang J, Zhou J, Hao Y, Zhang J, Youn CH (2018) 5G-smart diabetes: toward personalized diabetes diagnosis with healthcare big data clouds. IEEE Commun Mag 56:16–23
61. Chang SH et al (2016) A context-aware, interactive M-health system for diabetes. IEEE IT Profess 18(3):14–22
62. Ahmed HB, Serener A (2016) Effects of external factors in CGM sensor glucose concentration prediction. Proc Comput Sci 102:623–629
63. Bruen D, Delaney C, Florea L, Diamond D (2017) Glucose sensing for diabetes monitoring: recent developments. Sensors 17:1866
64. Rasyid A et al (2016) Implementation of blood glucose levels monitoring system based on wireless body area network. In: Consumer electronics-Taiwan (ICCE-TW), 2016 IEEE international conference, pp 1–2
65. Breton M et al (2018) Continuous glucose monitoring and insulin informed advisory system with automated titration and dosing of insulin reduces glucose variability in type 1 diabetes mellitus. Diabetes Technol Ther 20(8):531–540
66. Joubert M et al (2019) Remote monitoring of diabetes: a cloud-connected digital system for individuals with diabetes and their health care providers. J Diabet Sci Technol 13(6): 1161–1168
67. Wang N, Kang G (2012) A monitoring system for type 2 diabetes mellitus. Healthcom 2012: 62–67
68. Ahmad B, Ayu M, Abdullahi I, Yakubu Y (2017) Remote patient monitoring system architecture for diabetes management. In: International conference on computing, engineering, and design (ICCED), pp 1–6

69. Rushakoff R et al (2017) Remote monitoring and consultation of inpatient populations with diabetes. Curr Diab Rep 17(9):70
70. Cerina L, Notargiacomo S, Paccanit MG, Santambrogio MD (2017) A fog-computing architecture for preventive healthcare and assisted living in smart ambients. In: IEEE 3rd international forum on research and technologies for society and industry (RTSI)
71. Nandyala CS, Kim HK (2016) From cloud to fog and IoT based real-time U-healthcare monitoring for smart homes and hospitals. Int J Smart Home 10(2):187–196
72. Verma P, Sood SK (2018) Fog assisted-IoT enabled patient health monitoring in smart homes. IEEE Internet Things J 5(3):1789–1796
73. Azimi I et al (2017) HiCH: hierarchical fog-assisted computing architecture for healthcare IoT. ACM Trans Embed Comput Syst. https://doi.org/10.1145/3126501
74. Debauche O, Mahmoudi S, Manneback P, Assila A (2019) Fog IoT for health: a new architecture for patients and elderly monitoring. Proc Comput Sci 160:289–297
75. Paul A, Pinjari H, Hong WH, Seo HC, Rho S (2018) Fog computing-based IoT for health monitoring system. J Sens 2018:1386470
76. Awaisi KS, Hussain S, Ahmed M, Khan AA, Ahmed G (2020) Leveraging IoT and fog computing in healthcare systems. IEEE Internet Things Mag 3(2):52–56
77. Abdelmoneem RM, Benslimane A, Shaaban E, Abdelhamid S, Ghoneim S (2019) A cloud-fog based architecture for IoT applications dedicated to healthcare. In: ICC 2019–2019 IEEE international conference on communications (ICC)
78. Ghoneim A, Muhammad G, Amin SU, Gupta B (2018) Medical image forgery detection for smart healthcare. IEEE Commun Mag 56(4):33–37
79. Hossain MS, Muhammad G (2020) Deep learning based pathology detection for smart connected healthcare. IEEE Netw 34(6):120–125
80. Qadri YA, Nauman A, Zikria YB, Vasilakos AV, Kim SW (2020) The future of healthcare Internet of Things: a survey of emerging technologies. IEEE Commun Surv Tuts 22(2): 1121–1167
81. Open fog architecture overview. Open Fog Consortium Architecture Working Group. Accessed 20 Mar 2021
82. Hanada E, Kudou T (2018) Managing the electromagnetic environment of hospital IoT systems. In: IEEE international symposium on electromagnetic compatibility and IEEE Asia-Pacific symposium on electromagnetic compatibility (EMC/APEMC), pp 940–943
83. Mumtaj SY, Umamakeswari A (2017) Neuro fuzzy-based healthcare system using IoT. In: 2017 International conference on energy, communication, data analytics and soft computing (ICECDS), pp 2299–2303
84. Sun W, Cai Z, Li Y, Liu F, Fang S, Wang GS, Wang G (2018) Security and privacy in the medical internet of things: a review. Secur Commun Netw 2018:5978636
85. Aniket (2020) The role of IoT in healthcare: applications implementation. https://www.finoit.com/blog/the-role-of-iot-in-healthcare-space. Accessed 30 Jan 2020
86. Sloane EB, Gehlot V (2016) Improved population health surveillance and chronic disease management using secure email: application of the DIRECT, IEEE 11073, HITSP, and IHE standards and protocols. In: 2016 18th Mediterranean electrotechnical conference (MELECON), pp 1–3
87. Kalyankar GD, Poojara SR, Dharwadkar NV (2017) Predictive analysis of diabetic patient data using machine learning and Hadoop. In: 2017 International conference on I-SMAC (IoT in social, mobile, analytics and cloud) (I-SMAC), pp 619–624
88. Elmisery AM, Rho S, Botvich D (2016) A fog-based middleware for automated compliance with OECD privacy principles on the internet of healthcare things. IEEE Access 4:8418–8441
89. Baker SB, Xiang W, Atkinson I (2017) Internet of things for smart healthcare: technologies, challenges, and opportunities. IEEE Access 3:26521–26544
90. Gope P, Hwang T (2016) BSN-care: a secure IoT-based modern healthcare system using a body sensor network. IEEE Sensors J 16(5):1368–1376

91. Li C, Hu X, Zhang L (2017) The IoT-based heart disease monitoring system for pervasive healthcare service. Proc Comput Sci 112:2328–2334
92. Muhammed T, Mehmood R, Albeshri A, Katib I (2018) Ube-health: a personalized ubiquitous cloud and edge-enabled networked healthcare system for smart cities. IEEE Access 6:32258–32285
93. Farahani B, Firouzi F, Chang V, Badaroglu M, Constant N, Mankodiya K (2018) Towards fog-driven IoT eHealth: promises and challenges of IoT in medicine and healthcare. Futur Gener Comput Syst 78:659–676
94. Matthews K (2020) 5 challenges facing health care IoT in 2019. https://www.iotforall.com/5-challenges-facing-iot-healthcare-2019. Accessed 15 Feb 2021
95. Fotouhi H, Causevic A, Lundqvist K, Bjorkman M (2016) Communication and security in health monitoring systems – a review. In: 2016 IEEE 40th annual computer software and applications conference (COMPSAC)
96. Suryateja PS (2018) Threats and vulnerabilities of cloud computing: a review. Int J Comput Sci Eng 6(3):297–302
97. Touati F, Tabish R, Mnaouer AB (2013) Towards u-health: an indoor 6LoWPAN based platform for real-time healthcare monitoring. In: 6th Joint IFIP wireless and mobile networking conference (WMNC)
98. Sethi P, Sarangi SR (2017) Internet of Things: architectures, protocols, and applications. J Electr Comput Eng 2017:9324035
99. Jabbar S, Ullah F, Khalid S, Khan M, Han K (2017) Semantic interoperability in heterogeneous IoT infrastructure for healthcare. Wirel Commun Mob Comput 2017:9731806
100. Gia TN, Rahmani AM, Westerlund T, Liljeberg P, Tenhunen H (2015) Fault-tolerant and scalable IoT-based architecture for health monitoring. In: IEEE sensors applications symposium (SAS)
101. Reddy GT, Kaluri R, Reddy PK, Lakshmanna K, Koppu S, Rajput DS (2019) A novel approach for home surveillance system using IoT adaptive security. In: Proceedings of international conference on sustainable computing in science, technology and management (SUSCOM). Amity University Rajasthan, Jaipur-India
102. Domingo F, Josep O, Jordi R, David S (2019) Privacy-preserving cloud computing on sensitive data: a survey of methods, products, and challenges. Comput Commun 140:38–60
103. Gutub A, Nouf AJ, Khan E (2019) Counting-based secret sharing technique for multimedia applications. Multimed Tools Appl 78(5):5591–5619
104. Shi Y, Wei W, Zhang F, Luo X, He Z, Fan H (2020) SDSRS: a novel white-box cryptography scheme for securing embedded devices in IIoT. IEEE Trans Ind Informatics 16(3):1602–1616
105. Gull S, Mansour RF, Aljehane NO, Parah SA (2021) A self-embedding technique for tamper detection and localization of medical images for smart-health. Multimed Tools Appl 80(19): 29939–29964
106. Maiorana E, Campisi P, Neri A (2007) Biometric signature authentication using random transform-based watermarking techniques. IEEE Biometric Symp 2007:1–6
107. Cox I, Miller M, Bloom J, Fridrich J, Kalker T (2007) Digital watermarking and steganography. Morgan Kaufmann Publishers Inc., San Francisco, CA
108. Mondal S, Agarwal K, Rashid M (2019) Deep learning approach for automatic classification of x-ray images using convolutional neural network. In: 2019 Fifth international conference on image information processing (ICIIP). IEEE, New York, pp 326–331
109. Muhammad K, Sajjad M, Mehmood I, Rho S, Baik SW (2016) Image steganography using uncorrelated color space and its application for security of visual contents in online social networks. Futur Gener Comput Syst. https://doi.org/10.1016/j.future.2016.11.029
110. Khan AA, Shaikh AA, Cheikhrouhou O, Laghari AA, Rashid M, Shafiq M, Hamam H (2021) IMG-forensics: multimedia-enabled information hiding investigation using convolutional neural network. IET Image Process. https://doi.org/10.1049/ipr2.12272
111. Mehan V, Dhir R, Brar YS (2013) Watermarking for health management system. Int J Adv Res Comput Sci Softw Eng 3:224–228

112. Parah SA, Hurrah NH, Loan NA, Sheikh JA, Elhoseny M, Khan M (2019) Dual watermarking framework for privacy protection and content authentication of multimedia. Futur Gener Comput Syst 94:654–673
113. Kamili A, Nasir NH, Parah SA, Bhat G, Khan M (2020) DWFCAT: dual watermarking framework for industrial image authentication and tamper localization. IEEE Trans Ind Informatics 17:5108–5117
114. Singh KU, Abu-Hamatta HS, Kumar A, Singhal A, Rashid M, Bashir AK (2021) Secure watermarking scheme for color DICOM images in telemedicine applications. Comput Mater Continua 70(2):2525–2542
115. Gull S, Loan NA, Parah SA, Sheikh JA, Bhat GM (2020) An efficient watermarking technique for tamper detection and localization of medical images. J Ambient Intell Humaniz Comput 11(5):1799–1808
116. Puvvadi A, Venkata P, Kishore V (2018) An efficient medical image watermarking technique in E-healthcare application using hybridization of compression and cryptography algorithm. J Intell Syst 27(1):115–133
117. Anand A, Singh AK, Lv Z, Bhatnagar G (2020) Compression-then-encryption-based secure watermarking technique for smart healthcare system. IEEE Multimedia 27(4):133–143
118. Kaw JA, Parah SA, Sheikh JA, Bhat GM (2018) A new reversible stenographic technique based on pixel repetition method (PRM) and special data shifting (SDS). In: 2017 4th international conference on image information processing, ICIIP 2017, pp 199–204
119. Parah SA, Sheikh JA, Ahad F, Bhat GM (2018) High capacity and secure electronic patient record (EPR) embedding in color images for IoT driven healthcare systems. Springer, New York, pp 409–437
120. Loan NA, Parah SA, Sheikh JA, Akhoon JA, Bhat GM (2017) Hiding electronic patient record (EPR) in medical images: a high capacity and computationally efficient technique for e-healthcare applications. J Biomed Inform 73:125–136
121. Bhagat D, Bhardwaj R (2019) A survey on medical images for reversible data hiding techniques. In: The proceedings of Amity international conference on artificial intelligence, AICAI 2019, pp 811–817
122. Ayyappan S, Lakshmi C, Menon V (2019) A secure reversible data hiding and encryption system for embedding EPR in medical images. Curr Sign Transduct Therapy 15(2):124–135
123. Kaw JA, Loan NA, Parah SA, Muhammad K, Sheikh JA, Bhat GM (2019) A reversible and secure patient information hiding system for IoT driven E-health. Int J Inf Manag 45:262–275
124. Gull S, Parah SA, Khan M (2020) Reversible data hiding exploiting Huffman encoding with dual images for IoMT based healthcare. Comput Commun 163:134–149
125. Shah AA, Parah SA, Rashid M, Elhoseny M (2020) Efficient image encryption scheme based on generalized logistic map for real time image processing. J Real-Time Image Proc 17(6): 2139–2151
126. Manjula G, Mohan HS (2020) A secure framework for medical image encryption using enhanced AES algorithm. Int J Sci Technol Res 9(02):3837–3841
127. Khashan OA, Muath AS (2020) Edge-based lightweight selective encryption scheme for digital medical images. Multimedia Tools Appl. https://doi.org/10.1007/s11042-020-09264-z
128. Khan J, Li JP, Ahamad B, Parveen S, Ul Haq A, Khan GA, Sangaiah AK (2020) SMSH: secure surveillance mechanism on smart healthcare IoT system with probabilistic image encryption. IEEE Access 8:15747–15767
129. Vengadapurvaja AM, Nisha G, Aarthy R, Sasikaladevi N (2017) An efficient homomorphic medical image encryption algorithm for cloud storage security. Proc Comput Sci 115:643–650
130. Ahmed A et al (2020) Controlled alternate quantum walks based privacy-preserving healthcare images in the Internet of Things. Opt Laser Technol 124:105942

Part IV
Applications of Artificial Intelligence in Healthcare

Chapter 10
Low-Rank Representation Based Approach for Subspace Segmentation and Clustering of Biomedical Image Patterns

Ishfaq Majeed Sheikh and Manzoor Ahmad Chachoo

Contents

1 Introduction

Blood is a soft fluid that circulates through different parts of the human body. It is a combination of different components. The main constituents of blood are RBC, WBC, plasma, and platelets. These components perform several functions such as transporting oxygen to several organs of the human body, providing essential nutrients to the cells, removing several types of wastes from the human body, and giving protection to the different organs. These functions are essential for human survival. Blood cells are developed from hematopoietic stem cells that are formed in the bone marrow. A stem cell is a basic unit that can adapt the shape of any cell such as WBC, RBC, and platelets. These cells do automatic treatment of different diseases (leukaemia, infection, an autoimmune disorder, etc.). They circulate in the blood and bone marrow. Fifty-five percent of blood content is made of plasma, and the remaining 45% is of cells and platelets. These components are discussed as follows.

I. M. Sheikh (✉) · M. A. Chachoo
PG Department of Computer Science, University of Kashmir, Srinagar, India
e-mail: ishfaqmajeed.scholar@kashmiruniversity.net

S. A. Parah et al. (eds.), *Artificial Intelligence for Innovative Healthcare Informatics*,
https://doi.org/10.1007/978-3-030-96569-3_10

1. **Red blood cells or erythrocytes**: The structure of these cells is like a flattened disk. They perform the task of transporting oxygen. In 1 s around two million, RBC'S are produced in the human body. Its normal life is for 4 months. The number of RBC'S in 1 μL of blood is 4.5–6.2 million in men and 4.0–5.2 million in women.

   The growth of these cells is controlled by a hormone, produced from a kidney. The hormone is termed erythropoietin. This type of cell system is placed in the bloodstream after seven days because these types of cells are produced as immature cells by the bone marrow. They don't contain a nucleus inside them, which makes them easily adaptable to different shapes. This feature of flexibility helps them to travel in different vessels of the human body. A special type of protein called Haemoglobin enables them to carry oxygenated blood from the lungs to different parts of the body and carry carbonated blood from the body to the lungs. Blood appears red because of Haemoglobin present in its structure. The percentage of complete blood volume is called hematocrit, which is used to measure different levels of RBC'S.
2. **White blood cells, or leukocytes**: The WBC'S are fewer in number. Only 1% of these cells are found in the human body. The ratio of WBC to RBC is around 1 to 800. They act as an important component of the human immune because the leucocytes defend the human body from infections. These cells act as a measure defense system in the human body. The range of WBC'S in 1 μL of blood is between 3700 and 10,500. There are different types of WBC'S, that originate from the soft fluid of bone marrow. Figure 10.1 depicts the structure of different leucocytes. These cells are discussed as follows.

   (a) **Neutrophil**: The major type of WBC is neutrophil. Around 70% of leucocytes in the human body are neutrophil only. It is the responsive cell system that does the immediate reaction to different problems. The life of neutrophils is less than a day, our bone marrow consistently generates these cell types to defend the body from diseases.
   (b) **Lymphocyte**: Another important type of leucocyte is lymphocytes. There are two variants of the cell system, T and B lymphocytes. T cells help regulate other immune cells, whether they perform their functions appropriately or not. Whereas B cells defend the human immune from foreign substances, by making antibodies.
   (c) **Monocytes**: deal with the damaged cells and defend against many infectious organisms.
   (d) **Eosinophils**: kill parasites, destroy cancer cells, and are involved in allergic responses.
   (e) **Basophils**: generate responses to allergies.

3. **Platelets, or thrombocytes**: These cells stop bleeding by clotting blood. One microliter of blood contains around 150,000–400,000 platelets. Usually, small fragments of cells are called platelets. To prevent leakage of blood, they gather at the point of injury by making a fibrin clot, which forms a platform for blood

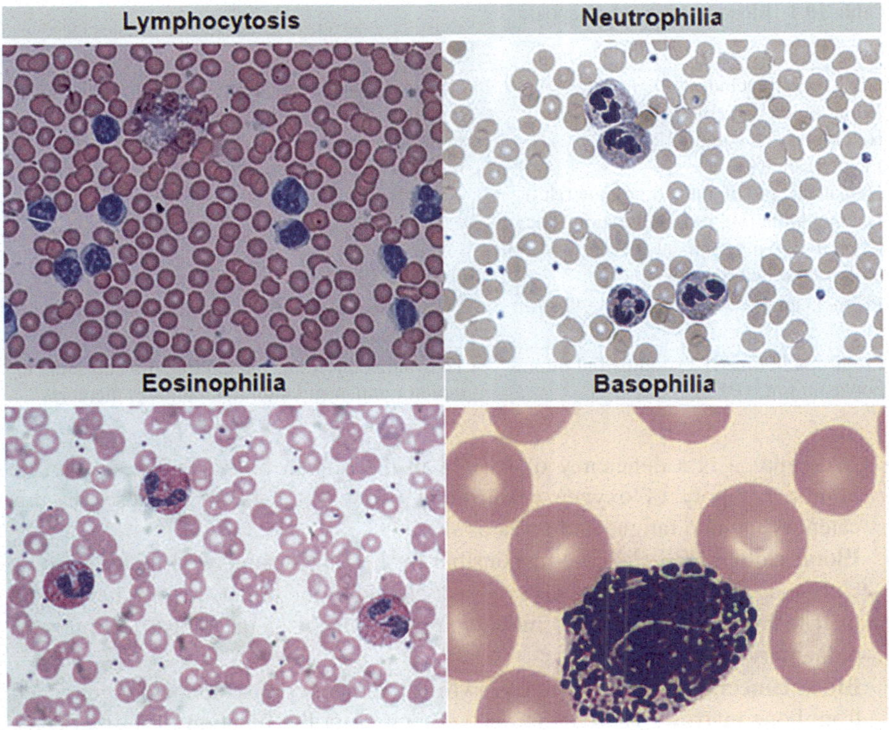

Fig. 10.1 Types of leucocytes

coagulation. If the number of platelets is higher than the usual count. It leads to unnecessary clotting of blood, which can cause brain strokes and heart attack. However, if they are less in number then it may lead to excessive bleeding from the wound.

4. **Plasma**: Ninety-two percent of plasma contains water and the remaining part contains the following components: carbon dioxide, glucose, hormones, proteins, mineral salts, fats, and vitamins.

1.1 Different Types of Blood Disorders

Blood disorder is a dangerous condition, in which the human body is unable to perform its basic functions [1, 2]. It spreads throughout the whole circuitry of the human body, which inflates other types of organs. The most common diseases associated with different types of blood disorders are mentioned as follows.

Table 10.1 Blood test-related diagnosis

Test	Uses
CBC, which includes: White blood cell count (WBC) Red blood cell count (RBC) Platelet count Hematocrit red blood cell volume (Hct) Haemoglobin (Hgb) concentration. The oxygen-carrying pigment in red blood cells Differential blood count	To aid in diagnosing anaemia and other blood disorders and certain cancers of the blood; to monitor blood loss and infection; or to monitor response to cancer therapy, such as chemotherapy and radiation
Platelet count	To diagnose and monitor bleeding and clotting disorders
Prothrombin time (PT) and partial thromboplastin time (PTT)	To evaluate bleeding and clotting disorders and to monitor anticoagulation (anticlotting) therapies

- **Anaemia**: it is a deficiency of RBC'S in the human body. This results in an improper supply of oxygen to different parts of the body. Diseases in this category include fatigue and pales of skin.
- **Blood clots**: blood clots are responsible for healing wounds and injuries. Some clots coagulate inside a blood vessel, which blocks the bloodstream. They can be fatal to human health, while moving from the heart to the lungs, leading to a pulmonary embolism.
- **Blood cancers**: it is an abnormal growth of the number of lymphocytes generated from bone marrow. These abnormal cells interrupt the function of normal cells. There are multiple types of cancers like Leukaemia, Myeloma, and Lymphoma.

To analyze blood-related disorders, doctors prescribe a commonly used test that is termed as complete blood count [3, 4]. It gives information about the range of various cell types present in the human body. The medical staff utilizes the results of CBC to diagnose various types of diseases. Table 10.1 lists different types of diseases associated with blood disorders.

1.2 Automatic Analysis of Biomedical Images

Blood images contain different types of structures that enable intelligent processing models to characterize their patterns. These sub-structures represent different types of blood components (WBC, RBC, Platelets, and Background). Each of the sub-component consists of parameters like eccentricity, perimeter, intensity, Major-Arc, Minor-Arc, and intensity. These parameters act as the base, for differentiating different types of blood components. The manual procedure of analyzing blood images is complex because its efficiency depends upon the knowledge of medical expertise. Which is time-consuming and prone to errors. Nowadays, machine learning is being utilized in the medical field for automatic disease detection, which will help the medical expert in the treatment methods. This approach of analyzing cell images will produce results at a very fast rate and without complexity overheads. Different machine learning algorithms have been proposed for subclass clustering of the cell images into the leukaemia and non-leukaemia class. However, the classification performance of the corresponding technique depends upon the robust segmentation of blood image components. The segmentation techniques have been classified into the boundary cell detection approach and the pattern-based analysis of cell structures. It has been observed in [5] that the threshold-based algorithm leads to an adverse effect on the geometric shape of the leucocytes. This is because the approach has particularly focused on the retention of the cell nucleus, based on the intensities of different image components. Which leads to distortion to the shape of WBC'S. The commonly used pattern-based cell image segmentation algorithms are k-means and fuzzy c-means.

The work in [6] has compared the segmentation performance of the concerned algorithms with the low-rank representation (LRR) model. The authors have used the following measures for comparisons such as under-segmentation rate (USR), over-segmentation rate (OSR), and overall segmentation rate (OVS). The results have shown that the OVS performance of LRR was very high in comparison to the k-means and fuzzy c-means. Also, it has been observed that the k-means algorithm suffers from USR, and fuzzy c-means has an OSR problem, on the segmentation of cell images. These points motivate us towards the utilization of the LRR approach for subspace segmentation of medical images. Which represents the global geometric structure of data, by doing a linear decomposition of very high dimensional data, into the low-rank meaningful patterns. That not only reduces the dimensional size of data but also the computational time required to process the data. Different types of data such as DNA microarray, biomedical images, RNA sequencing, vision data, and motion segmentation, can be well represented by low-rank subspaces. The basic assumption of the model is that the input data pattern lies near several subspaces. Each subspace is responsible for an independent data pattern in the image. Our objective is to segment the biomedical image into several components (WBC, RBC, and platelets). It is considered as one of the challenging tasks in machine learning because the biomedical data is subjected to different types of failures (environmental lighting factor of the image, angle of capturing the image, and microscopic quality). When the data is clean, subspaces can easily be constructed from the input blood image. The more challenging in this category include recovery of corrupted data from the errors (sample-specific corruptions, random noise, missed entries, and outliers) that exist in the data. The error represents the difference between the approximated and the actual value of the data. Our objective is to minimize this difference by reducing the sum of the square difference between the two values.

Some of the popular methods that follow the low-rank subspace segmentation approach are as follows principal component analysis (PCA), non-negative matrix factorization, and recovery of a corrupted data matrix. We have adopted the generalized PCA method that finds the low-rank subspaces of the data drawn from the union of multiple linear subspaces. It has found the best results on segmentation of image data, motion, and texture characterization. The algorithm performs segmentation of data, by using an affinity matrix, which encodes pairwise similarity between the data points. This class of algorithms is spectral. They are computationally inexpensive and are more robust to outliers present in the data. They have shown very good performance, as compared to the traditional clustering techniques, and are simple, which makes them easily understandable. There are different types of spectral clustering algorithms, that are used for subspace segmentation of data. They generally differ in the construction of the affinity matrix $A \in R^{N*N}$, which encodes the similarity between data points. The basic assumption is that $A_{ij} \gg 0$ when the data points are in the same sub-class, and $A_{ij} = 0$ when they are in dissimilar classes, where A_{ij} represents the entries of data points. One of the most powerful spectral clustering algorithms is sparse subspace clustering (SSC) [7]. It has dominated the subspace clustering algorithms in past, because of its superior data processing approach, which finds subspaces by exploiting the intra-strength of data. The objective of SSC is to obtain a block diagonal representation of Z. Which is computed by finding a linear combination of Z with a dictionary D. Its objective function is expressed in Eq. (10.1).

$$D = \mathrm{DZ} \tag{10.1}$$

Where D is the dictionary that also acts as an input matrix, and Z is the representation of the data. There exist different combinations of DZ, that can produce a resultant data matrix D. Among the different solutions, we are looking for an optimal one, that produces sparse Z. The condition depicted in (10.1) is for noise-free data. Solving such an objective is only useful when the data is known to be noise-free. Consider the case when the data is affected by outliers. This requires a reformulation of the objective function in Eq. (10.2), which incorporates constraints to deal with noise.

$$\min_{Z} \lambda \parallel \mathrm{Z}\|_1 + \frac{1}{2} \parallel \mathrm{D} - \mathrm{DZ}\|_F^2, \ \ s.t. \quad \mathrm{diag(Z)} = 0 \tag{10.2}$$

Where λ is the penalty parameter that controls sparsity of Z and D is the observed data matrix. $\| \,.\|_F^2$ is the squared Frobenius norm that minimizes the error in the data. The problem with SSC is that it computes the sparsest representation of individual data points, which may not generate global representation appropriately. It can also induce sparsity not only between clusters but also within a cluster.

To promote the global grouping effects of data we have utilized the LRR model [8]. It is more robust as compared to SSC because of its global representation power. The model works by representing the cell image pattern as the linear combination of dictionary and coefficient matrix. The dictionary generally acts as the resultant base matrix, which is generated from the input structure of the biomedical image data. Whereas the coefficient matrix is the representation of input data patterns which is obtained by computing the singular value decomposition (SVD). Each singular value is responsible for one independent pattern in the blood image. Computationally finding the minimal rank of a matrix is considered as NP (Non-deterministic polynomial)-hard problem, because it executes in an exponential amount of time. Keeping this in consideration we have chosen the closest convex envelope of the rank function i.e., nuclear norm, which is the regularized optimization problem that can be solved in polynomial time [9]. The final partitioning of data is performed by applying unsupervised clustering algorithms, k-means, or N-cut. The N-cut algorithm has shown efficient performance on connected data components [10]. Whereas, k-means perform well on compacted data patterns. Since the cell image contains connected data patterns, the partitioning of the data segments was performed by using N-cut. It works by generating a Laplacian Matrix L from the represented data patterns. Where matrix $\mathbf{L} \in \mathrm{R}^{N \times N}$ constructs different types of clusters in the data that are obtained by finding the least eigenvectors of the laplacian matrix.

2 Literature Survey

To analyze the pattern of different cell image components recent research has demonstrated different segmentation methods. The methodology differs from each other based on the approach that they follow for the discrimination of data. These methods can be divided into the following categories.

2.1 *Filter-Based Segmentation*

One of the most common approaches for the segmentation of blood images is the thresholding method. The algorithm works by finding a filter that differentiates between the leucocytic cell nucleus, and other blood components of the cell image. If the value of data points is greater than the filter they are retained in the image, otherwise, they are treated as noise thus removed from the biomedical image. The objective is to find the optimal value that can discriminate subcomponents appropriately. It is very difficult to obtain the optimal value of the threshold that can completely differentiate the foreground pixels from the background data points. The approach may act as the cause for destroying the shape of the nucleus because at times the intensity of the irrelevant data class matches with the cell nucleus magnitude [5]. Removing the data points of that magnitude value can distort the geometric shape of the nucleus.

2.2 *Region-Based Segmentation*

The region growing method follows the procedure of finding a group of pixels that have common properties (grey level intensity, geometric shape, color variation, etc.). It starts with a small set of data points that are also called seeds. The seeds grow gradually until all data points that satisfy common property are placed in a separate class. This approach does not produce well results on different types of WBC'S.

2.2.1 Region Splitting and Merging

The approach performs repetitive splitting of data points until all the data points that have particular properties are placed in a single class. Later we merge the classes that contain similar features.

2.3 Watershed-Based Segmentation

In image processing, the watershed is the most widely used approach for the segmentation of cell data. It treats the biomedical image as a topographic map, where different grey level intensities constitute the height of the topographic map function. The approach divides an image into the number of catchment basins based on the intensity of pixel values. The high magnitude pixel values are placed in a high topographical region, whereas low-intensity pixel values are placed in a lower region of a topographic map. The watershed approach is affected by the over-segmentation of data.

2.4 Cluster-Based Segmentation

These methods perform the segmentation of biomedical data content by computing membership values for each of the data points that exist in the blood image. The algorithm computes mean values for some k clusters present in the cell image. The more the data points are nearer to the mean value, the best will be their chance to appear in the particular cluster. The computation is performed by different types of distance measures (Manhattan distance, Euclidean distance, Minkowis-distance, etc.). There, exist different types of clustering methods (k-means, k-medoids, and fuzzy c-means) that can perform the partition of given data. Both the k-means and fuzzy c-means algorithms compute Euclidian-distance for the segmentation of data. The main difference between them lies in the assignment of a given data point to a particular cluster. The k-means algorithm uses a hard cluster-based approach, in which a data point is assigned to only one cluster at a time. Whereas fuzzy c-means use a soft clustering approach in which data points may belong to more than one cluster at a time. Instead of computing central means for data partition in K-medoids, we use data points as centers for subgrouping of data. Distance-based measures may not produce the best performance results on the segmentation of the cell images because the nature of leucocytes is irregular and non-specific to a particular location. These methods suffer from OSR and USR problems [6].

Garcia-Lamont et al. [11] have surveyed the most common recent approaches, for the segmentation of biomedical images. Since the color of the cell image acts as the base for discrimination of sub-components the authors have put their focus on the grey-level and color-based segmentation approach. The techniques that they have utilized are boundary cell detection, region growing, watershed segmentation for catchment basins, unsupervised segmentation using distance-based measures, and some deep learning methods. Anil-Kumar et al. [12] have done a review, on the recent segmentation methods used for the detection of leukaemia. The authors have highlighted most of the automatic disease detection-based approaches. The methods were categorized based on the procedure followed for the segmentation of cell images. Wang and Cao [13] propose a quick leukocyte nucleus segmentation method based on the component difference in RGB color space (B-G) because this difference of the color components (B and G) is very large in the leucocytes and platelets. Next, they retain the value of the WBC nucleus, by setting a filter that removes the content of platelets. Muntasa and Yusuf [14] have developed a model for the detection of leukaemia. They have computed different characteristics (energy, entropy, mean, variance, etc.) of the lymphocytes on the ALL-IDB dataset. The features were calculated by the different distance measures such as Euclidian distance, Manhattan, Canberra, and Chebyshev. They have reported the mean best accuracy of around 83% using the Euclidian distance measure. Acharya and Kumar [15] have developed a novel approach for the extraction of different cell features. Their objective was to develop an automatic solution, that will differ between abnormal and normal biomedical images. They have achieved their objective in two phases. First leucocytes were identified as a separate class in the blood image, next they have trained models on different characteristics of the leucocytes. They have classified leukaemia into three different classes of L1, L2, and L3. They have reported the mean best accuracy of 98%.

Considering the drawbacks of the recent literature, we have adopted an alternative solution (LRR) for analyzing biomedical image patterns. The approach works indirectly on the raw data [6]. Instead of distributing data points based on their distances, we are picking global representation for each of the independent data patterns present in the blood image. This avoids the need for placing all the related data points near the particular mean. There exist multiple approaches that can be used for subspace segmentation of biomedical image data. Recent work has used the following four methods for subspace segmentation of input data patterns. They are discussed as follows.

1. **A mixture of Gaussian** [16–18]: Gaussian is based on the probabilistic distribution of the set of input data points because the probabilistic distribution is Gaussian in nature. It divides the input set into the number of independent data patterns that is achieved by computing the distribution of statistical learning. Next, we do subspace segmentation of data. Which is performed by estimating the maximum likelihood of the expectation-maximization algorithm. Some follow iterative random sample consensus (RANSAC) that estimates the min-max value adopted by different subspaces. These methods perform well if the data is clean. However, their performance drops down if there are outliers (random noise, sample-specific) in the data. To improve the performance of the Gaussian approach, some have adopted Median flats and coding length characterization.

With the help of these refinements, somehow, we can improve the robustness, but the approach is difficult to optimize.

2. **Matrix Factorization** [19]: In the matrix factorization methodology the segmentation of a given data is computed by a matrix multiplication approach. Where the subspace segments are identified with the support pattern of the multiplicative matrix. To deal with outliers present in the data, we are modifying the methodology by incorporating regularized normal forms. With this modification, our objective function becomes non-convex. Which makes it difficult to optimize because the function may get stuck at local minima. It will degrade the performance of the model.
3. **Algebraic methods** [20, 21]: These methods describe subspaces by computing the gradient of the polynomial at each data point. Then the subspaces are identified by fitting data with polynomials. The most commonly used method in this category includes Generalized Principal Component Analysis (GPCA). The approach has shown good results on the clean data. Its performance degrades when the data is contaminated with noise because it becomes difficult to estimate the polynomial from the corrupted data. This cause may lead to the huge computational cost of GPCA. To resolve this issue some have utilized robust algebraic segmentation. But this approach performs well only on the low dimensional datasets in which subspaces are less in number.
4. **Spectral clustering-based approach** [22–24]: Some have picked subspace segmentation as a data partitioning problem. It works by constructing an affinity matrix from the given data. The matrix represents pairwise affinities between different data points. If the association between data points is high then they are placed in the same group, otherwise, they are placed in different groups. The final segmentation of the data is performed by the spectral clustering (Ncut, k-means) algorithm. There are several spectral clustering algorithms; sparse subspace clustering, spectral curvature clustering, spectral local best-fit flats, that have been used for subspace segmentation of data. The approaches differ from each other based on the construction of an affinity matrix. Most of them show good performance on noise-free data. If the data contains errors, sparse representation methods use l_1 regularization for subspace segmentation of data. Our objective is to obtain a coefficient matrix, where between class affinities are zero and within-class association is sparse. On some of the corrupted data sets, the l_1 regularization has not produced the best results. However, we can achieve this objective by minimizing ℓ_p $(p \leq 1)$. This condition makes objective function non-convex, thus we face difficulty in finding the optimal solution. This issue of convexity is addressed by the LRR approach, which reflects the global representation of data. Its objective function is convex that can be optimized in polynomial time.

3 Methodology

Blood cell image patterns are irregular and non-specific to a particular location. This requires the need for finding several independent structures at a more global level. This can be done by utilizing LRR that focuses more on the global representation of data. It does this by computing the lowest rank representation of the union of several input data structures. We start with the basic assumption that there are n number of data points in the biomedical image. Each of the data points has a close relationship with a particular sub-space because there exist different types of substructures in the image. Considering the point, we have observed that there are m number of sub-spaces $c_1, c_2, c_3 \ldots c_m$, each has a dimension of D_i, where $i = 1 \ldots m$. Data points are randomly distributed across different subspaces segments, where $dp = dp_1 \cup dp_2 \cup dp_3 \cup \ldots \cup dp_n$ is the partition of the input set. Our objective is to identify an appropriate class label, for each of the individual data points $[lb_1, lb_2, lb_3, \ldots, lb_N] \in \mathbb{N}^N$, where $lb_{i = 1 \ldots n}$ is the number of data points in the label i. The objective function of LRR is depicted in Eq. (10.3).

$$\min_{Z} rank(z), \quad s.t. \quad \mathrm{D} = \mathrm{DZ} \tag{10.3}$$

Where the rank penalty is responsible for creating a global grouping effect of data. This helps in discriminating substructures, in which data points that belong to a particular substructure are reflected with the same coefficient matrix. The rank penalty aims at creating a global grouping effect that reflects the underlying subspace structure of the data. In other words, data points belonging to the same subspace should have similar coefficient patterns. Direct rank minimization of the matrix is considered an NP-hard problem. It requires an exponential amount of time, for the convergence of objective function (10.3) to an optimal solution. We have avoided this computational complexity by using the heuristic solution that is a close convex surrogate to the rank function. That is done through the nuclear normal form function, which is the sum of singular values, where each singular value is responsible for different data patterns in the matrix. The nuclear norm reduces computational complexity because it is converged within a polynomial time. The reformulation of our objective function is given in Eq. (10.4).

$$\min_{Z} \| Z\|_*, \quad s.t. \quad \mathrm{D} = \mathrm{DZ} \tag{10.4}$$

Where $\|Z\|_*$ is the nuclear norm function. However, objective (10.4) is only useful when the data is known to be noise-free. As the quality of biomedical data depends upon several factors (environmental lighting conditions and resolution of the microscope). It is a rare case that the data is expected to be noiseless. Most of the time, the blood images are of medium to low quality. Which cannot make the appropriate discrimination of blood image sub-components. It indicates that there is a possibility of outliers present in the data (sample-specific and random corruptions). To deal with

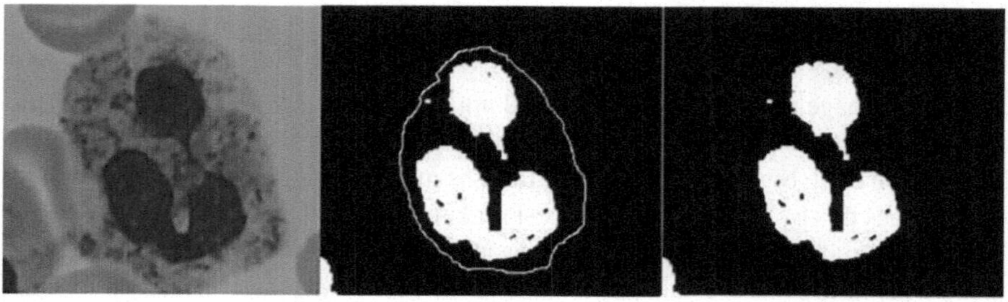

Fig. 10.2 (**a**) Blood image with single WBC cell. (**b**) Expected count should be single object. (**c**) Model counted three objects for the single nucleus

the matter, we need to reformulate our objective function, by incorporating noise-based normal forms (l_0, l_1, l_2 and Squared Frobenius Norm). It will induce regularization in the data so that we can minimize the impact of noise. This constraint changes the data point representation, to the objective function of $dp = x + n$. dp is the resultant data matrix that is decomposed into x and n. where x is noise-free data content of dp, it represents the underlying data content that is the union of subspaces, and n is used to represent noise in data. It has sparse column support. The resulting objective function is depicted in Eq. (10.5). The pseudo-code of LRR is depicted in Algorithm 10.1.

$$\min_{E,Z} \lambda \parallel E\parallel_F^2 + \parallel Z\parallel_*, \quad s.t. \quad \mathrm{D} = \mathrm{DZ} + E \tag{10.5}$$

This representation of data has addressed a number of new challenges in the recent work, and they are mentioned as follows.

- **Geometric shape retention of different blood components**: leucocytes are divided into two categories granulocytes and non-granulocytes. At the mature stage nucleus of granulocytes gets divided into several segments. During pre-processing recent approaches focus on retaining the leucocytic cell nucleus while the rest of the blood image components are removed as data noise. In [5] the authors have extracted the nucleus of a leucocytic cell given in Fig. 10.2. It produces the wrong count of the number of WBC'S. While doing manual count we have found there was only a single leucocytic cell nucleus but the automatic approach shows the count of three cells, for the single nucleus. The reason behind the multiple count problem is that the segmentation approach has focused on the local structure of data. This problem is addressed by the method, that will focus on the global structure of data. We have developed the LRR based solution. It has a focus on the global geometric representation of data. What we do, is that the problem is linearly decomposed into several independent patterns, in a joint coefficient matrix. The coefficient matrix is the global representation of the different data patterns, present in the biomedical image. It increases

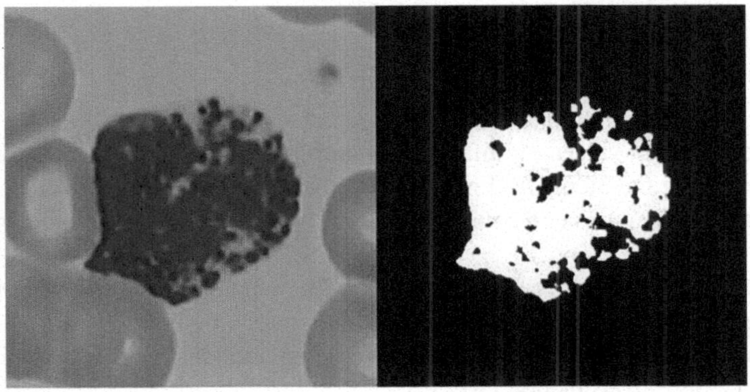

Fig. 10.3 (**a**) Input blood sample image. (**b**) Distorted WBC cell nucleus

sub-component representation, at a more global level. This results in addressing the multiple count problem of the boundary cell detection approach.

- **Recover the data from corrupted sub-samples**: to distinguish different types of data patterns present in the blood image, the data must be clean. If the data is affected by noise, it needs to be recovered from different types of corruption. To remove the noise from data, grey-level segmentation-based methodology sets some filters. Whereas filter is a constant value, and content that falls below the value of the threshold is removed from data. Sometimes the magnitude of noise class is very high that matches the cell nucleus intensity. Removing the data content of that filter value distorts the geometric structure of the nucleus. Its experimental result is depicted in Fig. 10.3. The approach that we are following handles noise indirectly. Which does not lead to impacts on the geometric shape of leucocytes. We have adopted regularization strategies that not only handle noise separately but also minimize its magnitude. The outliers that may affect the data include random corruptions, sample-specific noise, and outliers. We are considering three cases when dealing with noise.

  - If the input data pattern is clean, we consider the objective function depicted in (10.4). This is the rarest case because there always occurs some form of corruption in the data.
  - If there are random corruptions in the data, then we represent noise by matrix E. it has sparse column support. It is the most common type of noise, that persists in the data. This type of noise is difficult to judge because it has a random nature. We have incorporated a regularizer in Eq. (10.5) to handle the noise.
  - The final case that we are considering, is sample-specific corruption. These corruptions are limited to individual subspaces. The data becomes difficult to recover if there is an insufficient sampling of the input data pattern.

Algorithm 10.1 Low-Rank Representation

Input: A microscopic cell image dataset is read as input.

1. Set the input values for different parameters.

2. Represent the biomedical images in a joint matrix X, where rows represent different image features and columns indicate the number of blood samples in the dataset.

3. Perform the subspace segmentation of different cell image components.

(a) Generate the coefficient of the resultant data matrix by doing the linear decomposition of the dictionary D and the representation matrix Z. It is obtained by solving the objective function (10.5).

(b) Minimize the rank of the representation matrix by solving the nuclear norm.

(c) Handle the noise in the data by adopting the squared Frobenius norm as the regularization strategy.

4. Optimize the objective function (10.5) by the first-order method (LADMPSAP).

5. Perform the partitioning of the resultant data matrix by the Spectral clustering (NCUT) algorithm.

(a) Represent the data points in an undirected graph $X = (V, E)$.

(b) All the vertices that have high intra-strength are placed in the common set V_i and all those that are dissimilar to each other are partitioned into different sets V_i, V_j.

(c) Edges that show the highest degree of dissimilarity represent the cut of the graph.

(d) The optimal value of cut is obtained by finding association and disassociation measures between the different groups of data.

Output: Subclass label for each of the cell images.

3.1 *Global Optimal Convergence of LRR*

Since the objective function (10.5) is convex, it needs to be converged in polynomial time. Some of the well-known polynomial-time algorithms that can be used for optimization are discussed as follows.

1. **Interior point method**: these methods work best on small scale convex problems but when the data is scalable the algorithm lost its efficiency of producing optimal solutions. Most of the time our objective function has minimizing or maximization constraints, which makes it largely scalable. Consider the case of the following convex problems such as minimization of the nuclear norm, completion of matrix entries, low-rank coefficient representation, and principal component analysis. The interior-point methodology remains inefficient in solving the

mentioned problems because of the large-scale complex requirements ($O(q^6)$) for a single iteration. Where $q \times q$ represent the dimension of the matrix.

2. **First-order methods**: These methods are divided into constrained and non-constrained algorithms. The accelerated proximal growth (APG) is the most efficient, large scalable optimized non-constrained algorithm. It has a sufficient convergence rate of $O(K^{-2})$, where k is the number of iterations. To optimize large-scale constrained optimization algorithms, researchers mainly follow the alternating direction method (ADM). Here we place penalties in the objective functions that constrain the values of the coefficient matrix. Our objective is to minimize the distance between observed and estimated values. We penalize the representation matrix if there is an increase in the error. The said method of convergence is suitable for our objective function because the ADM provides the closest approximated result on the separable convex problems, and our objective function has adopted a similar behavior. Based on the unitary and non-unitary linear mappings of the representation matrices, multiple variants of the ADM have been designed. To produce global convergence solutions on the non-unitary mappings, a variant of ADM termed LADM (linearized alternating direction method) has been proposed. Both of the two methods work sufficiently on two block case i.e. n = 2. If the number of blocks is n > 2. The solution to the objective function may diverge because constraints on two block case are not sufficient for the multi-block case of n > 2. This does not guarantee the true convergence of objective function. The objective function that we are considering contains multiple blocks, which means there is a need for first-order methods that will do global convergence of multiple blocks in a polynomial time.

The program that suits best for convergence of our objective function is the linearized alternating direction method with parallel splitting and adaptive penalty (LADMPSAP). The approach is a combination of several methods (LADM, parallel splitting, and adaptive penalty). Where parallel splitting controls, the low rankness parameter of the coefficient matrix. Hence presents the global representation of the number of the independent pattern in low-rank format. The approach saves both storage and time of processing data because we do parallel distribution and execution of data. Whereas the adaptive penalty parameter enables the convergence of the objective function at a very fast rate because it adopts the penalty based on the least square error between the observed and approximated results. We don't need optimal penalty parameter values. The solution produced by LADMPSAP is the coefficient matrix, which represents the global grouping effect of data.

3.2 Partition of the Coefficient Matrix by Using Normalized-Cut

To perform the efficient partitioning of the data. We compute a linear decomposed block diagonal coefficient matrix from the input data pattern. The data patterns contain different types of components that are partitioned into the number of independent structures in a single coefficient matrix. The resultant data matrix is expected to be block diagonal. Considering this case, we form a similarity matrix of it. This symmetric matrix is passed as an input to the clustering algorithm. There were multiple provisions for the selection of the partitioning algorithm. Because of the high connectedness of data, we have chosen N-cut (Normalized cut) as our partitioning algorithm. It works similarly to the partitioning of the graph. The procedure works in a graph-based manner, in which we represent the data points as an undirected graph $X = (V, E)$. Where each point in the coefficient matrix is treated as a node and connectivity between each pair of data points is represented by an edge. The connection represents the weight $M(i,j)$ between nodes i and j. Our objective is to cluster the set of vertices $V_1, V_2, \ldots, V_n$. The measure that is used to partition the vertices is based on the similarity between the data points. All the vertices that have high intra-strength are placed in the common set V_i and all those that are dissimilar to each other are partitioned into different sets V_i, V_j. It means data points are placed in the same set if their within-cluster variance is low and they are partitioned into different groups if their between-class variance is high. Where the cut of the graph is an edge, whose removal increases the number of components. The cut is said to be normal if the weight associated with the edge is minimal. However, this has been considered as Np complete problem because there is an exponential number of ways through which minimal cut can be found. In (10.6) we have formulated the bi-partition (P, Q) of the graph $X = (V, E)$ that computes the degree of dissimilarity between two vertices. Edges that have the highest degree of dissimilarity need to be removed, in graph theory, this edge is called the cut of the graph.

$$cut(P,Q) = \sum_{i\epsilon P, j\epsilon B} \omega(i,j) \tag{10.6}$$

To find the optimal value of cut we use the measure of association and disassociation between the different groups of data. Where cut cost is the ratio of connection between two individual nodes to the edge connection of all nodes in the graph. This measure of disassociation is called N-cut. It is depicted in Eq. (10.7).

$$N_{cut}(P,Q) = \frac{cut(P,Q)}{asso(P,V)} + \frac{cut(P,Q)}{asso(Q,V)} \tag{10.7}$$

where $asso(P, V)$ is the link from nodes in P to all nodes in the graph, and $asso(Q, V)$ is the connection from nodes in Q to all nodes. We can use this to derive the optimal cut value that is the percentage of connections from a small set of nodes to the total of all the nodes in the graph. Total normalized connection within the group is defined by Eq. (10.8).

$$N_{asso}(P,Q) = \frac{asso(P,P)}{asso(P,V)} + \frac{asso(Q,Q)}{asso(B,V)} \tag{10.8}$$

where $asso(P, P)$ and $asso(Q, Q)$ are the edges that connect the nodes within A and B respectively. The relationship between association and disassociation can be reflected as follows:

$$\begin{aligned} N_{cut}(P,Q) &= \frac{cut(P,Q)}{asso(P,V)} + \frac{cut(P,Q)}{asso(Q,V)} \\ &= \frac{asso(P,V) - asso(P,P)}{asso(P,V)} + \frac{asso(Q,V) - asso(Q,Q)}{asso(Q,V)} \\ &= 2 - \left(\frac{asso(P,P)}{asso(P,V)} + \frac{asso(Q,Q)}{asso(Q,V)}\right) \\ &= 2 - N_{asso}(P,Q) \end{aligned}$$

Our objective is to minimize the within-cluster variation and maximize the between-class variation. The two measures can be solved simultaneously because they have a close relationship with each other. This can be done, by finding the minimal value of NCUT, but it is considered an NP-complete problem. We can solve this problem in polynomial time by finding the least eigenvectors of the laplacian matrix. The second least value of the eigenvector is considered as an optimal solution to the problem.

Computation of optimal values for NCUT Let the vertices of the graph, G, contain data from two components P *and* Q. The dimensional indicator $N = |V|$ of a graph is represented in s. The value of $s = 1$ if data points belong to P, otherwise $s = -1$. The relationship of node i, to other nodes, is represented by the weight matrix $w_i = \sum_j a_{(i,j)}$. With the help of *sandw* the equation of Ncut can be written as:

$$\begin{aligned} N_{cut}(P,Q) &= \frac{cut(P,Q)}{asso(P,V)} + \frac{cut(P,Q)}{asso(Q,V)} \\ &= \frac{\sum_{(s_i>0, s_j<0)} - \omega_{ij} s_i s_j}{\sum_{x_i>0} w_i} \\ &\quad + \frac{\sum_{(s_i<0, s_j>0)} - \omega_{ij} s_i s_j}{\sum_{x_i<0} w_i} \end{aligned}$$

Let Z be a block diagonal affinity matrix with z_i on its main diagonal and A be a symmetric matrix generated from Z. $A(i,j) = a(i,j), k = \frac{\sum_{s_i>0} w_i}{\sum_i w_i}$, and **1** be a column vector of all ones. The indicator vectors $\frac{1+s}{2}$ and $\frac{1-s}{2}$, are used to control direction for $s_i > 0$ and $s_i < 0$. The objective can be formulated as:

$$= \frac{(1+s)^T(Z-A)(1+s)}{k1^T Z1} + \frac{(1-s)^T(Z-A)(1-s)}{(1-k)1^T Z1}$$
$$= \frac{\left(s^T(Z-A)s + 1^T(Z-A)1\right)}{k(1-k)1^T Z1} + \frac{2(1-2k)1^T(Z-A)s}{k(1-k)1^T Z1}$$

The given equation can further be expanded by setting $\alpha(s) = s^T(Z - A)s$, $\beta(x) = 1^T(Z - A)s$, + $\gamma = 1^T(Z - A)1,\ and\ M = 1^T Z1$:

$$= \frac{(\alpha(s)+\gamma) + 2(1-2k)\beta(s)}{k(1-k)M}$$
$$= \frac{(\alpha(s)+\gamma) + 2(1-2k)\beta(s)}{k(1-k)M} - \frac{2(\alpha(s)+\gamma)}{M} + \frac{2\alpha(s)}{M}\frac{2\gamma}{M}$$

Constant terms from this can be dropped and the resultant equation from this can be represented as:

$$= \frac{(1-2k+2k^2)(\alpha(s)+\gamma) + 2(1-2k)\beta(s)}{k(1-k)M} + \frac{2\alpha(s)}{M}$$
$$= \frac{\frac{(1-2k+2k^2)}{(1-k)^2}(\alpha(s)+\gamma) + \frac{2(1-2k)}{(1-k)^2}\beta(s)}{\frac{k}{1-k}M} + \frac{2\alpha(s)}{M}$$

Setting $c = \frac{k}{1-k}\ and\ \gamma = 0$, the equation becomes,

$$= \frac{(1+c^2)(\alpha(s)+\gamma)+2(1-c^2)\beta(s)}{cM} + \frac{2c\alpha(s)}{cM}$$
$$= \frac{(1+c^2)(\alpha(s)+\gamma)}{cM} + \frac{2(1-c^2)\beta(s)}{cM} + \frac{2c\alpha(s)}{cM} - \frac{2c\gamma}{cM}$$
$$= \frac{(1+c^2)\left(s^T(Z-A)s+1^T(Z-A)1\right)}{cZ1}$$
$$+ \frac{2(1-c^2)1^T(Z-A)s}{c1^TZ1}$$
$$+ \frac{2cs^T(Z-A)s}{c1^TZ1} - \frac{2c1^T(Z-A)1}{c1^TZ1}$$
$$= \frac{(1+s)^T(Z-A)(1+s)}{c1^TZ1}$$
$$+ \frac{c^2(1-s)^T(Z-A)(1-s)}{c1^TZ1}$$
$$- \frac{2c(1-s)^T(Z-A)(1+s)}{c1^TZ1}$$
$$= \frac{[(1+s)-c(1-s)]^T(Z-A)[(1+s)-c(1-s)}{c1^TZ1}$$

Let the value of $f = (1 + s) - c(1 - s)$, the equation can be written as,

$$f^TZ1 = \sum_{s_i>0} a_i - c\sum_{s_i<0} a_i = 0$$

since $c = \frac{k}{1-k} = \frac{\sum_{x_i>0} w_i}{\sum_{x_i>0} w_i}$, then

$$\begin{aligned} f^TZf &= \sum\nolimits_{s_i>0} a_i + c^2\sum\nolimits_{s_i<0} a_i \\ &= c\sum\nolimits_{s_i<0} a_i + c^2\sum\nolimits_{s_i<0} a_i \\ &= c\sum\nolimits_{s_i<0} a_i + c^2\sum\nolimits_{s_i<0} a_i \\ &= c1^TZ1 \end{aligned}$$

Keeping the terms together we get:

$$min\ {}_sN_{cut(s)} = min\ {}_f \frac{f^T(Z-A)f}{f^TZf} \tag{10.9}$$

The condition $f(i)\epsilon\{1, -c\}$ and $f^TZ1 = 0$ is the Rayleigh quotient. Setting real values for f can minimize (10.9) by solving eigenvalue in Eq. (10.10).

$$(Z - A)f = \lambda Zf \tag{10.10}$$

Dimensional vector indicator, s has placed two different constraints on f. The constraint $f^T Z1 = 0$ can be satisfied by f. This is done by transforming Eq. (10.10) to the general eigenvalue system in Eq. (10.11).

$$(Z - A)Z^{-\frac{1}{2}}d = \lambda d \tag{10.11}$$

Let $d = Z^{\frac{1}{2}}f$, it can be verified that $d_0 = Z^{\frac{1}{2}}1$ is the smallest eigenvector of (10.11) with the eigenvalue 0. The second smallest eigenvector of (10.11) is d_1. It is perpendicular to d_0 because all eigenvectors of (10.11) are perpendicular to each other. The matrix $(Z - A)$ contains non-negative values. It is a positive semidefinite matrix that is also called a Laplacian matrix.

Rayleigh quotient basic fact Let s be a constraint on a real symmetric matrix H. Where s is orthogonal to $k - 1$ smallest eigenvectors $s_1, s_2, \ldots, s_k$. Its quotient $\frac{s^T Hs}{sTs}$ is minimized, by the second smallest eigenvector of s_k. Keeping this consideration, we get:

$$d_1 = arg.\,min_{\,d^T d_0 = 0} \frac{d^T Z^{-\frac{1}{2}}(Z - A)Z^{-\frac{1}{2}}d}{d^T d}$$

$$c_1 = arg.\,min_{\,c^T Z1 = 0} \frac{f^T (Z - A)f}{f^T Df},$$

From the analysis, we can conclude that the second smallest eigenvector is the optimal solution to (10.10). It is obtained by minimizing the Eq. (10.12).

$$inf_{\;f^T Z1 = 0} \frac{\sum_i \sum_j (f(i) - f(j))^2 \omega_{ij}}{\sum_i f(i)^2 a(i)} \tag{10.12}$$

4 Result and Discussions

We have evaluated our methodology on ALL-IDB (Acute Lymphoblastic Leukaemia-International Database) and biomedical image (Chest, Knee, and Brain-MRI) datasets. ALL-IDB is an international database. It contains microscopic cell images of leukaemia and non-leukaemia patients. The dataset is divided into two groups, segmented and non-segmented images. The segmented set contains around 260 blood images where 130 belong to leukaemia and the remaining 130 belong to normal patients. This dataset requires only classification because it is already segmented. The non-segmented set contains around 108 blood images, among

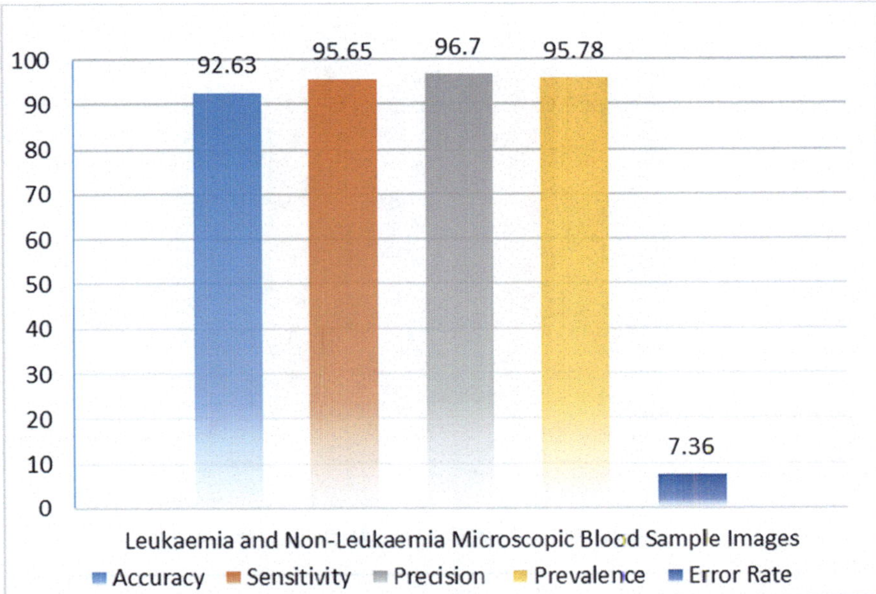

Fig. 10.4 Performance of the model on ALL-IDB dataset

them 46 belong to leukaemia and the remaining 62 belong to non-leukaemia patients. This subset needs, both the segmentation and classification of blood images. We have utilized a non-segmented ALL-IDB dataset for evaluation in which we have performed subspace segmentation and clustering. The blood images in a dataset are of non-uniform size. To make them in a particular dimension, we have resampled the size of each blood image, to the dimension of $1200 * 1200 * 3$. All the images of a dataset are placed in a joint data matrix of dimension $(1200 * 1200 * 3 * 108)$, where each image is represented as a single column vector in the joint matrix. The resultant data matrix is then used as input to the model where we obtain an independent representation of leukaemia and non-leukaemia images. The representation is performed by obtaining a singular value decomposition of data. Next, we have partitioned the coefficient matrix by using N-cut. The performance of the concerned methodology on the ALL-IDB dataset is depicted in Fig. 10.4. The formulation of the different performance measures is depicted in Eqs. (10.13–10.15).

$$Accuracy = \frac{TP + TN}{Total\ data} \tag{10.13}$$

$$Sensitivity = \frac{TP}{TP + FN} \tag{10.14}$$

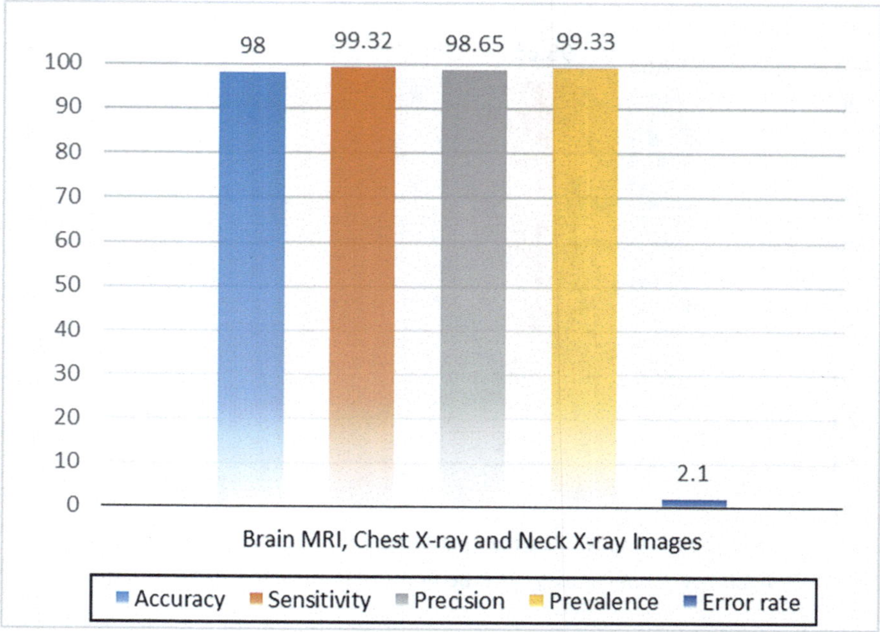

Fig. 10.5 Performance of the model on Biomedical image dataset

$$Precision = \frac{TP}{TP + FP} \tag{10.15}$$

To judge the efficiency of our adopted model, we have also evaluated it on the biomedical image dataset. It contains samples from three different classes of images such as chest X-ray, Knee X-ray, and Brain MRI images. We have collected a total of 150 images from different sources (Internet and Kaggle). The size of these input data patterns was resampled, to the dimension of $300 * 300 * 1$. Each of the biomedical images is represented in a joint matrix as a column vector, hitting the total dimension to the extent of $300 * 300 * 150$.

Our main objective was to address some of the challenging problems that exist in the recent literature. This has been done by utilizing a low-rank subspace segmentation-based approach. It classifies each of the biomedical images, in their appropriate groups by doing a representation and partitioning of data. Where representation generates different subspace segments in the data, and N-cut partitions these data patterns in their specified classes. The result of the LRR on the biomedical image dataset is depicted in Fig. 10.5. The model has shown efficient performance on the dataset as compared to the ALL-IDB. We have performed consistent experiments to judge the reliability of the model. We have reported mean performance measures for all the experiments.

We have compared the performance of our model with the different machine learning methods. The comparison was done with the studies of Thanh et al. [25],

Table 10.2 Comparison of different models with our adopted approach

Study	Dataset Used	Segmentation method	Classifier	Accuracy
Thanh et al. [25]	ALL-DB	NA	CNN	96.60%
Nizar Ahmad et al. [27]	ALL-DB ALL-DB ALL-DB ALL-DB ALL-DB	NA	CNN NB DT KNN SVM	88.25% 69.69% 62.94% 58.57% 50.09%
Rawat et al. [26]	ALL-DB	Threshold-based method	SVM	87%
Feilong Cao et al. [6]	ALL-DB	Hybrid-Low-Rank-Representation	NA	NR
LRR NA (Not Attended) NR (Not Recorded)	ALL-DB	Low-Rank-Representation	NCUT	92.63

Rawat et al. [26] Feilong Cao et al. [6] and Nizar Ahmad et al. [27]. The authors have adopted several different approaches for the segmentation and classification of cell images. They have followed the threshold-based, and low-rank representation approaches for the segmentation of blood cells. Whereas, for the subgrouping of biomedical data they have utilized classifiers like SVM (Support Vector Machine), NB (Naïve Bayes), DT (Decision Tree), KNN (k-Nearest-Neighbor) and CNN (Convolutional Neural Network). Table 10.2 depicts the comparison of the different literature studies versus our proposed work. Our developed approach has shown comparatively higher performance in comparison to some recent studies.

5 Conclusion

We have utilized a subspace segmentation-based approach for the segmentation and classification of cell images in their appropriate classes. It is performed, based on the similarity in the geometric pattern of different substructures of the blood cell image. The main intuition behind the utilization of low-rank representation-based models was to address some of the challenges that exist in the automatic disease detection process. This has been done by mapping the biological observation to the representation data matrices. Which is the minimal rank presentation of the input data pattern that not only reduces the dimensional size of the data but also reduces the computational time required to process the given dataset. Though the adopted approach has shown efficient results, some of the cell images were not discriminated appropriately. There is a need to improve the framework of the concerning methodology that will be more robust to outliers and varying structures present in the data.

References

1. The Leukemia & Lymphoma Society, New York. https://www.ils.org/facts-anstatistics. Accessed 16 Nov 2019.
2. Cancer Research UK. http://www.cancerresearchuk.org. Accessed 16 Nov 2019.
3. Blood diseases (1935) Br Med J 2(3907): 998–999. What are blood tests? National Heart, Lung, and Blood Institute (NHLBI). http://www.nhlbi.nih.gov/health/health-topics/topics/bdt/. Accessed 2 May 2012.
4. What are blood tests? National Heart, Lung, and Blood Institute (NHLBI). http://www.nhlbi.nih.gov/health/health-topics/topics/bdt/. Accessed 2 May 2012
5. Sheikh IM, Chachoo MA (2020) Advanced machine learning for leukaemia detection based on white blood cell segmentation. In: Badica C, Liatsis P, Kharb L, Chahal D (eds) Information, communication and computing technology. ICICCT 2020, Communications in computer and information science, vol 1170. Springer, Singapore. https://doi.org/10.1007/978-981-15-9671-1_17
6. Cao F, Cai M, Chu J et al (2017) A novel segmentation algorithm for nucleus in white blood cells based on low-rank representation. Neural Comput Applic 28:503–511
7. Elhamifar E, Vidal R (2009) Sparse subspace clustering. In: IEEE conference on computer vision and pattern recognition, pp 2790–2797
8. Tang K, Liu R, Su Z, Zhang J (2014) Structure-constrained low-rank representation. IEEE Trans Neural Netw Learn Syst 25(12):2167–2179. https://doi.org/10.1109/TNNLS.2014.2306063
9. Loan NA, Parah SA, Sheikh JA, Akhoon JA, Bhat GM (2017) Hiding electronic patient record (epr) in medical images: a high capacity and computationally efficient technique for e-healthcare applications. J Biomed Inform 73:125–136
10. Parah SA, Ahad F, Sheikh JA, Bhat GM (2017) Hiding clinical information in medical images: a new high capacity and reversible data hiding technique. J Biomed Inform 66:214–230
11. Garcia-Lamont F, Cervantes J, Lopez A, Rodriguez L (2018) Segmentation of images by color features: a survey. Neurocomputing 292:1–27. https://doi.org/10.1016/j.neucom.2018.01.091
12. Anilkumar KK, Manoj VJ, Sagi TM (2020) A survey on image segmentation of blood and bone marrow smear images with emphasis to automated detection of Leukemia. Biocybernet Biomed Eng 40(4):1406–1420. https://doi.org/10.1016/j.bbe.2020.08.010
13. Wang Y, Cao Y (2019) Quick leukocyte nucleus segmentation in leukocyte counting. Comput Math Methods Med 2. https://doi.org/10.1155/2019/3072498
14. Muntasa A, Yusuf M (2019) Modeling of the acute lymphoblastic leukaemia detection based on the principal object characteristics of the color image. Proc Comput Sci 157:87–98. https://doi.org/10.1016/j.procs.2019.08.145
15. Acharya V, Kumar P (2019) Detection of acute lymphoblastic leukaemia using image segmentation and data mining algorithms. Med Biol Eng Comput 57(8):1783–1811. https://doi.org/10.1007/s11517-019-01984-1
16. Lu C, Wang S (2020) Performance degradation prediction based on a Gaussian mixture model and optimized support vector regression for an aviation piston pump. Sensors (Switzerland) 20(14):1–21. https://doi.org/10.3390/s20143854
17. Frühwirth R (2020) Regression with Gaussian mixture models applied to track fitting. Instruments 4(3):25. https://doi.org/10.3390/instruments4030025
18. Budiarto A, Mahesworo B, Hidayat AA, Nurlaila I (2020) Gaussian mixture model implementation for population stratification estimation from genomics data Gaussian mixture model implementation for population stratification estimation from genomics data. In: International conference on computer science and computational intelligence
19. Shah S (2018) Introduction to matrix factorization for recommender systems. https://doi.org/10.5281/zenodo.3344938.

20. Moysisy L, Karampetakis NP (2018) Algebraic methods for the construction of algebraic-difference equations with desired behavior. Electron J Linear Algebra 34(1):1–17. https://doi.org/10.13001/1081-3810.3741
21. Bird R, Gibbons J, Mu S-C (2002) Algebraic methods for optimization problems. pp 282–309. https://doi.org/10.1007/3-540-47797-7_8.
22. Jia H, Ding S, Xu X, Nie R (2014) The latest research progress on spectral clustering. Neural Comput Applic 24(7–8):1477–1486
23. Qing H, Wang J (2020) Dual regularized Laplacian spectral clustering methods on community detection. ArXiv 2020:1–43
24. Rashid M, Singh H, Goyal V (2019) Cloud storage privacy in health care systems based on IP and geo-location validation using K-mean clustering technique. Int J E-Health Med Commun 10(4):54–65
25. Thanh TTP, Caleb V, Sukhrob A, Suk-Hwan L, Ki-Ryong K (2018) Leukemia blood cell image classification using convolutional neural network. Int J Comput Theory Eng 10(2):54–58
26. Rawat J, Sing A, Bhaduaria H, Virmani J, Devgun J (2017) Classification of acute lymphoblastic leukaemia using hybrid hierarchical classifiers. Multimedia Tools Appl 76(18): 1310–1317
27. Ahmed N, Yigit A, Isik Z, Alpkocak A (2019) Identification of leukaemia subtypes from microscopic images using convolutional neural network. Diagnostics 9(3):104

Chapter 11
Performance Comparison of Imputation Methods for Heart Disease Prediction

Shweta A. Tiwaskar and Prasad Gokhale

Contents

1 Introduction

Health care data is expected to increase at a compound annual growth rate (CAGR) of 36% by 2025 [1] but due to the recent pandemic, expert says Electronic Health Records/data adaption rates are higher than ever, at around 89% [2]. This increase in medical data also poses many challenges, the most important being the missing data. Handling missing data is crucial. According to researchers, the main consequences of not handling missing data are (a) loss of information (b) adverse effects on decisions. Missing data affect the efficient decision-making process due to (1) it might be the deciding factor in disease prediction, (2) It may affect the performance of the classifier, (3) it may negatively impact the analysis of the result, and (4) It can lead to a biased result. So precise data analysis needs correct filling of the missing data. However, this decision needs a correct understanding of the alternative options and their relative performances. In this study, we will evaluate the performance of

S. A. Tiwaskar (✉) · P. Gokhale
Department of Computer Engineering, Vishwakarma University, Pune, India
e-mail: shweta.tiwaskar-025@vupune.ac.in

S. A. Parah et al. (eds.), *Artificial Intelligence for Innovative Healthcare Informatics*,
https://doi.org/10.1007/978-3-030-96569-3_11

four methods: mean, median, KNNI, and Iterative imputation. This is the main motivation of this study.

In most of the classification studies of missing data, the performance of the classification method is evaluated only using accuracy. But accuracy can show overpromising and unreasonable results, particularly for imbalanced datasets. In this study relative performance will be evaluated using two performance metrics namely Accuracy and Mcoff. Mcoff is a more reliable evaluation measure as it gives a good score only if the prediction attains superior results in all groups of the confusion matrix. Missing data has three kinds of missing mechanisms [3] e.g. Missing Completely at Random (MCAR), Missing at Random (MAR), and Not Missing at Random (NMAR). In MCAR, the pattern of the missing value of an attribute is random and not related to that particular attribute or any other attribute in the dataset. In MAR, the probability of the missing value of an attribute is not related to that particular attribute, but the other attributes in the dataset. In NMAR, the probability of missing data relies on the missing data itself. According to earlier research, imputation techniques depend on the particular missing mechanism [4]. Researchers also say that knowledge of the missing mechanism is crucial in selecting the right data analysis method [5]. So it is necessary to identify the applicable missing mechanism when missing data occurs. This work is based on the MCAR type missing mechanism, as real data lies somewhere in between MAR and MCAR [6]. Also, verifications with MAR and NMAR mechanisms are very difficult as they depend on unobserved data. Missing data is handled by two types of methods i.e. deletion and imputation methods. The deletion method deletes the records so it may be used while dealing with medical data having less missingness in the medical records of patients [7]. However, loss of crucial data, creating invalid samples, and causing research deviation are some of the disadvantages of this method. Moreover, deletion should only be used for a very small percentage (5%) of missingness [8].

The contribution of this work is: It studies statistics-based and ML-based imputation methods. It gives a comprehensive empirical comparison of four imputation methods on a Cleveland heart disease dataset. The empirical evaluation of relative performance clearly shows the inferiority of some common imputation methods. One of the imputation methods, i.e. iterative imputation, clearly shows improved performance in both the evaluation criteria as compared to the other three imputation techniques. The following discussion examines the criteria under which these imputation techniques perform better or worse.

The rest of this chapter is organized as follows Sect. 2 describes various Imputation methods. In Sect. 3, we describe the related work done. Section 4 describes the experimental setup, dataset, and performance metric. Section 5 includes experimental results and analysis of the results using two performance metrics for various missing ratios. We conclude with a discussion on our results in Sect. 6.

2 Imputation Methods

Two statistics-based, and two ML-based, missing data imputation methods namely—Mean, Median, KNNI, and Multivariate Iterative Imputation are used to fill in the missing values in our dataset, and to create the corresponding four complete datasets.

Mean and median are simple and fast imputation methods. They are suitable for imputing numerical attributes. Mode imputation is generally used for imputing categorical attributes. In mean imputation, the average value of the attribute is used to impute the missing value. Mean imputation is very easy to implement and a popular technique. With this technique, the sample mean of the missing attribute does not change, however, it attenuates any correlation between the attributes that are imputed, and variability in the data is not represented correctly. Covariance between imputed and original data is misrepresented. This misrepresentation increases with an increase in MR [6, 9, 10]. In median imputation, the median value of the attribute is used to fill in the missing value. According to the researcher, mean and median are almost similar if the numerical attribute has a normal distribution. Median is a superior representation for skewed distribution. If the missingness in the data is of NMAR type Mean, Median, and mode imputation techniques are not preferred [11–13].

Generally, datasets have correlated attributes, which can be used for imputing missing data. Statistics-based methods—mean and median—do not consider the correlation of the attributes in the dataset, whereas ML-based methods use these correlated attributes to predict the missing data. One of the ML-based imputation methods is KNNI which finds K Nearest Neighbor, similar to the existing data, and imputes a value from them. The nearest neighbor is selected by some distance function. Euclidean distance, Minkowsky, cosine similarity measures, and Chi-square are some of the distance functions used in KNN. However, the most popular is the Euclidean distance. KNN is a supervised ML method. KNN is based on the fact that items which are near to each other are similar [14–16]. KNNI is suitable for both numerical and categorical attributes. In imputation of numerical attributes, the mean of the K Nearest Neighbors is taken, and in categorical attributes, the mode of the K Nearest Neighbors is taken [17]. When the number of attributes is large, an imputation method like KNNI is applied to impute the missing data, and it will help to reduce the cost of handling missing values. Mostly, the center of attention of current imputation research is focused on improving classification accuracy [4, 17].

Another dynamic ML-based method is Iterative Imputation. In iterative imputer, missing data is filled in with the rest of the features of the dataset. In iterative imputation, imputation is performed in ascending order of missingness, a feature with a minimum number of missing values is imputed first so that it can participate in predicting the subsequent features. This process is repeated multiple times. Generally, the Bayesian-Ridge model is used in iterative imputation, for estimating missing attributes, from the remaining attributes, in a dataset. The choice of the imputation method is influenced by the percentage of missingness and scenario [18].

3 Related Work

Literature mentions various works done on imputing missing values in the medical data. Zeng et al. [19], used Euclidean distance KNN, correlation coefficient KNN, and mean imputation technique to fill the missing medical data. They compared the performance of these imputation techniques using random forest, classification, and regression tree algorithms. However, they considered only accuracy as the evaluation criteria for classification, and the MR was from 1% to 40%. G. Madhu et al. [20], handled the medical dataset with MR 1.98% to 50.65%. They have used KNN, iterative, Miss Forest, and XGBoost imputation for filling the missing data, and performance is evaluated using the XGBoost classifier. However, the missing data approaches failed in cases with more than 50% MR. XGBoost works on the parallel tree boosting concept [21]. Anindita et al. [22], used multiple imputations and principal component analysis to fill missing values in the hepatitis dataset having 20 features and 155 instances MR was 48%. The classification was done by the Multilayer Perceptron algorithm. Performance was evaluated by accuracy and error rate. Instance selection was applied for selecting important attributes of the dataset. The aim was to enhance the accuracy of the analysis of the data which had missing values with the arbitrary pattern.

Hunt [23], used Pima and a cancer data set along with wine and Iris. Synthetic missingness was generated for 10–50% of MCAR type. Missing value was imputed using the R package and WEKA classifier with tenfold cross-validation. The authors observed that classifier accuracy decreases for mean, median and KNN imputation as the percentage of MR increases. The future direction of research is evaluating the consequences of imputation on the classification accuracy for the multiclass dataset. Purwar and Singh [24], analyzed various imputation techniques, on three medical datasets namely—breast cancer, hepatitis, and diabetes using Simple K-means clustering, and applied the number one technique to a data set. The authors used a combination of K-means clustering with Multilayer Perceptron. However, the authors did not handle noise in the dataset. The authors handled only binary datasets. Arasu and Thirumalaiselvi [25], proposed Weighted Average Ensemble Learning Imputation to fill the missing values in the kidney dataset, to improve the prediction of kidney disease. As per the study, most of the work is done on binary medical datasets and mostly accuracy is used as evaluation criteria. Analysis of the imputation techniques is shown in Table 11.1.

Table 11.1 Analysis of imputation technique

Study	Dataset	Sample size	No. of variables	Class	Technique used
Purwar	Pima	768	8	Binary	K-means clustering with multilayer perceptron
	Breast	683	9	Binary	
	Hepatitis	155	19	Binary	
Arasu	Kidney	400	23	Binary	Weighted average ensemble learning imputation
Anandita	Hepatitis	155	20	Binary	Multiple imputation and PCA
Hunt	Pima	768	8	Binary	Hot deck, iterative robust model-based, missForest imputation
	Prostate cancer wine	506 178	12 13	Binary Multiclass	
	Iris	150	4	Multiclass	
Madhu	Cleveland	303	13	Multiclass	KNN, iterative, Miss Forest, and XGBoost imputation
	Diabetes	768	8	Binary	
	Dermatology	366	34	Multiclass	
	Hepatitis	155	19	Binary	
	Mammographic	961	5	Binary	
	Wisconsin	699	9	Binary	
Zeng	TCM Medical dataset	531	43	Binary	Euclidean distance KNN, correlation coefficient KNN and mean imputation technique classifier is CART algorithm

4 Experimental Setup

The purpose of this experiment was to perform comparative analysis for MCAR Multivariate Missing pattern and evaluate the impact of four missing data imputation methods against four classifiers Machine Learning (ML) algorithms for 10–60% missing ratios (MR). The Relative Performance of the imputation methods with four classifiers was evaluated using two performance metrics.

4.1 Dataset

All the experiments were performed on the Cleveland Heart disease dataset taken from the UCI repository. This dataset contains 13 attributes namely Age, Gender, Chest pain type (CP), Resting Blood Pressure (trestbps), Cholesterol (chol), Fasting Blood Sugar (fbs), Resting ECG results (restecg), Maximum Heart Rate Achieved (thalach), Exercise-induced Angina (exang), Oldpeak, Vessels colored by Fluroscopy (ca), Thalassemia (thal) are used to predict heart disease and one target variable which indicates heart disease in the patient on various scales, from 0 to 4. 0 scale shows heart disease is absent. Values from 1 to 4 indicate the severity of the disease. We changed the values from 1 to 4 as 1. So, the dataset now shows only the presence and absence of heart disease.

The total number of samples in the UCI heart disease dataset is 303. Out of these 303 samples, 6 samples were having missing values in the input variables ca and thal, so those samples were deleted and processing was done with the remaining 297 samples. In 297 samples that are used for processing, 137 samples are of heart disease present cases and 160 samples are of heart disease absent cases. In these 297 samples, missingness is synthetically generated. All the experiments were conducted on Python 3.8 Anaconda Jupyter Notebook.

4.2 Performance Metrics

Relative Performance of four imputation methods with four classifiers namely—Decision Tree (DT), K-Nearest Neighbour (KNN), Linear Discriminant Analysis (LDA), and Logistic Regression (LR) were evaluated using two performance metrics namely—Accuracy and Mcoff. Many times we use classification accuracy as an evaluation criterion for our model, however, it is not enough to truly judge our model. Accuracy is the most common evaluation criteria in binary classification, but it can show overpromising and unreasonable results, particularly for imbalanced datasets. However, Mcoff is a more reliable evaluation measure as it gives a good score only if the prediction obtained good results in all of the four confusion matrix categories i.e. true positive, true negative, false positive, and false negative, proportionally both to the size of positive elements and the size of negative elements in the dataset.

4.3 Generation of MCAR Type Missingness in the Dataset

In these 297 samples of the heart disease dataset, synthetic missingness was generated using the MCAR mechanism. This missingness was generated randomly, in more than one variable of the dataset, called multivariate configuration, using a python program based on the binomial distribution. Binomial is a type of distribution as given in Eq. (11.1) which has two possible outcomes. It is discrete distribution having three parameters.

$$\mathsf{M} = \mathsf{np.random.binomial}\ (\mathsf{n}, \mathsf{p}, \mathsf{size})$$

1. n = Number of trials ($n \geq 0$)
2. P = probability of success
3. Size i.e. shape of the Output data

The probability density for the binomial distribution is

$$P(N) = \binom{n}{N} p^N (1-p)^{n-N} \tag{11.1}$$

The binomial distribution and the Bernoulli distribution have a close relation. As per Washington State University, "If each Bernoulli trial is independent, then the number of successes in Bernoulli trials has Binomial Distribution. Otherwise, the Bernoulli distribution is the Binomial Distribution with n = 1". Twala et al. [26] have used the Bernoulli trial for generating synthetic missingness in univariate as well as in multivariate configuration [27]. Synthetic missingness was generated for various missing ratios like 10–60% in the input features and the corresponding six incomplete datasets were generated. The target variable was never missing. Missing data in these six datasets were imputed (filled) using mean, median, KNNI, and iterative imputation methods to generate 6 datasets of mean, 6 datasets of the median, 6 datasets of KNNI, and 6 datasets of iterative total 24 imputed datasets. Experimentation was done on a total of 25 datasets, 24 imputed and one original dataset with a sample size of 297.

Experiments were performed on these 25 datasets, for heart disease prediction, using four classifiers namely—DT, KNN, LDA, and LR with mean, median, KNNI, and multivariate iterative imputation methods. For mean and median we have imported 'SimpleImputer' from "sklearn.Impute". KNNI imputation is done using KNNImputer and Iterative imputation is done using Iterative Imputer from "sklearn. Impute". For every experiment, tenfold cross-validation is used to assess the performance of all the models. Every experiment was run 10 times so that every sample of the dataset was tested. Finally, the mean of the results of all the ten experiments was considered as the final result. The performance of all the classifiers was evaluated using two performance metrics. In all the experiments, for LDA classifiers default settings are used. Whereas for other classifiers, settings are changed as follows, in LR, the solver is set to limited-Broyden-Fletcher-Goldfarb-Shanno (LBFGS), and the number of iterations to 2000. LBFGS relatively performs better compared to other methods, especially as it saves a lot of memory. In the DT classifier, entropy is used to measure the quality of the split, and the maximum depth of a tree is set to 3. In the KNN classifier, the nearest neighbor value is set to 5, and also the setting of other parameters algorithm, leaf size, weights, etc. are done.

5 Results and Discussion

Our experimental design is based on the desire to assess the relative effectiveness of the various imputation techniques. To achieve this, a comparative analysis of the performance of four missing data imputation methods, against four classifiers, using two performance metrics namely—Prediction Accuracy and Mcoff, for various missing ratios, is done.

5.1 Relative Performance Analysis of Prediction Accuracy for 10–60% Missing Ratio (MR)

Figures 11.1, 11.2, 11.3 and 11.4 shows the relative difference in prediction accuracy of original data versus imputed data. The formula for the relative difference in accuracy is given in Eq. (11.2)

$$\textit{Relative Difference Prediction Accuracy} = 100 \times (AO - AM)/AM \tag{11.2}$$

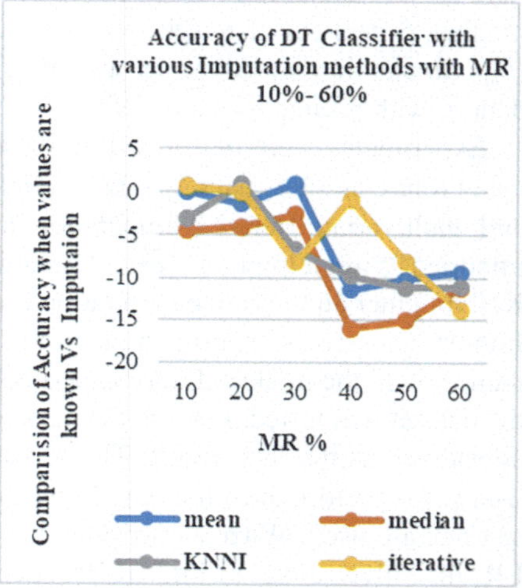

Fig. 11.1 Comparison of Relative Difference of Prediction Accuracy of Original vs. Imputed data for DT classifier

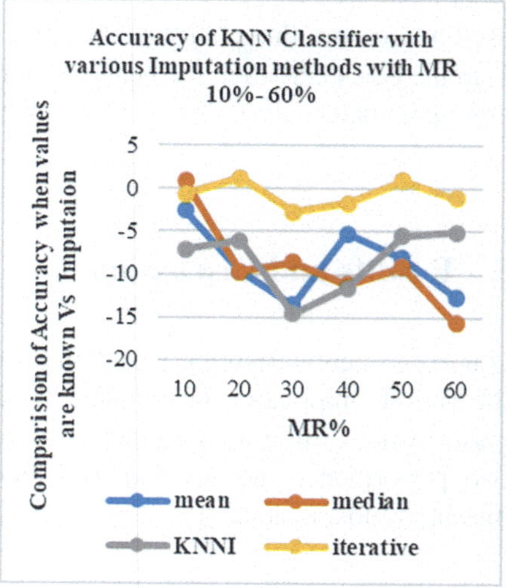

Fig. 11.2 Comparison of Relative Difference of Prediction Accuracy of Original vs. Imputed data for KNN classifier

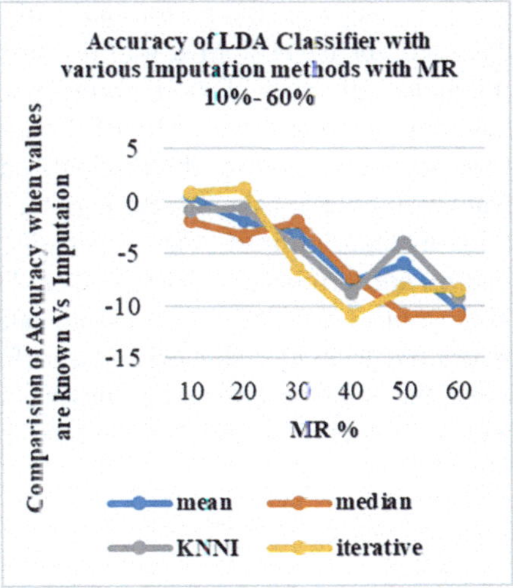

Fig. 11.3 Comparison of Relative Difference of Prediction Accuracy of Original vs. Imputed data for LDA classifier

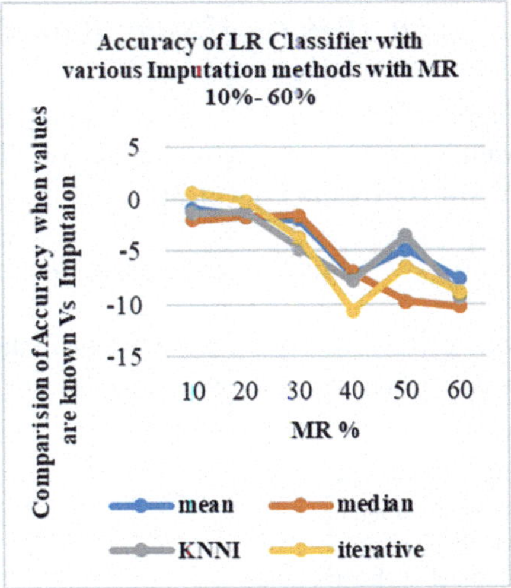

Fig. 11.4 Comparison of Relative Difference of Prediction Accuracy of Original vs. Imputed data for LR classifier

where *AO* is the prediction accuracy of the original dataset i.e. when all the features are known. *AM* is the prediction accuracy when the missing value is imputed by the corresponding imputation technique. In most cases, improvements are negative, which means missing data is degrading the prediction accuracy, even when the imputation is used. Positive values indicate that the corresponding imputation technique has increased the prediction accuracy, whereas negative values indicate that the imputation technique has reduced the prediction accuracy. Small negative values indicate that the corresponding imputation technique has brought a small reduction in accuracy, whereas larger negative values indicate a big reduction in prediction accuracy.

After analyzing the performance of four imputation techniques, with the four classifiers for 10–60% MR, we observed that when the MR is 10% and 30%, mean imputation gives prediction accuracy closer to the original accuracy, with DT classifier. However, with MR of 20%, 40%, 50%, and 60%, iterative imputation gives accuracy closer to the original heart disease dataset. This indicates that with evaluation criteria as accuracy, iterative imputation is the most suitable data imputation method, in most cases, especially if the MR is high. In the medical dataset, features are correlated with each other. As the iterative imputation technique uses all other features to estimate the missing values, in this heart disease dataset, imputation by iterative technique showed better performance in 4 out of 6 cases. KNN classifiers select the k nearest neighbor having similar values. Thus, the combination of iterative imputation and KNN classifier performs well, which is evident from Fig. 11.2.

5.2 *Relative Performance Analysis of Mcoff Score for 10–60% Missing Ratio (MR)*

Figures 11.5, 11.6, 11.7 and 11.8 shows the relative difference in Mcoff score, when values are known, versus imputation. The formula for the relative difference in Mcoff is given in Eq. (11.3)

$$\textit{Relative Difference Mcoff} = 100 \times (MO - MM)/MM \quad (11.3)$$

where *MO* is the Mcoff score, when all the features are known, and *MM* is the Mcoff score when the missing value is imputed. Positive values indicate that the

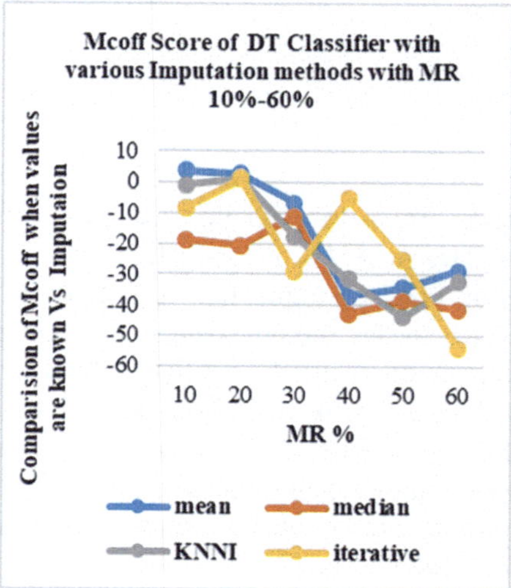

Fig. 11.5 Comparison of Relative Difference of Mcoff score of Original vs. Imputed data for DT classifier

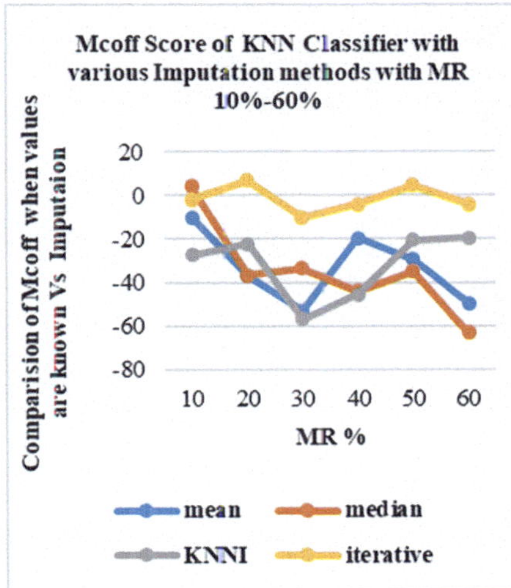

Fig. 11.6 Comparison of Relative Difference of Mcoff score of Original vs. Imputed data for KNN classifier

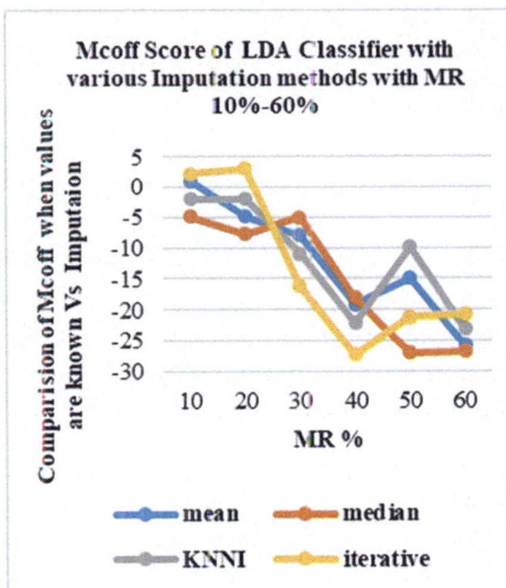

Fig. 11.7 Comparison of Relative Difference of Mcoff score of Original vs. Imputed data for LDA classifier

corresponding imputation technique has increased the Mcoff score, whereas negative values indicate that the imputation technique has reduced the Mcoff score.

So, this experimental study indicates that for evaluation criteria Mcoff, iterative imputation performs better than other imputation methods. It gives Mcoff score close to the original, in all the cases, except 10% and 30% MR, where KNNI and median give better performance. Iterative imputation gives the exact Mcoff score as the original with 20% MR. In Mcoff also, the combination of iterative imputation and KNN classifier performs better, as explained in prediction accuracy, and is also evident from Fig. 11.6. Table 11.2 shows the comparison of the overall best relative performance of mean, median, KNNI, and iterative imputation methods, and

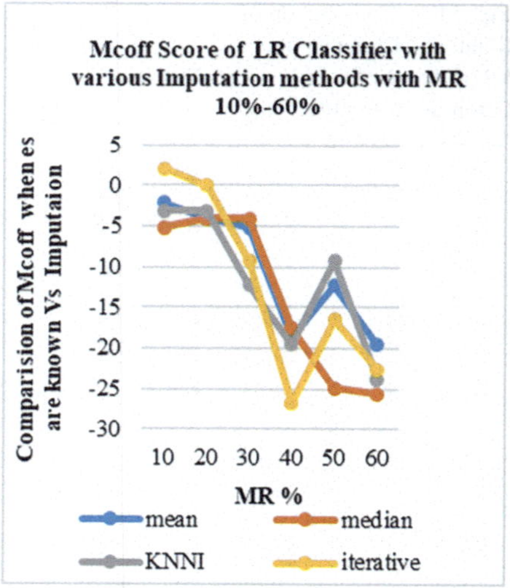

Fig. 11.8 Comparison of Relative Difference of Mcoff score of Original vs. Imputed data for LR classifier

Table 11.2 Comparison of overall best relative Performance of 4 Imputation Methods

	Accuracy		Mcoff	
MR%	Imputation	Classifier	Imputation	Classifier
10	Mean	DT	**KNNI**	**DT**
20	Iterative	LR	Iterative	LR
30	Mean	DT	Median	LR
40	Iterative	DT	Iterative	KNN
50	Iterative	KNN	Iterative	KNN
60	Iterative	KNN	Iterative	KNN

Table 11.3 Comparison of overall best relative Performance of four Imputation Methods in % of cases as per the data of Table 11.2

Accuracy%		Mcoff%		
Iterative	Mean	Iterative	Median	KNNI
66.66	33.33	**66.66**	**16.66**	**16.66**

Table 11.3 is constructed from Table 11.2, which shows the best relative performance of four imputation methods in % of cases.

6 Conclusion

MCAR type missing mechanism for the multivariate pattern is handled in the experiment described in this chapter. A comparative analysis of the impact of four missing data imputation methods, against four ML algorithms, for MR 10% to 60% with two evaluation criteria, is performed.

The experimental evidence confirms that relative performance of "Iterative Imputation Method" in prediction accuracy and Mcoff is at par with the original dataset in four out of six MR cases (i.e. 66% of cases) as compared to other imputation methods. Our study has several limitations i.e. our results are limited only to numerical data; we did not consider nominal data. We considered only MCAR type missing mechanism in the multivariate pattern. Future work will investigate the other missing mechanism and missingness in univariate patterns in nominal datasets.

References

1. Farrier H (2018) Seagate launches new data-readiness index revealing impact across four global industries as 30 percent of data forecasted to be real-time by 2025. https://www.businesswire.com/news/home/20181126005585/en/Seagate-Launches-New-Data-Readiness-Index-Revealing-Impact-Across-Four-Global-Industries-as-30-Percent-of-Data-Forecasted-to-Be-Real-Time-by-2025
2. Mansour RF, Parah SA (2021) Reversible data hiding for electronic patient information security for telemedicine applications. Arab J Sci Eng 46:9129–9144
3. Rubin DB (1976) Inference and missing data, Biometrika 63:581–592
4. Liu Y, Brown SD (2013) Comparison of five iterative imputation methods for multivariate classification. Chemom Intell Lab Syst 120:106–115
5. Hunt LA (2017) Missing data imputation and its effect on the accuracy of classification. In: Palumbo F, Montanari A, Vichi M (eds) Data science. Studies in classification, data analysis, and knowledge organization. Springer, Cham. https://doi.org/10.1007/978-3-319-55723-6_1
6. Beaulieu-Jones BK, Lavage DR, Snyder JW, Moore JH, Pendergrass SA, Bauer CR (2018) Characterizing and managing missing structured data in electronic health records: data analysis. JMIR Med Inform 6(1):e11. https://doi.org/10.2196/medinform.8960
7. Orczyk T, & Porwik P (2013) Influence of Missing Data Imputation Method on the Classification Accuracy of the Medical Data. Journal of Medical Informatics and Technologies, 22
8. Tsai CF (2018) A class center-based approach for missing value imputation. Knowl Based Syst 151:124–135
9. Pan R, Yang T, Cao J, Lu K, Zhang Z (2015) Missing data imputation by K nearest neighbors based on grey relational structure and mutual information. Appl Intell 43. https://doi.org/10.1007/s10489-015-0666-x
10. Xia J (2017) Adjusted weight voting algorithm for random forests in handling missing values. Pattern Recognit 69:52–60
11. Tang F, Ishwaran H (2017) Random forest missing data algorithms. Stat Anal Data Mining 10(6):363–377. https://doi.org/10.1002/sam.11348
12. Lai X, Zhang L, Liu X (2020) Takagi-Sugeno modeling of incomplete data for missing value imputation with the use of alternate learning. IEEE Access. PP. 1–1. https://doi.org/10.1109/ACCESS.2020.2991669
13. Rashid W, Gupta MK (2021) A perspective of missing value imputation approaches. In: Gao XZ, Tiwari S, Trivedi M, Mishra K (eds) Advances in computational intelligence and communication technology, Advances in intelligent systems and computing, vol 1086. Springer, Singapore. https://doi.org/10.1007/978-981-15-1275-9_25
14. Hu LY, Huang MW, Ke SW, Tsai CF (2016) The distance function effect on k-nearest neighbor classification for medical datasets. Springerplus 5(1):1304. https://doi.org/10.1186/s40064-016-2941-7

15. Lin W, Tsai C (2019) Missing value imputation: a review and analysis of the literature (2006–2017). Artif Intell Rev 53:1487–1509
16. Schafer JL, Graham JW (2002) Missing data: our view of the state of the art. Psychol Methods 7(2):147–177. PMID: 12090408.
17. Batista GEAPA, Monard MC (2003) An analysis of four missing data treatment methods for supervised learning. Appl Artif Intell 17:519–533
18. Soares J, Santos M, Henriques Abreu P, Araujo H, Santos J (2018) Exploring the Effects of Data Distribution in Missing Data Imputation: 17th International Symposium, IDA 2018, 's-Hertogenbosch, The Netherlands, October 24–26, 2018, Proceedings. https://doi.org/10.1007/978-3-030-01768-2_21
19. Zeng D, Xie D, Liu R, Li X (2017) Missing value imputation methods for TCM medical data and its effect in the classifier accuracy. IEEE 19th International Conference on e-Health Networking, Applications and Services (Healthcom) pp. 1–4, https://doi.org/10.1109/HealthCom.2017.8210844
20. Madhu G, Bharadwaj BL, Nagachandrika G, Vardhan KS (2019) A novel algorithm for missing data imputation on machine learning. In: International conference on smart systems and inventive technology (ICSSIT), pp 173–177. https://doi.org/10.1109/ICSSIT46314.2019.8987895
21. Gupta A, Sharma S, Goyal S, Rashid M (2020) Novel XGBoost tuned machine learning model for software bug prediction. 376–380. https://doi.org/10.1109/ICIEM48762.2020.9160152
22. Anindita N, Nugroho HA, Adji TB (2017) A combination of multiple imputations and principal component analysis to handle missing values with an arbitrary pattern. In: 7th International annual engineering seminar (InAES), pp 1–5. https://doi.org/10.1109/INAES.2017.8068537
23. Hunt L (2017) Missing data imputation and its effect on the accuracy of classification. https://doi.org/10.1007/978-3-319-55723-6_1
24. Purwar A, Singh S (2015) Hybrid prediction model with missing value imputation for medical data. Expert Syst Appl 42. https://doi.org/10.1016/j.eswa.2015.02.050
25. Arasu S, Thirumalaiselvi R (2017) A novel imputation method for effective prediction of coronary Kidney disease. 127–136. https://doi.org/10.1109/ICCCT2.2017.7972256
26. Twala B (2009) An empirical comparison of techniques for handling incomplete data using decision trees. Appl Artif Intell 23:373–405
27. Santos M, Pereira RC, Costa A, Soares J, Santos J, Henriques AP (2019) Generating synthetic missing data: a review by missing mechanism. IEEE Access. PP. 1–1. https://doi.org/10.1109/ACCESS.2019.2891360

Chapter 12
Ayurnano: A Solution Towards Herbal Therapeutics Using Artificial Intelligence Approach

Shridevi A. Desai and G. Mahitha

Contents

1 Introduction

Ayurveda, the oldest and traditional system of Indian medicine has significant importance in promoting customized medicines and treatments. Ayurveda drugs comprise herbal substances, animal origin, metals, or minerals for therapeutics. India is rich as the origin of many medicinal herbs and traditional treatments and so is a good source in identifying new medicines. Considering Ayurveda, an Indian traditional medicinal system (alternative medicine system) used even today for its ability in curing various kinds of diseases in a holistic approach. It focuses on complete coordination allying consciousness, mind, body, and soul.

Concern about herbal medicines and their treatments has propagated widely in developed, developing, and underdeveloped countries for many reasons. They are a

S. A. Desai (✉)
Department of Computer Science and Engineering, Dayananda Sagar University, Bengaluru, Karnataka, India

G. Mahitha
Department of Computer Science and Engineering, PES University, Bengaluru, Karnataka, India

S. A. Parah et al. (eds.), *Artificial Intelligence for Innovative Healthcare Informatics*,
https://doi.org/10.1007/978-3-030-96569-3_12

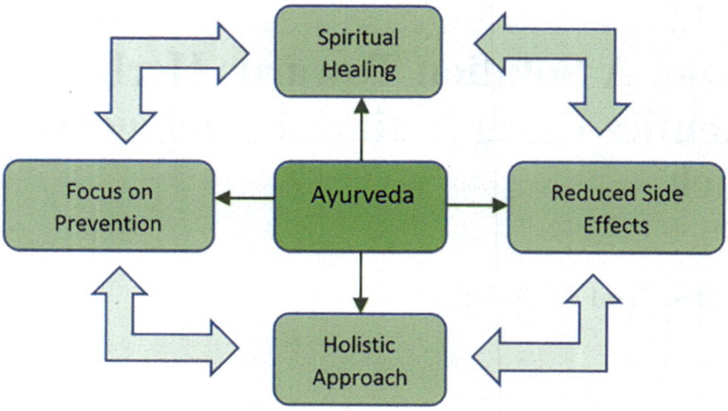

Fig. 12.1 Balanced representation of Ayurveda

study of the whole personality, no usage of chemical drugs, reduced side effects, and different techniques to manage drugs namely yoga and medication. Chief categories of traditional systems in the world are:

1. Ayurveda from India
2. Traditional Therapy from China
3. Unani medicines from Arab
4. Homeopathy and
5. Yoga

The chief principles of the Indian traditional system convey that the diseases are caused due to imbalance in three doshas such as Vata, Kapha, and pitta [1], and to maintain a good balance in all the above doshas for healthy living as shown in Fig. 12.1. The imbalance in any of the doshas leads to inflammation (sopha) and it treats the diseases at the site of the origin and not to the whole body. Today's diseases are not confined only to the body but also to emotional and mental levels. The herbal drug formulations need detailed information on the sources of its raw materials, safety, quality, etc. Today, the alternative system suffers from many facts like a supply of raw materials, recognition and extinction of herbal species, adulteration, and adverse effect of environmental factors.

Though modern medical science is centuries old in both practice and evidence. It finds its foundation from medicines and therapies of traditional medicines. It develops innovative compounds introduces novel drugs by synthesizing many chemicals and showcased spontaneity in the production of drugs. Hence, a victorious attempt by the modern medicinal system towards treating a wide range of diseases. This emergence of modern medicine (allopathy) in providing both technical and statistical analysis of data with evidence where on the other side traditional medicine suffered from updating and streaming of its resources [2–4]. The concern on the harmful issue of Ayurveda is that the drugs contain heavy metals such as mercury, iron, lead, and zinc. On consumption, it may lead to adverse effects on health. This is because the drugs cannot be clinically detected and toxicities may lead to global health issues.

Nanomedicine uses tools of 1–100 nm size which comprises physics, chemistry, biology, mathematics, medicine, and engineering to strive for success in improved drug delivery, detection of diseases, and imaging. Nanotechnology in Nanomedicine focuses on materials in the range of a few hundreds of nanometers that have the potential to cross biological and physiological barriers including cell membranes. The advantage of these nanometer particles is that they showcase distinctive biological and physical properties which in interaction provide a window for designing new nanoparticles for diagnostic and therapeutic approaches [5]. These nanoparticles persist in the circulation for a longer time and at the cellular level, they regulate the biological process. Nanomedicine developments are seen in nano-oncology, nano cardiology, nano neurology, and nano ophthalmology [6–17]. It also shines in the tissue engineering field. Thus, the technology provides a new path in customized treatment and medicine. Much needed is a blended approach of traditional medical systems and Nanomedicine to enrich the efficacy of healthcare.

The chapter proposes a system named "Ayurnano" to incorporate the current emerging technologies such as artificial intelligence and nanotechnology as a solution towards herbal therapies. The subdomain of artificial intelligence includes machine learning and deep learning techniques which have proved as an efficient method to classify many multi-class images. Many researchers have worked in implementing a different combination of machine learning algorithms on medicinal leaf images to classify its respective species. The classification from the images of herbs, roots, or even bark of a tree to its respective taxon includes the use of feature extraction approach to learn and extract the unique and valuable information from the image and lastly classify it using different classifier techniques. Once classified, the metals and minerals available in the medicinal plant can be extracted from the experts which can then be forwarded to perform different nanotechnology methods for the available metals or minerals to result in new drug formulation or for diagnosis purposes. The outcome will be a new bhasma that can be effectively used to cure many diseases and help society to attain a healthy herbal life. The whole process can be automated by integrating herbal plants, machine learning, and nanotechnology to provide nanoparticles that can be an efficient drug discovery in less cost and quick response towards healing without side effects. The recent contribution towards such an integrated medicinal system [18] is a first step in building a "nano-doctor".

The chapter is divided into sections where Sect. 2 describes the related works, Sect. 3 on the materials and methods and Sect. 4 presents the proposed method and Sect. 5 concludes the work.

2 Literature Survey

2.1 Ayurveda: An Alternate Medicinal System

The cogency of Ayurveda for sound health states to have balance in vital humor (Vata, dosha, and pita), the digestive fire (Agni), normal function of seven body tissues (dhatus), normal production, and elimination of waste products (mala) and blissful working of the mind, consciousness and senses (mana, Atma and indriya). Justification on promoting Ayurveda and not allopathy:

1. Prescribing synthetic drugs on symptomatic and on-mass whereas herbal medicines are holistic and individualistic.
2. Molecular-level of action as when compared to tissue level in traditional medicines.
3. Allopathy drugs are produced artificially having molecules of a single drug with high potential concentration while herbal medicines are at tissue level with their sources from natural resources with balanced content.
4. Many natural compounds cannot be duplicated to synthetic drugs.

Because of inflation, affordability, and the ability to cure many diseases without side effects, Ayurveda is slowly emanating by itself. The list of few alternative herbal medicines over synthetic drugs are:

1. *Morphine* is isolated from opium for relieving pain.
2. *Belladonna*—a perennial herbaceous plant cures asthma, whooping cough, cold, and many more. Used in treating ophthalmology problems and gastrointestinal disorders.
3. *Rauwolfia serpentina*, a flower species and a perennial undershrub for curing hypertension. This isolates Reserpine a constituent of tranquilizer but may lead to suicidal mania if unmonitored.

Few herbs, *Strychnos nux vomica*, *Rauwolfia serpentina,* and *Gloriosa superba* with rich healing strength are in extinction as it is listed in the red list of IUCN. One of the reasons for extinction may be the requirement of high dosages for few desired treatments. If the drugs are in nanoparticle carriers eventually doses will be minimized to a greater extent which also leads to saving many herbs at extinction.

Different forms of dosages are powder (churna), electuary (avlehas), and decoction (kwath) which are not good to taste and to be consumed in large doses. The drug dose in the form of decoction consists of various compounds which are active and impacts synergetic results on the diseases. But, includes continuous administration and higher dosage. The above drawback can be nullified if nanoparticles are integrated with Ayurveda. The other drawback of the herbal system includes the lack of scientific description of discrete components and their procedural actions which highlights the evolution of nanoparticles, liposomes, nanotubes, etc.

Application of nanoparticles has high potential in curing chronic diseases in herbal drugs as is based on unique size, high loading capacity by delivering more drug concentration, faster dissolution in blood as it is of nanometer size, persist to stay in a diseased area for a longer period, reduce side effect and dosage.

The nanoparticle form in Ayurveda, "Bhasma" is based on special mineral/metallic preparation. Referring to "*Charaka Samhita*"—an ancient text in traditional medicine. Bhasma is very close to a nanoparticle with dominating characteristics like bio-compatibility, bio-degradability, nature of ready absorbability, and non-antigenic and assimilate without being toxic. Example: *Swarna Bhasma* (Gold Ash) is of size 56 nm which is in contrast to gold nanoparticles by Transmission

Electron Microscopy (TEM). The issues in Ayurvedic medicines which motivates incorporating nanocarrier as an effective solution are:

1. Poor bio-availability
2. High doses
3. Continuous monitoring
4. Usage of metals
5. Issue of Stability

Nano Drug delivery would be an efficient and novel therapeutic system in a controlled manner without repeated monitoring, which is crucial as it helps to increase the availability of natural resources, reduce toxic effects, and consumption of mass dosage.

2.2 *Nanomedicine: Nanotechnology in Nano-health*

It is fact that nanoparticles are everywhere around us. Smoke, ashes, hemoglobin hold together the protein, DNA strand, and many more. Nanotechnology was first stamped in 1974 by T. Taniguchi. Nanoparticles range from 1 to 100 nm, proves capability in controlling the molecules and atoms, changes biological, physical, and chemical properties by processing [19], and target for safety, purity, and efficacy mainly for medical purpose. The big gap between the interaction of cellular response and the molecules is filled up by nanotechnology [20].

The nanomaterial size is comparable to that of most biological molecules and compositions. Nanomaterials can also be useful for both biomedical research and applications in vivo and in vitro. Nanotechnology has presented the possibility of using nanoparticles to deliver drugs to individual cells. Following are some of the possibilities of facilitating the nanoparticles.

- Reduction in overall drug consumption and side effects.
- Elimination of high price.
- Enhancement of bioavailability of medicines.
- Targeted action and customized medicine growth.

In a drug administration facility, drug delivery is the most important aspect, and the nanosystem design makes it more suitable and accordant. Nanoparticles bind effectively to the drug and skillfully spread the drug into the environment. The effectiveness of many drugs is also restricted by their ability to reach the therapeutic action site. Most of the time, only a limited amount of the administered dose reaches the target site while the remainder of the medicine is distributed following its physicochemical and biochemical properties to the rest of the body. It is therefore a demanding task to establish a drug delivery scheme that optimizes a drug's pharmaceutical action while its toxic side effects are reduced in vivo.

An important feature of drug administration is biocompatibility. Because of physicochemical characteristics, polymer nanoparticles represent notable effectiveness and efficiency. The use of polymers as binding agents in drug delivery increases the stability and precise dispersion of drugs. The polymeric nanoparticles have been specifically designed to channel them to deliver a higher pharmaceutical agent concentration to the desired location. The main focus of this chapter is to discuss the advantages of combining Ayurveda with Nanotechnology, where various nanoparticles are synthesized using different herbs and herbal compounds, which can reduce adverse effects by increasing the effectiveness of medicines against many diseases.

2.3 *Nanomaterial: Approaches*

Nanoparticles can be obtained either as mass material or discrete molecules using a top-down or bottom-up process to obtain specific nano-sizes and features as shown in Fig. 12.2. The techniques such as mechanical milling, spluttering and chemical etching are incorporated in a top-down approach with resulting nanoparticles used in fabricating nano-engineered systems. The synthesized materials from the bottom-up are carbon nano-tubes, polymeric nanoparticles, dendrimers, and many more resulting in a high degree end product hence used widely in biomedical applications. Nanoparticles in Nanomedicine overcome the downsides of capsules, tablets, etc. suffering from harm to healthy cells, bio-availability, and many more.

2.4 *Materials Used in Nano-health*

1. Nanomaterials: Bio-materials used for enriching bioavailability and biocompatibility of several materials [21].

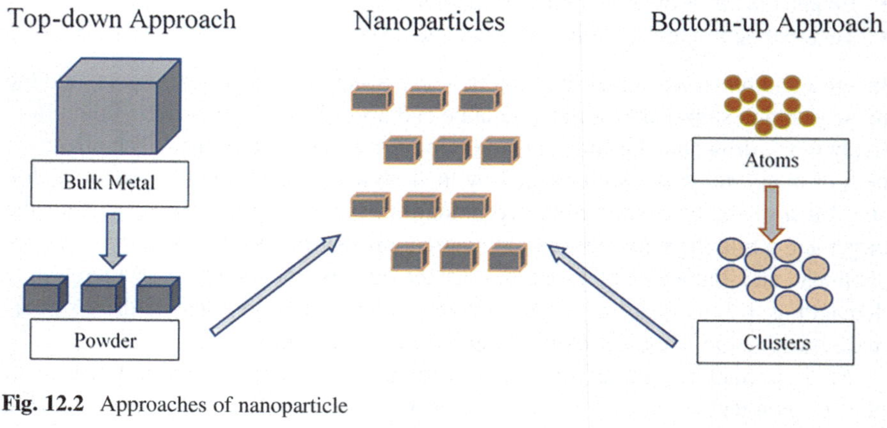

Fig. 12.2 Approaches of nanoparticle

2. Nanostructured: Processed forms used in micro and nanoelectromechanical systems.
3. Nanocrystalline: Manufactured to act as alternates to those which are poor in solubility and bioavailability featured materials.

2.5 *Types of Nanoparticles in Nanomedicine*

1. Polymeric: Nanosize ranging from 10 to 1000 nm used as carriers in sustained and controlled drug delivery providing complete protection of drugs as they are biodegradable and biocompatible [22, 23].
2. Metallic: Range of size is less than 100 nm with a huge surface area used in radiotherapy enhancement, sensitive diagnostic assays, etc. having stability and bioavailability features [24].
3. Dendrimers: Size less than 10 nm used in targeted and controlled delivery of drugs to the liver [25].
4. Polymeric micelles: Size between 1 and 100 nm used in passive and active delivery of drugs [26].
5. Liposomes: Size 50–100 nm range used in active and passive delivery of peptide and protein.

3 Materials and Methods

3.1 *Ayurveda: Bhasma (Incinerated Metal)*

Bhasma is of very small size with quick action and no specific taste. It is the outcome of Bhasmikarana where metals/minerals are transformed into microscopic form with

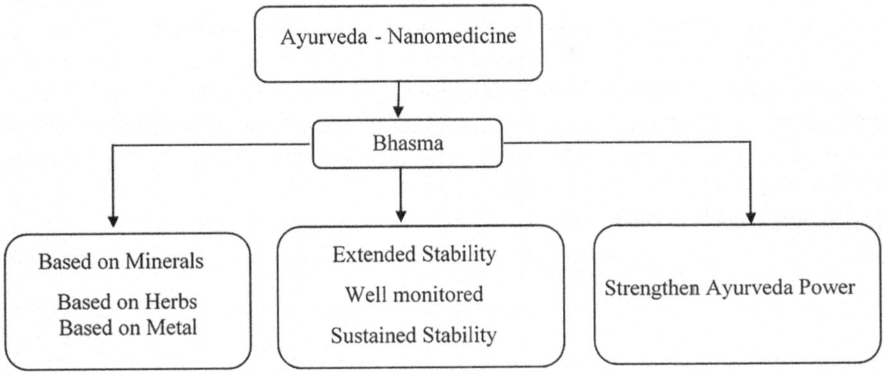

Fig. 12.3 Benefits of bhasma

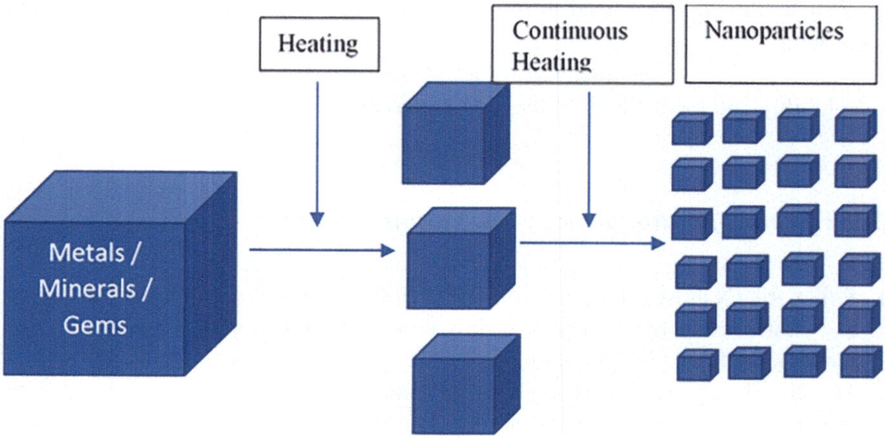

Fig. 12.4 Production of nanoparticles

therapeutic properties. Figure 12.3 shows the main benefits of bhasma in the Ayurnano world. The concept in preparation of Bhasma lies in heating and cooling of metals/minerals such as copper, lead, silver, gold, mercury, etc. later combining with necessary herbs and agents result in end-product known as Bhasma—free of toxic and side-effects. The process of continuous heating and cooling of minerals/metals show changes in both the chemical and physical properties of the metal. The resultant of this process is a nanoparticle as shown in Fig. 12.4.

The preparation of bhasma (Bhasmikarana) comprises breaking the metal/minerals in a sequence of the following steps i.e., Purification (Shodhana), Wet grinding (Bhavana), Heating (Marana), and the outcome is nanoparticle (Bhasma). The additional stages in Marana are addition of *Maraka gana* drugs, *bhavana* and *putapaka*. The quality of bhasma is determined in the Addition of *Maraka Gana* drugs which are the best quality bhasma (*Shreshta Bhasma*), *Madhyama Bhasma*, *Kanishta Bhasma*, and *Durguna Bhasma*. This complete process of purification and incineration is the result of a zerovalent state of metal transformed into a higher oxidized state by eliminating the toxicity and increasing the medicine value.

The branch of Ayurveda which deals with bhasma is known as *Rasa Shastra*. The chemical characteristics of bhasma are inefficient to regain back the original metallic form, very fine powder which should easily get into lines and crevices of the fingers and float on the surface of the water. The physical characteristics include color (specific to parent metal), light and fine (based on the law of surface tension), size of the particle, and lusterless.

3.2 Herbs and Its Compounds Used for Bhasma

There are multiple reasons why patients turn to herbal therapies. Many chronic or incurable diseases like diabetes, cancer, arthritis or AIDS, are treated using herbal medicines. Herbs are used as home remedies to treat acute conditions such as the cold, sore throat or bee sting as often professional care is not available immediately or it may be costly and time-consuming. In rural areas, various cultural factors and religious beliefs encourage the use of herbs to a greater extent, as natural plant products are considered healthier compared to manufactured medicines. Herbal medicine has the potential to treat mental illness and restore mental stability. There are many medicinal herbs known as *Medhya* drugs (*Ashwagandha*, *Brahmi*, *Shankapushpi*) that can be used as functional leads to treat mental illness.

Ashwagandha (*Withania somnifera*) commonly known as "*Winter Cherry*" is found widely in the Northwestern part of India. This is the prominent herb of Ayurveda which mainly promotes physical and mental health. It also helps to enhance the learning ability of children. *Brahmi* (*Bacopa monnieri*) is widely found all over India in wetlands and marshy tropical regions. This is used as a reinstating herb that strengthens brain function and memory. *Shankapushpi* (*Convolvulus pluricaulis*) is an herb found in India and Burma. This is used as a brain tonic and helps in solving a wide range of issues. It helps in the reduction of serum cholesterol, lipoprotein cholesterol, and triglycerides. It also exhibited a thyroid suppressing effect when it was administered to mice with hypothyroidism. *Convolvulus pluricaulis* functions as an anxiolytic, antidepressant, antistress, antiamnesic, and antioxidant agent [27].

Hence, to cure diseases, recognizing the desired herbs among available thousands of herbs and synthesizing nanoparticles from these herbs, plays a vital role. Properties of metals, when considered in bulk form, differ from the properties in the nanoscale dimension. Metals and their nanoparticles exhibit the active potential of the herbal compound when they are combined with biologically active herbal compounds. Herbs and herb compound extracts that have medicinal values are selected for the synthesis of nanoparticles.

Herbal nanoparticles are considered a better option to overcome the limitations of traditional herbal drugs. Nanoparticles are used to increase the solubility of the herbal drug and also help to localize the drug in a specific area thus increasing the efficiency. It also decreases the side effects. Nanoparticles deliver a high concentration of drugs to disease areas because of their unique size and high loading capacities. The drug is delivered in small particle size which will enhance the entire surface area of the drugs which further facilitate quicker dissolution in the blood. Nanoparticles can be produced using various herbs and herbal compounds. Table 12.1 shows the biological activity of the nanoparticle produced, details of herbal compounds, and where those herbs are found/grown [28].

Herb named *Cassia angustifolia*, which grows in south India throughout the year mainly in Tirunelveli, Madurai, Tiruchirappalli, and Mysore, is used in the synthesis of silver nanoparticles. The silver nanoparticles exhibited good antibacterial

Table 12.1 Nanoparticle synthesized using herbs and herbal compounds

Nanoparticles	Herb and herbal compounds	The region where herbs are found/grown	Medicinal properties	Reference
Silver	Carica papaya leaf extract	Native to Mexico and northern South America, found in tropical and sub-tropical regions of the world	Anticancer	Surya P. Singh et al. 2020 [29]
	Cassia angustifolia	South India throughout the year mainly in Tirunelveli, Madurai, Tiruchirappalli, and Mysore	Antibacterial	T. Peter Amaladhas et al. 2012 [30]
	Cocos nucifera (inflorescence)	Grown in tropical regions of the world	Antimicrobial	Mariselvam et al. 2014 [31]
Zinc oxide	Aloe vera extract (leaf)	Native to North Africa, South Europe, and the Canary Islands but grown in tropical climates worldwide	Nano antibiotics against multidrug-resistant clinical bacterial isolates	Khursheed Ali et al. [32]
Gold Nano	Couroupita guianensis (flower)	Native to tropical forests of Central and South America found in tropical areas throughout the world, has cultural and religious significance in India	Anticancer	Geetha et al. 2013 [33]
Iron oxide	Lawsonia inermis (henna)	Southern areas of the Middle East and South Asia	Anticancer, anti-microbial, antibacterial	Manoranjan Arakha et al. 2015 [34]

potential against *Escherichia coli* and *Staphylococcus aureus*. *Carica* leaf extract and *Cocos nucifera* can also be used in the synthesis of silver nanoparticles which exhibit anticancer and antimicrobial properties respectively.

Aloe vera leaf extract native to North Africa, Southern Europe, and the Canary Islands, can be used to synthesize the zinc oxide nanoparticles which can be used as nano antibiotics against multi-drug resistant clinical bacterial isolates. Today, *Aloe vera* is grown in tropical climates worldwide. *Couroupita guianensis* flower extract found in tropical areas throughout the world can be used to synthesize gold nanoparticles that exhibit anticancer properties. *Lawsonia inermis* is used in the synthesis of iron oxide nanoparticles which exhibit antimicrobial, anticancer, and antibacterial properties.

3.3 *Recognition of Herbs Using Machine Learning Techniques*

To synthesize the herbal nanoparticles, the selection of proper herbs with the best medicinal properties is an important step. Even though herbs are the main source of traditional ayurvedic medicine, a lot of herbs are endangered and neglected as most of the population is not aware of their existence. Identifying the herbs manually is time-consuming and requires meticulous training for achieving higher accuracy. The techniques of computer vision and machine learning can accelerate the process of herb identification thereby reducing the time and effort required in manual process.

Until recent times, the classification of herbs is performed manually which results in consumption of both time and energy. No commercial device is used for the identification of herbs, hence developing an automatic system using machine learning techniques will be widely accepted. Classification of herbs is quite challenging due to their similarity in color and shape and the huge variety of available species. Herbs can be classified according to smell, leaf shape, and leaf color. Leaves are widely used for the classification of any plant as they possess distinct characteristics. Features extracted from the leaf image show significant results compared to its other parts such as stem, seed, fruit, or flower. There are many approaches for the extraction of features in machine learning. Some of them are texture, shape, color, scale-invariant feature transform, histogram of gradients, and many more. The extracted features are further classified by several classifiers such as support vector machine, k nearest neighbor, naive Bayes, decision trees, ensemble classifier, and many more [35].

The fundamental procedure for the identification of herbs has different stages namely, image acquisition, image pre-processing followed by feature extraction and classification. Generally, an herb sample image is captured by the webcam as part of the image acquisition stage. In image pre-processing, the query image is cleaned to remove noise for further processing. In the feature extraction phase, a single feature many times lead to a low recognition rate, as a result, multiple features are combined to increase the detection rate. The classifiers use the extracted features to identify the correct variety of medicinal plants.

The shape of the leaf is the main feature for plant classification. Scale Invariant Feature Transform (SIFT) descriptors can extract both vein and shape features of the leaf and hence is a better feature extraction technique when compared to others such as texture, color, and shape. It is useful to match images with different scales and rotations. There are two important steps as part of SIFT i.e., detection of key points and extraction of a descriptor for each key point detected. The outline of the overall SIFT is organized into these steps. Firstly, construction of scale-space by blurring the original image. Secondly, generate another set of images called Difference of Gaussians (DoG) for finding key points from the blurred image. The key point detection is itself a two-step process, which includes locating minima and maxima from previous DoG images and finding subpixel minima and maxima. Lastly, unwanted key points which are of low contrast and those lying on the leaf edges are removed and then the orientation is assigned to the key points.

The model is built by extracting SIFT features and classifying using classifiers such as SVM, KNN, Naïve Bayes. Good results for the classification of Indian herbs are obtained by clustering the extracted SIFT features using K-Means followed by an SVM classifier [36]. Usage of enhanced, clear, and high contrast leaf images are essential to train and test any machine learning model. This type of dataset helps to extract various unique features which are valuable and non-redundant. A good medicinal leaf dataset (Indian herbs) [37] can be used to develop any automatic identification system for medicinal plants. Not many medicinal leaf datasets are available online, this motivates researchers and scientists to build new medicinal leaf datasets of their region to increase the knowledge and awareness of herbs among common people. The current available general leaf dataset may not be sufficient to build an automated system for medicinal plants.

3.4 Types and Uses of Ayurvedic Bhasmas

1. *Swarna Bhasma* (Gold Ash): Prepared from gold and used in treating tissue wasting, asthma, infertility, and cardiac toner.
2. *Varatika Bhasma*: Prepared from cowries and used to treat eye disorders, boils, indigestion, bronchitis, etc.
3. *Muktashukti Bhasma*: Prepared from pearl oyster and useful in urinary calculi, cardiac disorders, abdominal colic, etc.
4. *Mandura Bhasma* (Iron): Prepared from iron oxide and treats to cure jaundice, anemia, improve strength and immunity, etc.
5. *Naga Bhasma*: Prepared from lead and helps in curing skin disorders, liver disorders, asthma, diabetes, etc.
6. *Tamra Bhasma* (Copper): Prepared from copper and used to eradicate piles, asthma, obesity, skin diseases, etc.

Ayurvedic Bhasma as shown in Fig. 12.5 should be consumed under strict medicinal supervision. Hence, it is prominent that in nano health—Ayurvedic bhasma as nanomedicine is a safe, economical, and efficient treatment for many chronic diseases including non-communicable diseases.

3.5 Applications of Nanoparticles

1. Diagnosis: Imaging, protein to protein interaction, and cellular metabolism
2. Drug delivery system: Overcome the drawbacks of conventional delivery systems such as patient poor compliance, the requirement of high dose, and many more

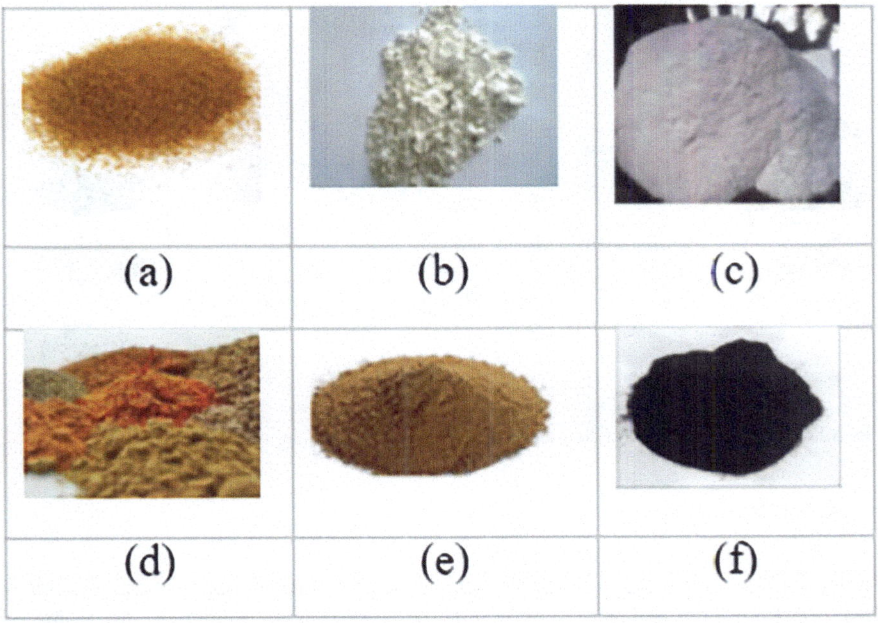

Fig. 12.5 Types of ayurvedic bhasma: (**a**) *Swarna Bhasma*, (**b**) *Varatika Bhasma*, (**c**) *Muktashukti Bhasma*, (**d**) *Mandura Bhasma*, (**e**) *Naga Bhasma*, (**f**) *Tamra Bhasma*

3. Discovery of new drugs: Determining drugs by improving in bioavailability and solubility

4 Proposed Model

In this chapter, the proposed system is "Ayurnano", a blend of Nanotechnology and Ayurveda for health care as shown in Fig. 12.6. Various herbs and herb compounds are identified and are classified as medicinal plants using techniques of machine learning and image processing. These herb compounds are further synthesized to form nanoparticles/bhasma which helps to cure many diseases.

This system provides holistic approach treatment to many chronic diseases assuring the medicines are toxic-free, soluble, and have less dosage. Thus, overcoming the main drawbacks of Ayurveda through nanotechnology. Eliminating the other forms of traditional doses such as "churna", decoction and directing to bhasma for drug formulation in curing the non-communicable and chronic diseases is much needed for the current scenario. Bhasma—a much affordable drug for society. If even today India's ancient Ayurveda shows its presence, this portrays that it is an effective system and it widely accepts the incorporation of modern technology for its betterment and global acceptance.

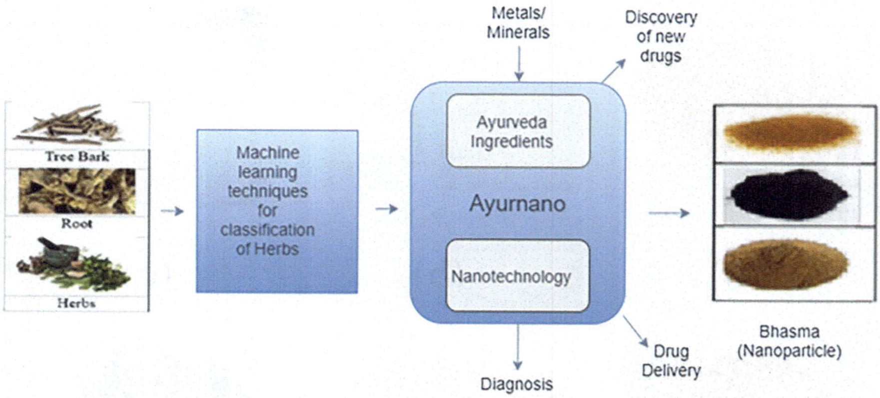

Fig. 12.6 Proposed schematic diagram of Ayurnano

5 Conclusion

Ayurveda, the oldest and yet alive truly because of its effectiveness in treating many diseases. Poor knowledge of it is mainly because it lacks evidence and forms of dosage which are bitter and sour, long duration of consumption, bulk dosages, and many more. One of the Ayurvedic dosage—Bhasma, the evidence of nanoparticle can be improved by standardizing in its manufacturing process using nanotechnology techniques by increasing its medicinal value, quality, and nano properties so that it is toxic-free, safe in mass production, and others. The study of assimilating Ayurveda combined with machine learning and nanotechnology (Ayurnano) creates a new era in the medical system. Ayurnano indeed provides a huge scope of encouragement for a healthy and content lifestyle. Ayurnano—A combination of nanosystem and herbal solution, free from adverse side effects is the need of the hour to treat many chronic ailments or incurable diseases. This would renovate and restore the ancient riches present in the field of Ayurveda.

References

1. Chopra A, Doiphode VV (2002) Ayurvedic medicine: core concept, therapeutic principles, and current relevance. Med Clin 86(1):75–89
2. Mans DR (2013) From forest to pharmacy: plant-based traditional medicines as sources for novel therapeutic compounds. Acad J Med Plants 1(1):101–110
3. Rashid M, Goyal V, Parah SA, Singh H (2019) Drug prediction in healthcare using big data and machine learning. In: Hidden link prediction in stochastic social networks. IGI Global, Hershey, PA, pp 79–92
4. Kamboj A (2012) Analytical evaluation of herbal drugs. Drug Discov Res Pharmacogn 3:23–55
5. Bhattacharya R, Mukherjee P (2008) Biological properties of "naked" metal nanoparticles. Adv Drug Deliv Rev 60(11):1289–1306

6. Gull S, Loan NA, Parah SA (2020) An efficient watermarking technique for tamper detection and localization of medical images. J Ambient Intell Human Comput 11:1799–1808
7. Bae KH, Chung HJ, Park TG (2011) Nanomaterials for cancer therapy and imaging. Mol Cells 31(4):295–302
8. Jain KK (2010) Advances in the field of nanooncology. BMC Med 8(1):1–11
9. Gull S, Mansour RF, Aljehane NO, Parah SA (2021) A self-embedding technique for tamper detection and localization of medical images for smart-health. Multimed Tools Appl 80(19): 29939–29964
10. Ranganathan R, Madanmohan S, Kesavan A, Baskar G, Krishnamoorthy YR, Santosham R, Venkatraman G (2012) Nanomedicine: towards the development of patient-friendly drug-delivery systems for oncological applications. Int J Nanomedicine 7:1043
11. Hurrah NN, Loan NA, Parah SA, Sheikh JA, Muhammad K, de Macedo ARL, de Albuquerque VHC (2020) INDFORG: industrial forgery detection using automatic rotation angle detection and correction. IEEE Trans Ind Informatics 17(5):3630–3639
12. Gull S, Parah SA, Khan M (2020) Reversible data hiding exploiting Huffman encoding with dual images for IoMT based healthcare. Comput Commun 163:134–149
13. Sarosh P, Parah SA, Bhat GM, Heidari AA, Muhammad K (2021) Secret sharing-based personal health records management for the Internet of Health Things. Sustain Cities Soc 74: 103129
14. Cyrus T, Wickline SA, Lanza GM (2012) Nanotechnology in interventional cardiology. Wiley Interdiscip Rev Nanomed Nanobiotechnol 4:82–95
15. Jha N, Prashar D, Rashid M, Shafiq M, Khan R, Pruncu CI, Saravana Kumar M (2021) Deep learning approach for discovery of in silico drugs for combating COVID-19. J Healthc Eng 2021:6668985
16. Khan AA, Shaikh AA, Cheikhrouhou O, Laghari AA, Rashid M, Shafiq M, Hamam H (2021) IMG-forensics: multimedia-enabled information hiding investigation using convolutional neural network. IET Image Process. https://doi.org/10.1049/ipr2.12272
17. Yadav D, Suri S, Choudhary AA, Sikender M, Hemant K, Beg NM (2011) Novel approach: herbal remedies and natural products in pharmaceutical science as nano-drug delivery systems. Int J Pharm Technol 3:3092–3116
18. Bodunde OP, Ikumapayi OM, Akinlabi ET, Oladapo BI, Adeoye AO, Fatoba SO (2020) A futuristic insight into a "nano-doctor": a clinical review on medical diagnosis and devices using nanotechnology. Mater Today Proc. https://doi.org/10.1016/j.matpr.2020.11.232
19. Godin B, Sakamoto JH, Serda RE, Grattoni A, Bouamrani A, Ferrari M (2010) Emerging applications of nanomedicine for the diagnosis and treatment of cardiovascular diseases. Trends Pharmacol Sci 31(5):199–205
20. Ibtehal S, Omaima EG, Arwa EH, Ahmed AB (2012) Preparation of zaleplon microparticles using emulsion solvent diffusion technique. J Pharm Drug Deliv Res. https://doi.org/10.4172/2325-9604.1000108
21. Parteni O et al (2016) The release of tacrolimus from a cotton biomaterial to dermis. J Pharm Drug Deliv Res 5:1
22. Orji JI et al (2015) Physicochemical properties of co-precipitate of plantain Peel cellulose and gelatin. J Pharm Drug Deliv Res 4:4
23. Radu CD et al (2015) Comparative study of a drug release from a textile to skin. J Pharm Drug Deliv Res 4:2
24. Solomon AO et al (2015) Making drugs safer: improving drug delivery and reducing side-effect of drugs on the human biochemical system. J Pharm Drug Deliv Res 4:4
25. Satyavathi K et al (2015) Formulation and in-vitro evaluation of liposomal drug delivery system of Cabazitaxel. J Pharm Drug Deliv Res 4:2
26. Kumar R, Lal S (2014) Synthesis of organic nanoparticles and their applications in drug delivery and food nanotechnology: a review. J Nanomater Mol Nanotechnol 3:4

27. Margret A (2017) Stratagems of nanotechnology augmenting the bioavailability and therapeutic efficacy of traditional medicine to formulate smart herbal drugs combating. In: Pharmaceutical sciences: breakthroughs in research and practice. IGI Global, Hershey, PA, pp 1367–1392
28. Gomes A, Ghosh S, Sengupta J, Datta P, Gomes A (2014) Herbonanoceuticals: a new step towards herbal therapeutics. Med Aromat Plants 3(3):162
29. Singh SP, Mishra A, Shyanti RK, Singh RP, Acharya A (2021) Silver nanoparticles synthesized using Carica papaya leaf extract (AgNPs-PLE) causes cell cycle arrest and apoptosis in human prostate (DU145) cancer cells. Biol Trace Elem Res 199(4):1316–1331
30. Peter AT, Devi AT, Ananthi N, Velammal PS, Sivagami S (2012) Biogenic synthesis of silver nanoparticles by leaf extract of Cassia Angustifolia. Adv Nat Sci Nanosci Nanotechnol 3: 045006
31. Mariselvam R, Ranjitsingh AJA, Nanthini AUR, Kalirajan K, Padmalatha C, Selvakumar PM (2014) Green synthesis of silver nanoparticles from the extract of the inflorescence of Cocos nucifera (Family: Arecaceae) for enhanced antibacterial activity. Spectrochim Acta A Mol Biomol Spectrosc 129:537–541
32. Ali K, Dwivedi S, Azam A, Saquib Q, Al-Said MS, Alkhedhairy AA, Musarrat J (2016) Aloe vera extract functionalized zinc oxide nanoparticles as nanoantibiotics against multi-drug resistant clinical bacterial isolates. J Colloid Interface Sci 472:145–156
33. Geetha R, Ashokkumar T, Tamilselvan S, Govindaraju K, Sadiq M, Singaravelu G (2013) Green synthesis of gold nanoparticles and their anticancer activity. Cancer Nanotechnol 4(4–5): 91–98
34. Arakha M, Pal S, Samantarrai D, Panigrahi TK, Mallick BC, Pramanik K, Jha S (2015) Antimicrobial activity of iron oxide nanoparticles upon modulation of nanoparticle-bacteria interface. Sci Rep 5(1):1–12
35. Kaur PP, Singh S, Pathak M (2020) Review of machine learning herbal plant recognition system. Available at SSRN 3565850
36. Roopashree S, Anitha J (2020) Enrich Ayurveda knowledge using machine learning techniques. Indian J Tradit Knowl 19(4):813–820
37. Roopashree S, Anitha J (2020) Medicinal leaf dataset. Mendeley Data, V1. https://doi.org/10.17632/nnytj2v3n5.1

Chapter 13
Artificial Intelligence in Biomedical Education

Samreen Fayaz, Vishal Jagota, and Shaik Kamaal

Contents

1 Introduction to Artificial Intelligence

Artificial Intelligence is replacing work techniques and the living. This text will give how to steer the advancement of AI, the definition of buzzwords that people can use either for personal or incorporation research. Firstly, we will provide the exposure to give the realistic perspective of Artificial Technology [1]. As per the study conducted by research arm McKinsey Global Institute by the year 2030, AI will

S. Fayaz (✉)
Department of Computer Science and Engineering, Chandigarh University, Mohali, Punjab, India

V. Jagota
Department of Mechanical Engineering, Madanapalle Institute of Technology & Science, Madanapalle, Andhra Pradesh, India

S. Kamaal
School of Computer Science & Engineering, Lovely Professional University, Jalandhar, India

S. A. Parah et al. (eds.), *Artificial Intelligence for Innovative Healthcare Informatics*,
https://doi.org/10.1007/978-3-030-96569-3_13

appraise to 13 trillion US dollars. Although AI is already doing massive changes into the software industries, more to be produced in the future which is out of the software companies, fields such as transportation, education, healthcare, traveling, and manufacturing [2–4].

Artificial intelligence is very challenging as AI robots can speak in the audience with eye contact on the stages but how to use a robot to do automatic hairdressing? This discussion is of much hype and there are two separate ideas in AI, the former is Applications like automatic cards, web searching, AI technology in factories, smart speakers all come under artificial narrow intelligence (ANI), these applications can do even more than human intelligence [5]. However, ANI makes people think like there are vast changes and AI will take over all the human activities but in actual lots of work is required to be done in Artificial General Intelligence (AGI) which is the latter one. This work will explain why we need to study AI, what is Machine learning then what data is valuable, where to need accurate prediction using the technology, how deep learning is also known as Neural Network has driven. AI has a tremendous impact on people, also mentioned that there can be biases using AI technology and how to improve the systems to remove biased predictions, how it's going to provide more jobs and going to affect the economy, by the end you will understand and get the ability to navigate the progress [6].

Motivation In this chapter diverse fields have been surveyed by the authors in one single document where AI plays a vital role in medical education, authors want to enlighten the various ailments where AI is acting as a cure and is providing techniques which when incorporated into the biomedical education will be proving to perform laurels to wrestle the fatal diseases and easing the sufferer.

1.1 AI Techniques: Machine Learning

Several techniques enable the software machines to imitate the nature of human intelligence with the use of logic, decision trees, if-then rules, and machine learning. Machine learning is a part of a type of artificial intelligence that learns to map from input to output. Machine learning is also known as supervised learning, below is an example to understand the concept, here A is input to software and B is the result after processing.

$$A \rightarrow B \tag{13.1}$$

Let's input A as a voice message or any speech translating input into B a text transcript is going to use the core AI and application called speech recognition. Similarly, other examples are given in Table 13.1.

All these inputs are different types of data which is paramount in AI system building. If a person wants to purchase or trade a rope then you may start collecting the information regarding the size of rope in some units like meters or centimeters,

Table 13.1 Method to understand supervised learning

Input A	Response B	AI application
English Sentence	Hindi Sentence	Language Translation
Email	Spam or not?	Spam Filter
Picture	Are human faces available in pictures? (1 or 0)	Photo tagging
Car Sensors and Camera	Location of other cars on the road	Self-driving cars

and the second important thing for you is charges of the rope. Thus if you are starting to make a Machine learning system that helps you to find the price according to your requirement of rope length you can think of the rope length as an input and the price of rope is output and the mapping is done by a system of supervised learning. Now it's not just rope size because the price depends on many other parameters like the color of rope and quality or fabric of rope, in such cases, the input can be together length and fabric type and the outcome is charges of the product. Thus, it depends on the system or can say on the business to filter the output according to the given input and people can also search or check the rope length approachable according to their budget. So, for such situations, the input can be the amount a person can spend and output can be the size of rope. Importantly, the main concern is data should be correct, there are different types of data text, visual videos, voice tracks, and all these types are intercepted by humans easily and come under unstructured data, but the AI techniques to work on structured and unstructured data are different accordingly [7].

As of now, AI can do, is looking for data input and output mapping but some inflated the expectations of AI that some things are not possible by AI. The challenge is from academic literature reports they are all positive results stories without any failure thus people always think that everything is possible using AI. Therefore, in companies, there might be the intuition of handling more and can be less optimistic. For example, speech recognizant, the position of other cars in driving training all these things is possible by AI in seconds the same as humans can observe in less than 1 s, in contrast, like in the analysis of any report of 100 pages humans can't do this within seconds. Here is an example, if you have ordered a gift from an online e-commerce website on your friend's birthday, you want to surprise only on his special day but your order has not reached on that particular day but after 2 days it reached your given address, and some questions raised in our mind like can I return now?. If in such a situation, you mailed to the company's customer support center, your mail will be the input A in the AI system and output can be a refund request, there was a shipping problem or there was another issue or request. These three are the possibilities of output B. It's what AI can't do, if you text A as input to the AI system A is not able to automatically generate a reply like Sorry to hear this. We hope your friend had a wonderful birthday. For an AI system, it is difficult to send this type of test by analyzing the text that it was a friend's birthday. For every single type of mail creating an intelligence reply, not the automatic reply such as we are using nowadays, we have received your mail please wait for 24 h. Thus the AI systems taking input and emails and creating such responses that are according to the written text are not under the category of can't do. It is difficult to say that after 10,000 examples of such mails will it be possible for the AI to reply automatically and do well in other sender's context and show the concern by this much data.

1.2 Deep Learning

Deep learning and Neural networks are two replaceable words to each other in Artificial Intelligence. Here we will discuss the deep learning concept. In our market let's see a shopping store if you want to sell your products, first, there will be some data based on facts applicable to data a person can take interest in your shop products for example if the price is more the demand of that particular product is lower which is shown in graph in Fig. 13.1 that the demand drops when prices increases.

In Fig. 13.2 we can see the first factor which we are going to compare and consider is the price whenever you have to purchase anything, by looking at the price you will get to know is it in my budget so affordability is checked and based on this person is making a decision and thus it acts as a neuron, in the same way, second, this will come is marketing. It also affects the demand of people. Marketing convinces people to purchase a particular company according to weight, fabric, and size. The person will check the fabric of the product quality wise and will check if the same quality in the market is available at a lesser price, thus for one product, there are different neurons awareness, quality of the product in the range of charges these all make neural network and results in fluctuation in demand. Neurons in Artificial

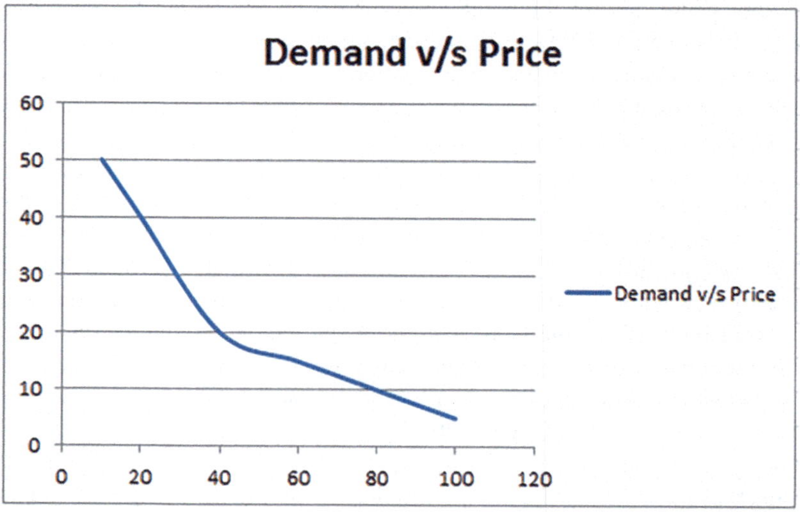

Fig. 13.1 Demand on y-axis and Price on the x-axis

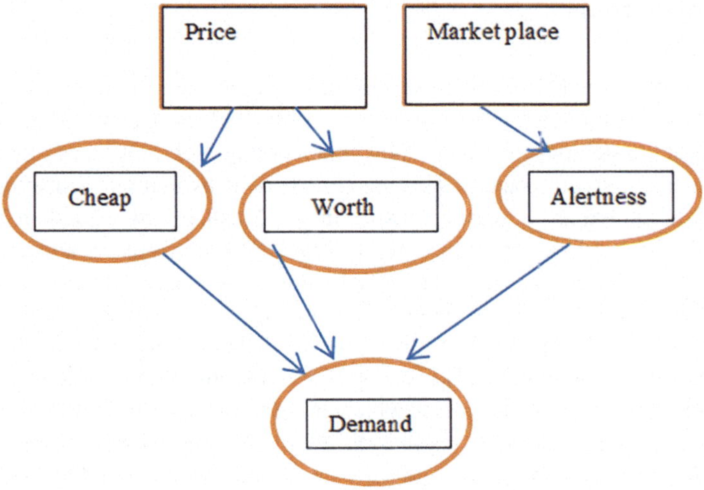

Fig. 13.2 Small neural network

intelligence are also known as Artificial Neurons and these small neurons create a network called a neural network. Thus a neural network computes one function with the help of neurons like demand predictions [8].

Examples: understanding the audio, recognizing the voice, identifying the person in pictures, and are the common intelligence used in our daily life from smartphones. There are a lot of surveys of computer visions in different areas and for different applications. The major area is image classification and object detection.

AI Image Classification/Object detection: By taking a picture as the input your system will detect that it is a human picture or a dog in the picture. This type of classification is used vastly. This is what we are using regularly on our smartphones, smart doors known as face recognition. We first register our face pic and then whenever we look by our face in front of the camera, it gets unlocked by recognizing that this is the same person's registered face. Not only classification or recognition, but object detection is also possible by deep learning algorithms. The next step after detection is image segmentation. It is creating boundaries on the actual shape of the object. This same concept of Image Segmentation is used in the Medical field in X-ray scans and some other image processes of the human body. These scans or images are given as the input to the image segmentation algorithms and the system will detect and segment the body parts and boundary the other suspected objects. Therefore, deep learning plays an important role in the health field.

In this chapter, Sect. 2 discusses related work. Section 3 contains AI techniques in Biomedical imaging. Section 4 is about the uses of AI in Detection and Prioritization. Section 5 will be about Virtual High Throughput Screening in AI, segment. Section 6 is discussing the improvement of the treatment process in AI, followed by Sect. 7 which is about healthcare in AI and the last module is the conclusion section.

2 Related Work

A lot of research has been done in several fields of education to obtain information on how AI is incorporated in various stages of life. Nelson A et al. [9], in his paper explained the basic concept of how Machine learning works. It takes input as data and will map the input to output. This mapping is done by neurons is inspired by the human brain known as the neural network in AI. All such things are done by AI in less than 1 s. For Individuals in the coming years it's a job displacement and it's not only this, it will progress as the work by AI automation is vast than before, thus this is not ending. In this article, different healthcare fields like ophthalmologists collaborate with the intelligence system to work the diabetic system by deploying the image classification automatically in seconds. Fundus photography in computing is a way to remove blindness in adults which is seen worldwide by monitoring and checking if early treatment is possible on a patient's stage identification. Several tasks of diagnosis and taking decisions are overtaken and improved by AI systems. Table 13.2 describes the diverse fields of the survey.

3 Techniques of AI that Are Employed in the Biomedical Field

Computer visualization, or machine revelation, is tremendously growing and extensively employed in biomedical productiveness and health care. Computer visualization or machine vision is the facility that enables the computers towards the arena of recognition, interpretation, analyzing, and comprehending the aspects contained by a visual. Computer Visualization can practice the prior knowledge, outlining, quality, and profile beside the contextual evidence in the images, to make visual comprehension enhanced in the humans. Health Productiveness is spilling over the norm of MRI, CT, PET, and USG practices that delivers a huge diversity of ironic data to be processed through computer Visualization [18–20].

3.1 AI Techniques to Treat the Hefty Datasets

The mammoth volume of visual data is being manufactured through the healthcare and biotechnical setups. As the apparatuses for catching genetic and curative images are attaining betterment, it enhances the data gathering to propagate exponentially. In the core of the data, we may attain the prized intuitions in a condition of a patient, disease enlargement in his body including the cell arrangement at the molecular level [21, 22]. Though, the potentials of traditional investigation are outshined with the opportunity obtained from the data. Meanwhile, certain evidence commencing the imaging data can be snubbed or misinterpreted which is a noteworthy challenge to

Table 13.2 Research work

Year	Reference of title	Conclusion
2019	[9]	It is essential to measure the technical accuracy of quality results to patients using Robust clinical valuation (AI Algorithms). Future work is needed on the improvement of interpretability and generalization of predictions using machine learning.
2019	[10]	This paper describes the prediction that could be biased into the healthcare sector by algorithms like in genetic findings when there was genetic study availability in a particular population as per the analysis of AI algorithms used in non-medical fields. This kind of discrimination in the health field is to foresee. There should be ethical rules that could guide the determination, methods to predict for patients whose data is not recorded and need to reimage the confidentiality first instead of supporting the biased electronic records.
2019	[11]	This study focuses on the different applications of AI in the Health field namely Diagnostics, Therapeutics, population health management systems, Administration, and regulations. Algorithms work based on patient information which is nowadays present electronically and the accessibility of the records will help in decision making to the patient's health for remote monitoring, physicians, registries on hospitals systems, used for surveys in Regulatory bodies.
2019	[12]	The work shows a Knowledge Cycle from Tacit to explicit knowledge implemented using AI tools. It represented the Information by modeling as input as explicit to do the Analysis of intelligent data to make a knowledge representation. This is completed by the management cycle Care flow Management System (CfMS) to make information again from the next analysis. Thus the creation of knowledge is an important part of organizational learning.
2018	[13]	In this paper, the representation form derived consists of several non-linear, primitive operations and in medicine, it helps in imaging and movements as seen in radiology, dermatology, ophthalmology, and pathology diagnosis in result enhancing the ML phenotype predictions. Deep learning can be used in improving the quality of analysis of genomic data. Genomic data like DNA cell-free are usually noisy and require advanced study and measurements for identification.
2018	[14]	This article gives the views on how ML can Augment the work of Clinicians. A model was constructed and all the tasks with the treatment and for diagnosis were explained.
2018	[15]	This paper reviews that it would use more instead of customer interaction algorithms like now the AI promises but works low on the data proof. The Ability of performance in medicines on the data-driven and by intercepting the resources of humans.
2020	[16]	In between the predictive behavior of algorithms and human specifications of algorithms have one mark which is the machine learning spectrum, One more study depicted that to ensure valid results there should be the practice of clinical experts with original risky statistics for the decisions on dependent and independent variables and their interactions.
2021	[6]	This paper explains the progress of the role of NLP and ML in Oncology. Notable results have been seen from AI Genetic Diagnostic Analysis Practices with Watson's initiative to collaborate with Quest Diagnostics.

(continued)

Table 13.2 (continued)

Year	Reference of title	Conclusion
		Further work required firstly to use data from the real world to get performance justification and to get low-risk customer products by general wellness of AI products. Secondly, Machines are tested in a simulated environment based on historical data but data updating is necessary for continuation which is a major issue as organizations are putting incentives that create hurdles in data exchange.
2019	[17]	AI investments are growing vastly, Not only is AI on top of the technology edge but outside the computer world also it's on an experimental stage. This paper exhibits the investment in AI in the deployment of AI products, by the corporation to develop the AI application. It depicts the investment in travel and tourism, retails, media, account services, Transportation, and telecommunication with an overall index of assets, usage, and labor.

take care of. AI may assist us to achieve information out of voluminous data in the same way as the human brain does [23, 24].

3.2 Medical Advances Through AI Medical Diagnosis

AI embedded with medical diagnosis expertise assist in the conductance of mechanized and universal findings to detect the health state with a trifling error occurrence [25] and is shown in Fig. 13.3.

1. **Digital Imaging**: The role of artificial intelligence in testing the lab is no doubt more in the use of machines where these are embedded in programs for imaging. These programs are skilled with the expertise of the medical field and their usage is required in the identification of numerous ailments that can be recognized with digital imaging techniques. More precautions need to be taken for minimizing the miscalculations while designing the digital imaging machines therefore AI techniques can be incorporated within the machinery for optimum ailment detection. Hence assimilating Artificial Intelligence in devices of medical analysis results in attaining the turnaround time which is minimal compared to the conventional analysis.
2. **Automated Diagnosis**: To increase the productivity and reduction in manual processing of pathology reports, the mechanized behavior of pathology in a digital way is involved with the brainpower by embedding the AI abilities in these instruments. The intelligent machine supports the speedy result and Machine learning makes diagnosis more accurate and proper.
3. **AI incorporation in Lab testing**: With the association of artificial intelligence in Lab testing there is conversion to intelligent algorithms which can find the general and particular patterns that can provide accurate prediction and offer methods to

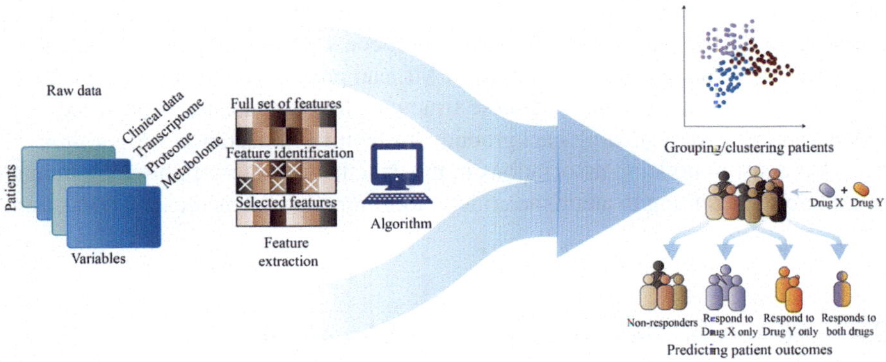

Fig. 13.3 Software solution of medical diagnosis using AI

cure the syndromes in a different patient. The medical diagnosis association with AI makes the usage of programmed devices for the investigation of ailments in the fatalities to offer a turnaround time shorter than outdated examinations.

4. **Analyzing through Images**: The medical identification through AI produces an instantaneous renovation, which enables the pathologists to play digitally with no more dealing through glass, but through digital images while dealing essentially through pixels which can be examined over a globe by any expert. Incorporating algorithms by using the image investigation enhances the mechanized exploration of AI in medical analysis which allows the generation of results concluded over research and detailed records in the software.
5. **Dealings through Cloud-based policy**: In medical diagnosis Over AI, research enhancement and collaborative diagnosis are possible by sending documents as well as scanned reports to diverse consultants around the globe, by which there is no need to physically present them from one place to another location. AI in pathology has many features, including AI for testing, less manual involvement in results that are often found in physical inquiry.
6. **Predictive Analysis**: Preceding the inception of the vulnerable ailments the technique of the predictive analysis that is significant resolutions of AI promotes the clinicians to identify the chances of fatal disease happening. Thereby crafts the belief of precautionary care as conflicting to curative care. With the acknowledgment of machine learning intelligence, susceptibility in the patients for certain disorders is highlighted and consequently, the devotion of the pathologist is seized in advising them for long-term attention.

3.3 Enhancement in the Medical Analysis Accuracy

Medical experts from various scans like Magnetic Resonance imaging to X-rays are obligatory to survey the compound imaginings to scrutinize the health of a patient to initiate its identification. AI resolutions can be employed by medical doctors to meet the answers to the patient's requirements and constrict the diagnosis varieties by enriching the accuracy. The algorithms of ML can progress and gain the new tricks for recognition arrangements of disease structures like breast cancers presence over mammograms and evaluating backgrounds for textural appearances. Algorithms of ML also assist in noticing associations in the data that is imperceptible for a human eye, therefore resulting to attain the critical 'tool' for superior medical identification.

3.4 AI Aids in Time and Resources Managing

For ailment analysis AI may assist by cutting down the overheads in careful conveyance, it supports healthcare consultants by cutting the time overheads for ascertaining a lethal condition. AI techniques can train models with the intelligence with which they can predict the slimmest deformities, which can create significant challenges in saving or mislaying a patient.

3.5 Enhancing Artificial Intelligence Processes

Artificial Intelligence practices can be enhanced by implementing them in various applications such as follows:

1. **Radiology usage**: AI advances and implementation in radiology are scattering speedily. It has been assessed that in the United States in the radiology arena an algorithm every month is approved by Food and Drug Administration.

   Example: Google has established an algorithm to control a cardiovascular threat in a patient by observing their retinas scan.
2. **Usage in drug detection**: In the arena of drug detection, enormous value is brought by AI. It's been challenging to deal with microscopic imageries, as imageries formed may vary in testing from one set to the next. Temperature Instabilities, component bunches, and revelation time may be producing ambiguous fluctuations unrelated to the reading which alters the drug complex. Charging the track by sorting out the properties is challenging in data-bound drug detection. Therefore AI blocks all these tasks, exclusively throughput screening stage, resulting in a competent, inexpensive, and quicker drug detection process.
3. **Usage in surgery optimization**: Enhanced pre-operative arrangement of surgeries may be associated with the usage of AI that enables the doctors to strategize the surgical method from prevailing medical accounts. At this point, imaging is vital for the victory of the surgery and it can be obtained using various scanning techniques. With the involvement of AI, specialists are capable to fix superior surgeries. AI improves anatomic organization, discovery, segmentation, and

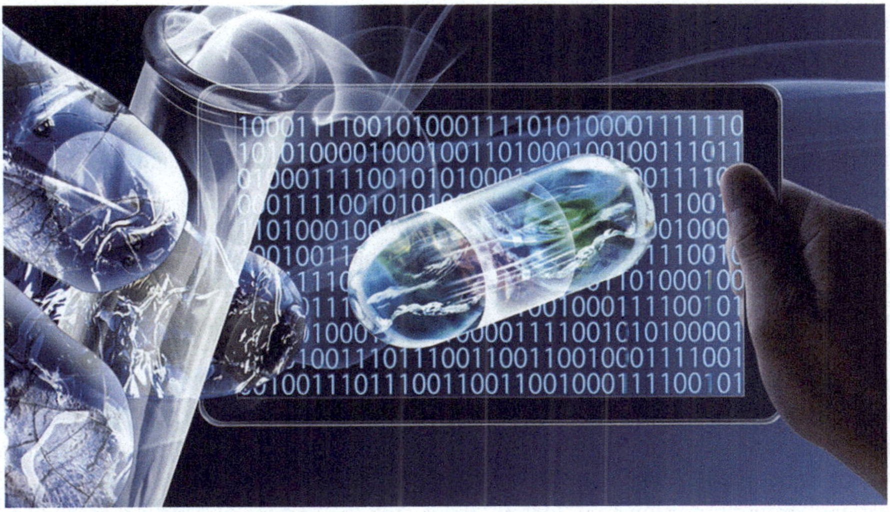

Fig. 13.4 Improvement of radiology with AI

cataloging between medical imageries. Usage of AI also assists the intra-operative supervision for enhancing surgical procedures.

3.6 *Benefits of Applying AI to Radiology*

Figure 13.4 represents AI with radiology. The benefits of applying Artificial Intelligence to Radiology are used for the detection and prioritization through radiological imaging.

The AI in the context of clinical workflows on imaging is as follows:

1. **Triage**: Artificial Intelligence Screens the Investigations for the possibility of illness to govern the sequence of the elucidation.
2. **Auxiliary**: Artificial Intelligence is employed to produce the output that regularly outperforms social radiologists.
3. **Optional**: Artificial Intelligence maintenances the conventional medical pathways in controlling the time-demanding activities.

Certain capabilities can assist the radiologists which are:

1. **Productive**: The productivity can be done through robotics and ranking of jobs along with the data feeds.
2. **Computable**: By the supply of requests and tools to half-automatic or full automatic abstract may compute the information.
3. **Precise**: the right to evidence is available, that can be manipulated and offered sustenance of the analysis, as well as certifying the repeatability of the quantification practices.

4 AI Used for Prioritization and Discovery

In medical care revealing is the artwork for AI, but several techniques can be supplementary as a showing tool. It is very intricate and composite to express the margin in a proper way between a common and an anomalous image. With automated detection, radiologists view images based on the reading priority which speeds reporting and improves patient outcomes. With the addition of retrieval services, the AI pulls similar images from a database for review when it encounters unusual or complex cases [26, 27]. Artificial intelligence technique deals with time reserves, enrich performance, and prioritize the former concealment of fatal ailments like cancers. In the varied range of lethal diseases, breast carcinoma in females is the most frequently spotted carcinoma in European countries, with over 36,000 women, detected to be its victim in 2020 following by colorectal cancer 340,000 i.e. 12.7%, prostate cancer 335,000 which figures to 12.5%, followed by lung cancer where the victim ranges to 320,000. With the expansion of European inhabitants the older patients grow proportionately, thereby increasing the victims of cancer disease like lungs, prostate, etc. correspondingly With the present-day scarcity of radiologists in European countries is likely to stay in the upcoming times. It has been investigated that more than 330,000 scans have been in a queue for above 30 days therefore there is a great demand for the development of AI in this field to secure many breaths. Lunit is an Intelligence software company in the medical field that works for the development and enhanced digital medical scanning, analytical plus records driven from the biological markers by cutting-edge in the technique of deep learning. Lunit's operation is to supply numerous AI resolutions to expose a new period of record-driven correctness medicine, to resolve the utmost critical concerns in cancer care ailments currently [28].

4.1 AWARENESS of Lunit Mammary Gland Scan

Awareness of Lunit mammography (MMG) assists the various authorities ranging from breast experts to general experts and non-expert radiologists by incremental the cancer recognition ratio and decreasing the ratio of false positives by inferring selection mammograms. The accuracy of this software is 96% that can enhance significantly the interpretive skills of radiologists by more than 10%. Incorporating AI in the investigation of mammogram imaginings could assist in reducing the false positive/negative recalls and efficaciously triage up to 60% of all circumstances devoid of human interpretation, minimizing the reading job by more than half. Additionally, it advances diagnostic correctness of mammograms for thick and blubbery breasts up to 9% and 22%.

4.2 Lunit AWARENESS in Chest

Plunging into chest X-rays i.e. chest CXR has supported radiologists in handling challenging circumstances of chest oddities, aiding them in diminishing the danger of unused cases. The Lunit CXR has enhanced the accuracy of 97% to 99% has increased with the aid of intelligent techniques. Workflow effectiveness of it is diminishing the total report of chest abnormalities. It enables customization of Radiologists in detecting the verdicts and their imagining methods over the scientific environs. Lunit CXR insight discovers the nodules, cardiomegaly, atelectasis, pneumothorax, fibrosis, calcification, pleural effusion consolidation, and widening. It also provides maintenances for the selection in tuberculosis.

AI provides the potential that enables several radiologists with the enhanced skills by providing the diverse concept to disease detection in modern times and has made many advents in diverse congresses. Therefore AI is providing a gap for the researchers to enhance the various educational fields.

4.3 Profits of Applying AI in Discovery of Drugs

The AI usage in the discovery of drugs has the prospective to transform the current time including the opportunity of drug detection. Based on understanding benefits are as under:

1. **Increase precision**:

   To elaborate significant dealings Artificial Intelligence has a sophisticated predictive control in a drug screening comparatively to the customary approaches of drug detection. For example, it can be used to identify novel drug structures/ compounds and helps in improving the skill of that unique substance to occupy its goal. Ultimately, AI help's to increase precision, reduce false positives, and improve the design of the parameters of the assay in question.
2. **Find new drugs cheaper and faster**:

   Because of the advancements in processing power, AI-based algorithms can make drug discovery a much cheaper and much faster process. For Example, AI can screen a compound library of several billion molecules, and significantly reduce the time needed for in vitro efforts and for preclinical candidates to be identified.
3. **Empower Virtual Labs**:

   It is not uncommon for companies to not have in–house laboratory plants, equipment, and instruments needed to run experiments. Fortunately, AI has the potential to move drug screening to a virtual lab, where the results of a screen can be obtained with greater speed, and without the need for extensive costs and long manpower hours.

5 AI in Virtual High Throughput Screening (HTS)

The traditional drug discovery process is a high-risk, high-return approach that is costly and time-consuming. For that reason, Artificial Intelligence has been attracting attention in this field as an innovative technology that can increase the possibility of success, while dramatically reducing costs and time for research and development.

5.1 Why Is AI Spreading to Drug Discovery?

New drug discovery is a field that requires vast resources, is time-intensive, and requires an integration of a wide variety of specialized skills in each step of the method. It's assessed that one in ten minor molecules, jobs turn into applicants for experimental judgments, and about one in ten of these combinations will provide the clearance efficaciously through medical trials. Our virtual HTS solution transforms the drug development process, by speeding up to hit discovery, from weeks to hours.

We developed our state-of-the-art solution for drug discovery. This early-stage technology is highly effective for virtual high-throughput screening. The technology has provided performances superior to common virtual screening tools and methods, thanks to our novel algorithm that keeps on improving every day.

5.2 Business Benefits in Drug Discovery

Discovering new and successful drugs is a hard and time-consuming process. Our virtual HTS solution can improve drug development by:

1. Ascertaining more auspicious drug applicants.
2. Hovering the percentage or "hit rate" of drug applicants which creates it over the scientific trials gains the governing the authorization.
3. Flying up the whole procedure.
4. Focusing HTS effort on promising compounds and bioassays.
5. Reducing time and costs (expensive reagents, expensive bioassays).

Our virtual HTS solution can help companies make their search for new pharmaceuticals quicker, cheaper, and more effective.

5.3 *Increase Speed and Reduce Costs*

Substance screening and making Artificial Intelligence saves 40–50% of the period, saving up to $26 million in screening costs per year. Our solution can process and analyze extremely large libraries in a fraction of time and money. Hence increasing the speed and efficiency of the drug development process and decreasing the time to shop. To bring a novel drug the normal cost in the marketplace is assessed to be $2.6 billion. Our solution enables biopharma organizations to dedicate their resources to the most promising compounds and save considerable resources. It also increases their chances to find new promising compounds or generate new insights on existing compounds.

6 How Artificial Intelligence Is Improving the Process of Treatment

The best entity in relating Artificial Intelligence with health maintenance is its progress in several domains from collecting and handing the valued information out of data to implementing in programmed specialist robots. There are different ways that AI can be used for medical purposes which are discussed below:

6.1 *Usage of Artificial Intelligence in Detecting Diseases*

In sprouting healthcare productiveness application of Artificial Intelligence delivers abundant benefits to medical identification. Before the apparent indications, Artificial Intelligence embedded software can envisage several issues in the health of a patient. The examples of detecting diseases through AI are as follows:

1. Detection of lung carcinoma and strokes on basis scans.
2. Classifications of skin lesions using skin imaginings.
3. Discovering the signs of eye imaginings to detect diabetic retinopathy.
4. Evaluating the threat of unexpected cardiac expiry or other heart sicknesses on basis of electrocardiograms as well as cardiac arrests through MRI imaginings.

6.2 *Cataloguing Diseases*

The opportunity of deep learning technologies to analyze images and recognize patterns opens up the potential for creating algorithms to help doctors diagnose specific diseases faster and more accurately. AI-driven software can be programmed to accurately spot the signs of certain diseases in medical images such as MRIs,

X-rays, and CT scans. Similar solutions already use AI for cancer Diagnosis by processing photos of skin lesions. Using such tools doctors can diagnose patients more accurately.

6.3 Improvement in the Process of Decision-Making

Diagnostics and treatment have always been tricky processes. The reason for this is that doctors need to simultaneously consider the symptoms of the patients, the possible research mistakes, all the existing treatment methods, potential side effects, diseases with similar signs, and many more aspects. The solutions based on AI technology already help doctors to overcome research obstacles, process vast amounts of health data fast, and ensure a holistic understanding of a patient's health.

6.4 Treatment Resolutions on Basis of AI

Even when the disease is detected and classified, the treatment process can cause additional issues. Not only, a treatment plan includes prescribing medicines and exercises, but also coordinating care plans, helping patients manage their treatment programs, and considering the risk of an adverse event. AI algorithms already help doctors arrange a comprehensive approach to disease management. They are often used to improve surgical robots that execute highly complex operations.

6.5 Making People to Breathing Longer

AI is a ruling technique that assists in forecasting the life of people and shrink the necessity of hospitalization. Algorithms embedded with AI process each evidence related to healthiness, existence, and atmosphere we proceed in. They can predict our biological age and offer measures we need to take to stay healthy. AI is already combined with aging research to create an aging clock, which is going to help track immune senescence levels and identify new interventions designed to boost the immune system in the elderly.

1. **Sequential age**: Sequentially, the number of years you survived and when a person expires, the total becomes the time of death. This normal cast-off the determination in universal logic of life probability, however, it's agreeable to have somewhat to shoot beside it.
2. **Biological age**: The stage of development is numeric perceptions that consist of the standard of living, genetic temperament, and background. A super-healthier individual is one whose descendants naturally lived to 100 years of age.

7 AI in Healthcare

It depicts capability in software programs towards work the mode human beings are identifying the patterns, symptoms in different situations based on real-life changes. It is changing the method of getting the information and using it to develop and invent the systems for the healthcare of people. Artificial Intelligence is the yield of input supply: big data requires scrubbing, structuring, and integration. Big data is well-defined in veracity, velocity, volume, variability, variety, and complexity. These expressions are referred to as the quantity, speediness, range sources, correctness, and accuracy of data.

7.1 *Deep Learning to Diagnose Diseases*

A field in which machine learning cutting-edge the health maintenance area profits in the utmost surprising in the arena of diagnosis. Primary stage identification is a significant point to cure the health of a patient. Deep learning AI algo's are used to simplify the time to detect critical disorders. Methods of Artificial Intelligence rapidly practice and works on bulky quantities of data and attains in resulting the foundations of signs that considerably make a lower period on diagnosis, treatment, and recovery cycle for many patients.

7.2 *Automating Administrative Tasks*

The health is one should always be on the top and while working in our life we have to pay the extra charges on administrating and time consuming administrative tasks. With intelligence systems, these administrate tasks without wasting time and hiring people possible within less time and the same resources can be used on diagnosis and cure by helping with that charges on health care providers and on research which is required more than other tasks.

7.3 *Reducing Operational Costs*

The working cost of healthcare companies and especially the private one for employees working for manual entries is reducing and providers at each level in medical fields embed the intelligent software programs for fast results and for less manpower which manage the budget and improve the work efficiency.

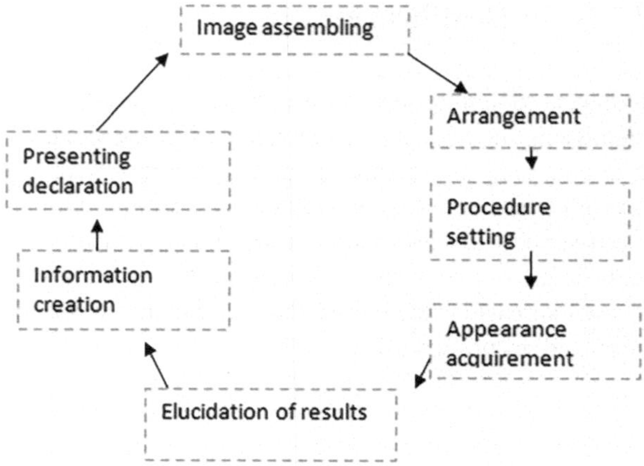

Fig. 13.5 Procedure AI in radiology medicines

7.4 *Artificial Intelligence in Medicine*

Siri, Alexa, and Cortana are the corporate usages of Artificial Intelligence. IBM Watson oncology in the medication field has chosen preparations for handling the cancerous patients with efficient tips comparatively to the human authorities Hanover project of the Microsoft's at Oregon has examined curative exploration to tailor bespoke options in cancer management. National health services used Google's deep mind stage for distinguishing wellbeing threats by evaluating mobile app information and medicinal descriptions aggregated from NHS patients. Stanford's radiology procedure selected pneumonia enhanced than social radiologists, while in diabetic retinopathy task; the processor was as worthy as expert ophthalmologists for creating a referral assessment (Fig. 13.5).

7.5 *Detecting Blood Cancer Using Artificial Intelligence*

The latest research has depicted that an important and most arising type of cancer in blood—is severe myeloid leukemia that can be detected, identified using Artificial Intelligence systems. AI can diagnose such blood cancer form by high reliability. The researcher's technique was based on the gene motion of cells present in plasma. They showed that this can accelerate the start of therapy and could enhance conventional diagnostics. The symptoms seen of AML in the starting level, are similar to individuals having a bad cold but AML should be cured as quickly as possible as it is a life-threatening disease.

The patient is advised to visit a specialist only when the suspicion is confirmed. The diagnosis could happen much earlier leading to early therapy. The researchers focused on a kind of fingerprint of gene activity, called the "transcriptome". Only a few categories of genes in every body cell, on its state, are essentially moved to that reflection of their gene motion. In the current study on AML, the same data were acquired from chambers of blood trials, and crossing several thousands of protein sequences was evaluated. The trials have been taken from around 4100 individuals whom they had detected using AML, and the rest have been obtained from beings who are healthy and or from individuals who have other symptoms and are facing the other diseases. Furthermore, data is analyzed and based on the pattern recognition which is followed and the particular algorithms are classified into two categorical samples without AML and AML containing samples. Conventional diagnostics could be supported by this method using artificial intelligence when it is used, and it can help save costs.

Artificial intelligence can detect one of the most common forms of blood cancer AML with high-reliability researchers at the German Center for neurodegenerative diseases and the University of Bonn, Artificial intelligence is a much-discussed topic in medicine especially in the field of diagnostics. Numerous studies have been carried out on the topic and the results are available through databases. Thus there is an enormous data pool.

7.6 *Fingerprint in Gene Activity*

Schultze and his colleagues focused on the transcriptome which is a kind of fingerprint of gene activity. Every cell of a body is depending on its condition. Then only certain genes are switched on which is reflected in the profiles of their gene activity. Then such data derived from cells in the blood samples and spanning many thousands of genes were analyzed.

The transcriptome holds important information about the condition of cells. However, classical diagnostics is based on different data. The current study focused on AML without adequate treatment, this form of leukemia leads to death within weeks. AML is associated with the proliferation of pathologically altered bone marrow cells, which can ultimately enter the bloodstream. Both healthy cells and tumor cells drift in the blood. All these cells exhibit typical gene activity patterns, which were all considered in the analysis. The data has been taken from more than 12,000 blood samples that came from 105 different studies. Approximately 4100 of these blood samples are derived from individuals diagnosed with AML.

8 Conclusion

In this chapter, the authors discussed the various fields of Bio-medical education where Artificial intelligence is going hand in hand, a wide range of ailments need to be addressed when considering artificial intelligence. The rising construction of massive amounts of data related to health care will vitally change biomedical care. We firmly believe that soon will be the time when all the biomedical practitioners whether in the medical field or education field will be incorporating the various models of Artificial intelligence for decision making to out care the billions of patients to cure the dreadful diseases and to outshine in the field of biomedical education to perform various research to address the solution to the unreachable corners in this field.

References

1. Mahadevaiah G, Prasad RV, Bermejo I, Jaffray D, Dekker A, Wee L (2020) Artificial intelligence-based clinical decision support in modern medical physics: selection, acceptance, commissioning, and quality assurance. Med Phys 47(5):e228–e235. https://doi.org/10.1002/mp.13562
2. Gull S, Loan NA, Parah SA (2020) An efficient watermarking technique for tamper detection and localization of medical images. J Ambient Intell Human Comput 11:1799–1808
3. Lång K, Hofvind S, Rodríguez-Ruiz A, Andersson I (2021) Can artificial intelligence reduce the interval cancer rate in mammography screening? Eur Radiol 31(8):5940–5947. https://doi.org/10.1007/s00330-021-07686-3
4. Gull S, Parah SA, Khan M (2020) Reversible data hiding exploiting Huffman encoding with dual images for IoMT based healthcare. Comput Commun 163:134–149
5. Sarosh P, Parah SA, Bhat GM, Heidari AA, Muhammad K (2021) Secret sharing-based personal health records management for the Internet of Health Things. Sustain Cities Soc 74:103129
6. Diaz O, Guidi G, Ivashchenko O, Colgan N, Zanca F (2021) Artificial intelligence in the medical physics community: an international survey. Phys Med 81:141–146
7. Shah AA, Parah SA, Rashid M, Elhoseny M (2020) Efficient image encryption scheme based on the generalized logistic map for real-time image processing. J Real-Time Image Proc 17(6):2139–2151
8. Sarosh P, Parah SA, Bhat GM (2021) Fast image encryption framework for medical images. In: 2021 2nd International conference on intelligent engineering and management (ICIEM). IEEE, New York, pp 149–154
9. Nelson A, Herron D, Rees G, Nachev P (2019) Predicting scheduled hospital attendance with artificial intelligence. NPJ Digit Med 2(1):26
10. He J, Baxter SL, Xu J, Xu J, Zhou X, Zhang K (2019) The practical implementation of artificial intelligence technologies in medicine. Nat Med 25(1):30–36
11. Rajkomar A, Dean J, Kohane I (2019) Machine learning in medicine. N Engl J Med 380(14):1347–1358
12. Sidey-Gibbons JAM, Sidey-Gibbons CJ (2019) Machine learning in medicine: a practical introduction. BMC Med Res Methodol 19(1):64
13. Vayena E, Blasimme A, Cohen IG (2018) Machine learning in medicine: addressing ethical challenges. PLoS Med 15(11):e1002689
14. Char DS, Shah NH, Magnus D (2018) Implementing machine learning in health care—addressing ethical challenges. N Engl J Med 378(11):981–983
15. Rajkomar A, Oren E, Chen K, Dai AM, Hajaj N, Hardt M, Liu PJ, Liu X, Marcus J, Sun M, Sundberg P, Yee H, Zhang K, Zhang Y, Flores G, Duggan GE, Irvine J, Le Q, Litsch K, Dean J (2018) Scalable and accurate deep learning with electronic health records. NPJ Digit Med 1(1):18
16. Garg T (2020) Artificial intelligence in medical education. Am J Med 133(2):e68
17. Watanabe AT, Lim V, Vu HX, Chim R, Weise E, Liu J, Bradley WG, Comstock CE (2019) Improved cancer detection using artificial intelligence: a retrospective evaluation of missed cancers on mammography. J Digit Imaging 32(4):625–637

18. Kamili A, Fatima I, Hassan M, Parah SA, Vijaya Kumar V, Ambati LS (2020) Embedding information reversibly in medical images for e-health. J Intell Fuzzy Syst 39:8389–8398
19. Nazeer I, Rashid M, Yousuf MM, Wani UI, Kaur A (2019) Medical diagnosis cloud model for detection of kidney diseases. In: 2019 Fifth international conference on image information processing (ICIIP). IEEE, New York, pp 315–320
20. Rashid M, Yousuf MM, Ram B, Goyal V (2019) Novel Big Data approach for drug prediction in health care systems. In: 2019 International conference on automation, computational and technology management (ICACTM). IEEE, New York, pp 325–329
21. Parah SA, Kaw JA, Bellavista P, Loan NA, Bhat GM, Muhammad K, Victor A (2020) Efficient security and authentication for edge-based internet of medical things. IEEE Internet Things J 8: 15652–15662
22. Jan A, Parah SA, Malik BA (2020) A novel Laplacian of Gaussian (LoG) and chaotic encryption based image steganography technique. In: 2020 International conference for emerging technology (INCET). IEEE, New York, pp 1–4
23. Gull S, Mansour RF, Aljehane NO, Parah SA (2021) A self-embedding technique for tamper detection and localization of medical images for smart health. Multimed Tools Appl 80(19): 29939–29964
24. Sethi GK, Ahmad N, Rehman MB, Dafallaa HMEI, Rashid M (2021) Use of artificial intelligence in healthcare systems: state-of-the-art survey. In: 2021 2nd International conference on intelligent engineering and management (ICIEM). IEEE, New York, pp 243–248
25. Kumar I, Alshamrani SS, Kumar A, Rawat J, Singh KU, Rashid M, AlGhamdi AS (2021) Deep learning approach for analysis and characterization of COVID-19. Comput Mater Continua 70: 451–468
26. Rathour N, Alshamrani SS, Singh R, Gehlot A, Rashid M, Akram SV, AlGhamdi AS (2021) IoMT based facial emotion recognition system using deep convolution neural networks. Electronics 10(11):1289
27. Khan AA, Shaikh AA, Cheikhrouhou O, Laghari AA, Rashid M, Shafiq M, Hamam H (2021) IMG-forensics: multimedia-enabled information hiding investigation using convolutional neural network. IET Image Process. https://doi.org/10.1049/ipr2.12272
28. Mondal S, Agarwal K, Rashid M (2019) Deep learning approach for automatic classification of x-ray images using convolutional neural network. In: 2019 Fifth international conference on image information processing (ICIIP). IEEE, New York, pp 326–331

Chapter 14
The Emergence of Natural Language Processing (NLP) Techniques in Healthcare AI

Rakesh Kumar Attar and Komal

Contents

1 Introduction

Natural Language Processing, a specialized branch of AI, aims on the interpreting and manipulating of human generated written or spoken data. NLP mainly focuses on inference of meaningful data by analyzing speech and text data. Natural language processing (NLP) can be termed as the ability for computational machines to better understand the human spoken terms and written text. NLP is extensively used in modern technology to provide assistance for privacy of spam email, personal voice assistants and application of language translation. NLP is a very demanding and appealing research domain in linguistic informatics. NLP has the capability of analysis and extraction of information from distinct unstructured sources, rendering question answer process in automatic manner and summarization of textual data and conducting analysis on sentiments. NLP is often used to include a set of methods

R. Kumar Attar (✉)
Department of Computer Science, University College Miranpur, Patiala, India

Komal
Department of Computer Science, M.M. Modi College, Patiala, India

S. A. Parah et al. (eds.), *Artificial Intelligence for Innovative Healthcare Informatics*,
https://doi.org/10.1007/978-3-030-96569-3_14

involving the processing of unstructured texts. However, some methods make use of less semantic knowledge, and are purely based on the occurrence of words in text. The semantic knowledge required in these is the knowledge of what comprises a word; these methods rely on the approach of bag-of-words or a keyword. One instance of a method is a search engine, which make use of only words, extracting all the records containing the occurrence of a mixture of words in a group, although these words may totally differ from each other in the extracted documents. For instance, a method of machine learning that make use of words independently to build a statistical model. Generally, more advanced semantic methods of NLP pursue to ascertain all or some of the linguistic structure in text and to construe meaning of related information in text. Natural language processing is being utilized to portray the methodology of exploiting computer algorithms for identification of main elements in everyday language and extracting meaning from unstructured written or spoken input. NLP needs special skills in AI, computational linguistics, and other disciplines of machine learning [1].

Natural Language Processing, being formulaic, makes easy reason for computational methods to process it. Being formulaic, it contains discrete words, and grammar rules defining how diverse semantic elements can be joined to create or build a sequence of words representing a well-formed phrase or sentence that is capable of conveying a specific meaning. NLP is emerged from AI that is purely devoted for development of algorithms and designing models capable of using natural language of the human beings [2]. It is extensively used in searches and translations made using Google or in virtual personal assistants like "Alexa" and "Siri". NLP is capable of analyzing and extracting information from various unstructured sources, automating question answering process and conducting analysis on sentiments and summarization of text data [3]. As public healthcare and medical institutions acquire and exchange knowledge with natural language as main source of communication, NLP can play a vital role to unlock the potential of artificial intelligence in biomedical sciences. In modern scenario, techniques of machine learning are extensively used to build most of NLP platforms [4]. The main aim of Natural Language Processing (NLP) is for automation of tasks with help of computing techniques that are capable of representation of the specific information in the textual or written form reliably. Machine learning models consists of four main components: a model; input data; a data fitting function; and a training algorithm for model [5]. Recent developments in these areas have paved the way to improve NLP models largely with use of deep learning techniques, emerging from machine learning [6]. New innovations and developments in the diverse types of models, such as convolutional neural network-based (CNN), recurrent neural network-based (RNN), and attention-based models, has facilitated capturing and modelling of more complex semantic associations and concepts than simple keyword presence using recent NLP systems [7]. The approaches of vector embedding has this effort for preprocessing the data that is capable of encoding the words before passing data into a model. These approaches are capable of recognizing that different meaning of word in different contexts (e.g. the meanings of "shot", "patient," "virus", and "disorder," may change according to context) and treating them as points in a conceptual space rather than separated entities. The advent of transfer learning has augmented the performance of these models as once a model is trained its output can be fed to another model as input for training the model in a related task. The performance of NLP models has received a great boost with advancements in hardware and steep rise in freely available databases [8]. Novel evaluating tools and yardsticks such as GLUE, BioASQ and superglue are providing help to a great extent in broadening our understanding information type as well as scope these novel models can capture [9, 10].

This chapter is structured around the concepts of the emergence of Natural Language Processing (NLP) techniques in healthcare AI. Firstly, an in-depth detailed introduction of Natural Language Processing in healthcare are presented in Sect. 1. In the subsequent Sect. 2, the background and motivations behind use of Natural Language Processing is given. Section 3 presents a detailed study on use of NLP in healthcare. NLP techniques and role of deep learning and NLP is presented in Sect. 4. Section 5 is focused on NLP and COVID-19 information. Finally, in Sect. 6 we conclude our findings on emergence of NLP techniques in healthcare and present its future directions.

2 Background and Motivations

Natural Language Processing (NLP) aims for rendering support for the advancement of the basic aims of biomedical and healthcare informatics, which comprises the new discovery and supporting scientifically validation of available knowledge, enhancement in the quality and expenses of healthcare facilities, and full backing to health professionals and patients. In healthcare and biomedical fields, a large scale of data and knowledge are circulated in the literature of scientific nature in text form as articles, as text fields in large distributed databases, and as administrative nature or technical reports or articles on the Internet. In healthcare centers, patient health records mostly generates in the form of handwritten narrative notes and large computerized reports. The pervasive acceptance of electronic health records (EHR) in clinics, hospitals, nursing homes, medical centers and other healthcare facilities is the main source of generation of huge real-world health information, which is very beneficial for carrying out clinical or medical research. From the last many years, electronic health records (EHR) systems are being greatly welcomed by hospitals clinics, medical centers and other healthcare facilities. Analysis of giant volumes of data is the underlying principle for providing patients improved and better healthcare facilities. Nevertheless, manual review process of this huge amount of data procuring from multiple sources is very expensive and sluggish creating many challenges while reviewing this healthcare data in a meaningful or intelligible form.

Because of the increasing acceptance of electronic health records (EHRs), it is a trend nowadays for patients to make available their health records at more than one healthcare facilities, and the involvement of several notes in the health chart of a single patient at one healthcare facility. These days' scientists and medical professionals are finding it very difficult to keep them up to date or vigilant about the latest discoveries or research studies due to the easy availability of huge volumes of online textual health information. As a result, they are feeling dire need of help for the acquiring, managing, and analyzing the huge amounts of knowledge and data available online. On the Internet, people are keen on finding and exchanging exchange health-related available information, and patients and health professionals are often flooded by the huge volume of the health related information accessible to them procuring from wither health related websites or through online socially health forums or communities. A lot of information is also occurring verbally through scientific or medical interactions at workshops or conferences, in health related lectures at hospitals and medical centers, and in doctor-patient consolations meetings.

In this chapter, we are concentrating on the written or textual form of health data. While there is very vital information communicated in textual form, it is not in a conducive format to further computerized processing. The intrinsic characteristics and diversification in languages renders the job of text processing very challenging. Mostly automated applications prefer the use of systematic regulated data so a notable quantity of manually work is particularly designed to map text or written health information into a structured, coded or systematic representation: in the healthcare domain, for example, professionally trained programmers allocate billing number/codes analogous to diagnoses and rules and regulations to healthcare facilities admissions; and database designers extracting genomic and phenotypical type information on organisms from the available literary works. Moreover, the large availability for tons of text or written information makes the manual work expensive, sluggish and very arduous task to keep vigilant and up to date. Hence, the role of Artificial Intelligence (AI) techniques are emerging as very vital in enhancement of clinical or medical research and healthcare. Natural Language Processing (NLP) mainly aims to automate the tasks using computerized techniques or methods that can represent the pertinent information in the textual form with higher reliability and validity.

As a huge numbers of electronic health records (EHR) are entwined in clinic written notes, the use of Natural Language Processing (NLP), Machine Learning (ML) and Deep Learning (DL) techniques have been exploited for mining or extracting information [11]. As for medical imaging the techniques of computer vision (CV) are preferred but to analyze the unstructured data or information contained in the electronic health records (EHR) NLP techniques are mostly used; and for robotics-assisted operations, techniques of reinforcement learning are used. During text analysis and determination of relationship among phrases grammatically, NLP algorithms are mainly used for identification of clinically phenotypes. To obtain highly sensitivity such as to identify true cases on a large scale and getting prediction value positively very high in healthcare records, NLP techniques using rule based approach can be more useful.

Healthcare being the most preferable domains where computer science is acting as supportive of diverse tasks. Artificial Intelligence is very willingly accepted across the healthcare domains covering from very basic level activities to moderate ones, and moderates to specialization practices, and a great number of appealing AI applications using Natural language processing (NLP) to maximum extent. These AI techniques being potentially capable to identify the distinctive medical or clinical features among patients that further offers new ventures for clinic care and reducing methodological variations in medical or clinical research concentrating on diverse health diseases. The availability of giant volumes of textual information through published works related to science, clinical or medical care or on the internet can be used to maximum extent to obtain and documenting well knowledge procuring from the information expressed or communicated in textual form, and paving way for promotion through discovery of new occurrences [12, 13]. To cite an example, the information communicated through patient text notes, while not initially prepared for purposes to discover new things, but originally aiming rather for the better care of patients individually, can be analyzed, collected and extracted to find new or similar patterns across different patients.

For health professionals and doctors accessing electronic health records for treatment of a specific patient, Natural Language Processing can be supportive in healthcare domains: when studying and analyzing the patient information sheet, NLP can be influenced to collect and integrate information distributed across various health notes and summary reports, and to accentuate relevant details of the patient. Information contained in health notes extracted through NLP can impart to the decision support systems in the electronic health records at the time of actual health care and decision-making [14]. At the time of making report of patient information by health professionals, NLP oriented methods can contribute in generating qualitative health quality notes and reports. Eventually, Natural Language Processing can be supportive to patients and healthcare professionals seeking informative notes of a specific disease or treatment, with question understanding that can then provide easy availability of related information, meeting their needs, and enhancing their health education levels analyzing information contained in document and the lexis used in the health notes.

3 Natural Language Processing in Healthcare

The acceptance and application of natural language processing in healthcare sectors is increasing on a great extent due to its identified potential for searching, analyzing and interpreting huge amounts of patient health databases [15]. With the use of ever-advanced medical models, machine learning along with NLP technologies in healthcare have the ability to exploit associated concepts and insights from data that was previously taken as buried in textual form [11]. NLP in healthcare media can precisely bring life to the unstructured data of the healthcare world, delivering unbelievable insight into quality of understanding, gaining improvement in methods, and providing better outcomes for patients [16].

Healthcare professionals takes a lot of time entering the possible reasons behind, the happening and what's happening to their clients into handwritten chart notes.

These chart notes are not in a form that data available in these can be easily extracted and analyzed by a computational machines or computers. When the doctor listen your ailments at the time of appointment, and records your appointment in a chart note, these narrations becomes the part of the electronic health record systems (EHRs) and get stored as free form textual data [17]. Although, mammoth volumes of unstructured patient health data is entered daily into EHRs, but it is a very cumbersome task for a computer to assist healthcare professionals gather that crucial data [18]. Structured data like CCDAs/claims/FHIR APIs may give assistance to ascertain disease burden, but provides us a restrained view of the actual patient health record.

According to big data analytics in healthcare demonstrates that around 80% of healthcare records are unstructured, and therefore remain mostly unutilized, since text mining and extracting of information of this health data is arduous and resource consuming. Without the use of NLP, this healthcare data is not in a read to use format for latest computer-oriented models to retrieve. Natural Language Processing in Healthcare utilizes dedicated engines capable of cleansing huge amounts of unstructured healthcare data for discovery of previously ignored or inappropriately recorded patient health conditions [19]. NLP healthcare records with use of machine learning models [20] can help in uncovering diseases that could not have been identified previously, fundamental characteristics to make discovery of HCC disease. Electronic health records and healthcare professionals do not always follow same direction. The additional load of entering data responsibilities brings many challenges, and can lead to frustration and fatigue. Researchers comes with a conclusion, some healthcare professionals endure torture of EHR burnout and willing to get retired from job much earlier rather than enduring torture through the many clicks and computer screens needed for navigation of the electronic health records [18]. NLP in medical sector is steadily becoming as a solution to this problem since tools of NLP healthcare can easily use and correctly extract meaning from clinical records.

The availability of large amounts of learning data directly lead to an increase in the accuracy of NLP models in healthcare. The regular use of NLP models in healthcare helps us getting more accurate and efficient NLP systems as these systems are capable of learning from their experiences and training data. Even some suppliers of NLP systems for healthcare demonstrates the capability and functionalities system can offer in healthcare with a particular medical group fulfilling the needs of that specific group. NLP models in healthcare also provide the advantage of synthesizing and summarizing all the information contained into lengthy chart notes into some pertinent points. In the past, thus process of synthesizing and summarizing all information could vary from several weeks to even years following the manual process for reviewing and processing piles of chart notes from patient health records, just to extract the vital information. NLP systems in healthcare sector can easily look through medical textual data within seconds and find out the relevant that should be retrieved from these records. This help in getting some leisure time for healthcare professionals and focusing more intensively on the complex issues and minimizes the time eaten in frequently occurring administrative tasks [19, 21]. When computers can become self-sufficient in understanding doctors' notes correctly and does processing tasks on extracted data accordingly, these systems can prove very beneficial in delivering valuable decisions. This can lead to carrying out drug and medicinal research in near future providing greater assistance to health professionals and patients.

All the doctors do not "speak the same way", and should be vigilant enough that their chart notes and narratives will likely be consumed by their colleagues, patients and even computational systems, adhering to data privacy policies of their organizations. The use of standard natural language in creation and maintenance of chart notes and narratives is very pertinent. Many of the NLP systems in healthcare are designed and developed with the aim to serve a wide variety of notation terminologies used in healthcare [22]. However, the use of nonstandard and uncommon notations can lead to confusions among readers of these chart notes and NLP systems. In last 3 years, the developing system for gaining improvement in NLP healthcare data has proven a very arduous task. If the outcomes of NLP systems in healthcare suggests too many results, or artificial results that are not correct, users will have been forced in ignoring the intelligence and move towards a system that is capable of minimizing overall business output. NLP systems in healthcare should focus around least noised and robust signal data outcomes about what healthcare professionals intended to do. Medical NLP provide a great opportunity for computers to center around the things that they meant to do.

3.1 Challenges in NLP

Despite the recent developments, hurdles to extensive use of NLP methods and technologies still exist. Similar to other AI techniques, Natural Language Processing is very much dependent on the easy availability, qualitative and natural orientation of the training datasets [23]. Smooth access and easy availability of appropriately annotated datasets (using supervised or semi-supervised learning in effective manner) are basic for training as well as implementation of powerful NLP models. For instance, the development and use of algorithms that are capable of carry a well-organized synthesis of reported research work on a specific topic or a comparative study and extraction of data from electronic health records (EHRs) needs access without any imposed restrictions to publisher or healthcare/primary care databases [18]. Although in recent years, the number of datasets in biomedicine and healthcare that are easily accessible without any hindrance and pre-trained learning models has been arising, but the number of dealing persons with public healthcare concepts stays very limited [24, 25]. The ability to remove biasness from data (i.e. by offering the ability for inspecting, explaining and adjusting data in ethical manner) indicates another major issue for the training purpose and using NLP models in public healthcare sectors.

The Failure for accounting for biasness present in the developing (e.g. annotating data), deploying (e.g. using pre-trained systems) and evaluating of NLP based models could lead to compromising of the model outcomes and reinforcing existing health prejudice [26]. However, it is worth mentioning that even when annotated datasets and its evaluations are a modified for biases, this does not provide guarantee for an equivalent impact across morally applicable stratum. For instance, using healthcare data provided through social platforms must be considered the particular age group and socio-economic groups using this health data [27]. A monitoring system trained on data obtained from social media application Facebook is no doubt to have biasness towards healthcare data and semantic quirks specifically related to a set of population older than system trained on data obtained from another social application Snapchat [28]. In the recent times, many model unbiased tools have been developed to identify and bring unfairness in machine as well deep learning models according to the efforts imitated by the government agencies and academic organizations for defining unacceptable artificial intelligence development [29, 30]. At present, one of the main hindrance for further development of NLP platforms is limited access of data in public healthcare sectors [31, 32].

In a recent study at Canada, data related to public health are generally maintained and controlled on the regional basis and, due to confidentiality and security issues, there is hesitation for providing freely access to these NLP systems and their incorporation with other available datasets (e.g. data linkage) [23]. There are also some other challenges with public perception of privacy and freely access of data. A recent survey, conducted on users of social media platforms, demonstrated that the major chunks of the users have taken into account comparative analysis of data on their social platforms account for identification of health issues related to mental condition "intrusive and exposing" and they would not be willing to give their consent to this [33]. Prior to main NLP public health related activities could be ascertained at large scale, such as the comparative analysis in real-time of trends in disease nationwide, judiciary will require to jointly ascertain a reasonable scope and effortless access to public healthcare data sources (e.g. data related to health and administration). In order to prevent and eliminate privacy violations and misusing of data, NLP applications, in near future, to analyze personal healthcare data are contingent on the capability for embedment of distinguished privacy into learning models [34], both during at stages of training and after the deployment of model. Access to vital data is also restrained through the methods used currently to freely access full textual oriented publications. Unhindered and freely access to databases containing journal publications or novel models for storage of data is the basic need for realizing fully automatic PICO-oriented knowledge extraction and synthetization [35].

Eventually, meeting the requirements of new technologies, more intention must be given for identification and evaluation of Natural Language Processing based models for ensuring their working with intention and pace according to the society's ever changing views about ethics. These NLP models and technologies are required to be analyzed for ensuring their functionality according to their expectation and accounting for biasness [25]. Although in the present time improved or equivalent to human scores on text analysis tasks are posted by many approaches, the equating high scores with true natural language understanding is not of too much importance.

However, it is also equally of very much significance not to visualize a lack of true natural language understanding as a lack of utilization. NLP Models with a "relatively poor" in-depth understanding can still be of very much effective at the time of extracting information, classifying and predicting tasks, specifically with the enhanced availability of data of labelled type [11].

3.2 Opportunities for NLP in Healthcare

Public healthcare organizations work with the motive to gain optimum health results within and across diverse sets of populations, mainly by focusing on the development and implementation of interventions that are meant for alterable causes of poor health condition [8, 15]. The success solely relies on the capability of quantifying the impact of disease in effective manner or its risk factors within the population and also identifying clusters that are influenced in disproportionate manner or at the verge of risk; detect best practices (i.e. optimum prevention or therapeutic procedures); and measure results [23]. There is a decision making model based on evidence-informed that uses "PICO concept (patient/problem, intervention/exposure, comparison, outcome)" [36]. This PICO concept based model offers a strategy to identify optimum knowledge for framing and answering particular clinical or public health queries [37]. The decision-making based on evidence-informed is typically well grounded on the thoroughly and well-organized comprehensive review and synthetization of data according to the PICO concept elements.

In present scenario, information is being generated and published (e.g. technical reports, science literary text, medical information, surveys, socially media generated data, and other well documented data) at incredible rates [38]. NLP is capable of rapidly analyzing huge amounts of unstructured data or semi structured data, thus paving the way to open up tremendous opportunities for proof-informed decision-making process and text-based research [17, 37]. NLP has emerged as a potentially robust tool to support the rapidly identifying populations, interventions and results of interest that required for surveillance and prevention of disease and promoting health. For instance, the use of NLP systems that can identify specific characteristics of individuals in unstructured medical documents or social media content can be utilized for enhancement of existing surveillance structures with real-world testament [39].

One latest study revealed the capability of NLP methods to assess the existence of depression much before it appeared in health related records. The ability of NLP to carry out real-time text mining of scientific research publications or reported articles for a specific "PICO (Patient/Problem, Intervention, Comparison, and Outcome)" concept [36] creates enough opportunities for decision makings to rapidly offer recommendations and provide suggestions on the prevention of disease or management that are made aware of latest body of evidence when timely recommendations and suggestions are sought, such as during an outbreak of disease or epidemic. NLP enabled Chatbot's and question-answering systems [36] also possesses the much required potential to gain improvement in health promoting activities by creating environments for individuals to get engaged in theses health activities and offering personalized assistance or advice.

3.3 NLP Applications in Healthcare

Natural language processing (NLP) has a very vast range of possible applications. The following are some very important applications of Natural language processing technology for healthcare:

1. **Information Extraction**: It is the process of locating and structuring particular information in text, most widely used application of NLP in field of biomedicine, and usually carried out without having semantic analysis of the text, but focusing and finding on the patterns present in the text. Once task of extraction and structuring of text information is completed, then textual information can be utilized for various diverse tasks [11]. In the field of bio surveillance, for example, symptoms from a main complaint field in a handwritten note can be extracted when a patient was directed to get admitted in the emergency wards of a healthcare facility [40] or from handwritten notes of electronic health records meant for ambulance services [41]. The gathered data from a number of patients after extraction can provide help in understanding the prevailing and progressive stages of particular epidemic or pandemic. In the field of biology, bio molecular conservations as well as interactions between patients and health professionals on written notes can be extracted (if taken from one single note) or merged (if taken from multiple articles) for construction of pathways of bio molecular type. In the clinical sector, NLP can be employed on large number of health records of patients for obtaining structure data to be used in pharmacovigilance systems for discovery of adverse drug happenings [11]. In named-entity recognition process, the information extraction techniques may be used to the identify names of persons or places, numerical expressions, and dates, or to several types of terms present in text (e.g. mentioning of proteins or medications) and then can be transformed into standardized or canonical forms. This process of transformation is termed as named-entity normalization. More well organized and reliable techniques are used for identification and representation of the modifiers related to a named entity. Such advanced techniques are needed for reliable extraction of information because the accurate meaning of a term typically associated and may vary in association with other terms in a provided sentence. For example, the term pain has different meanings in no pain, high pain, pain lasted 3 days, and low pain. Another important method of information extraction is to identify relations among named entities. For instance, when locating and finding adverse events in association with a medication, the phrases "the patient developed a rash from ciprofloxacin" and "the patient came in with a rash and was given benadryl" must be differentiated. In both sentences, a relation between a

rash and a drug is showing, but the first sentence indicates a possible adverse drug happening whereas the second sentence indicates a treatment for an adverse happening. As extraction of entities takes place from multiple sources, need for one very crucial step of reference resolution arises. Reference resolution is the process to recognize two mentioning in two different source locations referring the same entity [19]. In some cases, Reference resolution is a very arduous task. For instance, mentions of fracture in two different articles related to same patient could indicate the same fracture or two very distinguished fractures; some more contextual information and additional domain knowledge is often required to resolve this complex problem.

2. **Information Retrieval**: Information Retrieval (IR) and Natural Language Processing coincide in many of the methods in use. The methods of Information Retrieval (IR) are aimed for providing support to user for gaining access of documents in huge databases, such as the scientific research literature, electronic health records (EHRs), or the WWW. This is a very important application in health and biomedicine, due to the outburst of vast information present in electronic form. The fundamental aim of information retrieval is to check a user's question against a collection of documents and retrieve an organized list of related documents [11]. A search operation is conducted on an index of the large collection of documents. The most fundamental form of indexing separates simple terms and words, and therefore, utilizes very less semantic knowledge. Many of modern approaches makes use of Natural Language Processing (NLP) oriented methods of same kind which are used in information extraction, finding entities of complex nature and ascertaining their associations in order to increase the accuracy level of information retrieval. For example, one could look out for Cough and have the search being operated at the conceptual level, retrieving documents mentioning the phrase Asthma in addition to the phrases that mentions cough only. Furthermore, one could look out for cough in a particular context, such as study of the disease or treatment.
3. **Question Answering**: Question Answering (QA) is termed as a process in which a user submits a question expressed in natural language and answer is then automatically presented by a QA system. The easy availability of required information in published articles or works and on the Internet empowers these type of systems increasingly very significant as healthcare professionals as well as consumers, and researchers in biomedical field frequently explore the Web to procure information about a disease/medical condition, its cure, or a clinical procedure. A question answering system can be very beneficial for procuring the answers to factual questions, like "In children with an acute febrile illness, what is the efficacy of single-medication therapy with acetaminophen or ibuprofen in reducing fever?" The answer to above query produced by QA system is like "Ibuprofen provided greater temperature decrement and longer duration of antipyresis than acetaminophen when the two drugs were administered in approximately equal doses" [36]. QA systems enriches an Information Retrieval

(IR) system with additional capabilities. In an IR system, a query is generated after user translates a question into a list of keywords, but a Question Answering (QA) system performs this step automatically. In the addition, user obtains an actual answer (often more than one passages mined from the original documents) presented by a QA system, in the place of a list of related original documents. A QA has aimed to focus on the scientific literature thus far [36].

4. **Text Summarization**: It is the process of producing a single output file containing rational text synthesizing the basic points from one or multiple documents taking as input. Using text summarization users are able to derive sense of a mammoth amount of data, by finding and reporting the essential points in retrieved texts in automatic manner. Text summarization can be either question-focused or general purpose (i.e. focusing on a specific information need into consideration when choosing significant content of inputted documents). Question-focused text summarization can be regarded as a post-processing stage of information revival and question answering: the relevant paragraphs or documents related to an input query are further refined into a standalone, rational text. Text summarization process consists of several steps such as selection of relevant content (recognizing essential points of information in the inputted documents), organization of content (recognizing duplicity and contradictory issues present among the selected passages of information, and placing them into order so the final summarization is coherent), and regeneration of content (presenting natural language from the organized passages of information). Following the similar way of question answering, text summarization has aimed to focus on the scientific literature [11, 19].
5. **Text Generation**: It is the process of formulating sentences of natural language from a provided source of information that human are not able to read directly. Generation can be employed for creation a text from a well-organized database, such as summarizing patterns and in data procured from laboratories [11].
6. **Machine Translation**: It is the process of transforming text in one source language (e.g. Hindi) into another target language (e.g. English). These applications could prove very beneficial in multilingual environments in which translation by humans is either very time consuming or too expensive.
7. **Text Readability Identification and Text Simplification**: Text Readability Identification and Text Simplification is proving very beneficial to the healthcare sectors, as health professional as well as consumers and patients search and explore more and more health related information on the WWW [19]. However, they lacks in their literacy levels according to the health documents available on the Web and seeks support for easy readability.
8. **Emotion Detection and Sentiment Analysis**: Emotion Detection and Sentiment Analysis are latest applications of Natural Language Processing and responsible for making the process of content analysis automatic. There are encouraging research outcomes revealing that patients' discourse can be studied analytically in automatic manner for identification of their mental states [30].

Table 14.1 enlists some examples of possible applications of NLP in public healthcare that have showed at least some success.

Table 14.1 Some possible Applications of NLP

Activity	Objective of Public Healthcare	Examples based on using NLP
Identifying populations at risk	To measure the occurrence and pervasiveness of diseases and risk factors related to diseases continuously (i.e. monitoring)	A comparative analysis of semi structured or unstructured textual data from social media or EHRs [33]
	To detect and find highly vulnerable and at-risk individuals in population	A comparative analysis of risk behaviors using social platforms [42]
Identifying of health related interventions	Developing the optimum suggestions/interventions	Automatic systematic literature review and comparative study of the information conveyed through scientific research published as well as unpublished articles [33]
	Identifying best practices	Recognition of potential public healthcare interventions through comparative analysis of online available peer reviewed and grey literature
Recognition of healthcare outputs with use of real-world evidence	To assess the gains of healthcare interventions	A comparative analysis of semi structured or unstructured textual data from online social media, EHRs and publications to ascertain the impact of public healthcare suggestions and interventions [23]
	To recognize unforeseen adverse outputs related to health interventions	A comparative analysis of semi structured or unstructured textual data from online social media, EHRs and publications to assess possible adverse happenings of health interventions
Generation and Translation of Knowledge	To provide assistance to public healthcare research	A comparative analysis of semi structured or unstructured textual data from EHRs and scientific research published articles for generation of knowledge
	To provide assistance to decision making process using evidence information	Use of questioning answering systems, chatbots and text summarization systems by providing personalized information to people needing advice for improvement of their health and prevention of disease [23]
Scanning of Environment and awareness of situations	To carry risk assessments related to public healthcare and providing situational awareness	A comparative analysis of online available content for detecting and mitigating critical events in real time [26]
	To observe activities that can affect decision making in public healthcare	A comparative analysis of decisions of national and international stakeholders [32]

4 Role of Deep Learning Techniques Based NLP Systems in Healthcare

Most of the NLP based systems are developed with separate or dedicated components that take care of different functionalities offered by these systems. The dedicated components typically roughly occur simultaneously with the semantic levels. Generally, the outcomes of each lower level is fed to the next higher level as input [43]. To exemplify, the outcomes of tokenization process coverts a text string into separated tokens that will have to bear lexical analysis for determination of their parts of speech (POS) and other linguistic properties as inscribed in a lexicon; the POS tags along with the equivalent semantic definitions will then serves as the input to syntactic analysis phase that will ascertain the structure of the sentence; the structure of sentence will be then serves as input to semantic analysis phase for the interpretation of the meaning [7]. Each NLP systems bundles these stages of processing differently. At each processing stage, the component meant for that stage works with the aim for regularizing the data in some aspect to minimize variety at the time of perseverance the informative data as much as possible.

There are two approaches to Natural Language Processing:

- A rule-based approach in which systems have to follow predefined rules in the algorithms.
- Machine Learning approach in which learning method based on supervised and unsupervised are used for training of the systems. In supervised Learning, the machines are able to learn according to predefined rules under the guidance of human while in the case of unsupervised learning machine learns without any human guidance or interaction [44, 45].

Firstly, the information contained in electronic health records is extracted by NLP algorithms, which is then processed for classification of patients into a sub categories according to the predefined rules and learners. The Nature of NLP procedures NLP is very complicated due to combination of various techniques together. NLP systems in healthcare will associates words or phrases to concepts of interest, and it requires very cautious approach to pre-process the extracted text and it needs to be transformed into document from the human form [46].

Following are few instances of low-level Natural Language Processing tasks (pre-processing of text):

- Detection of sentence boundary (usually a period indicates sentence boundary)
- Tokenization (partitioning a sentence into separated tokens)
- Stemming (deriving the root form of a word)
- Lemmatization (applying Lemma rules on tokens)

Following are few instances of high-level Natural Language Processing tasks:

- Recognition of Named entities
- Formulating rules for negation

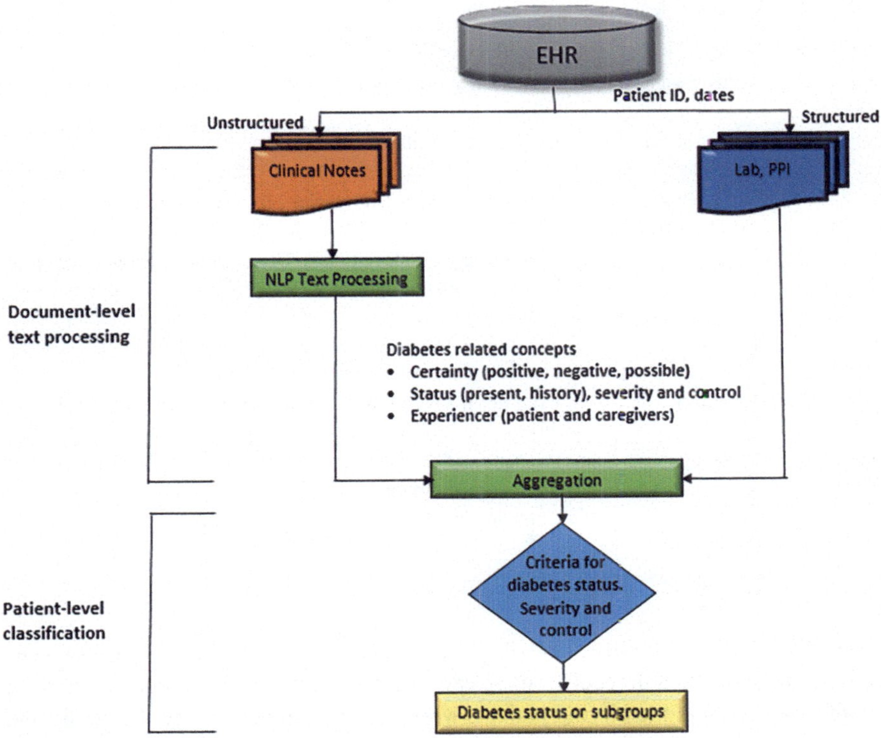

Fig. 14.1 Document-level processing of text and patient-level classification using NLP algorithms

Figure 14.1 demonstrates the preprocessing and classification of text of a diabetes patient.

The healthcare information can originates from four sources in terms of users such as Physicians, Patients, Staff members of paramedical team and Pharmaceuticals. Proper diagnosis of a disease directly relates to post-process stage of a disease. Patients can receive proper and timely treatment if the disease is detected timely and properly. Sometimes, delays in decision-making can lead to worse condition of patients. Deep learning is an approach consisting of a big network that is able to take a wide variation of inputs data types such as image, text, time-series data, audio etc. learns related features in its low-level networks corresponding to each data type. The data from each tower is combined to make it passes through higher levels, providing the provision to the Deep Neural Network in reaching to result based on evidence and reasoning across data types [11].

NLP can provide assistance to healthcare in extraction of information, transformation of unstructured to structured data, categorization of documents, and summarization of text. Eventually it will help in reducing administrative costs by means of efficient billing and correct prior authorized permission. It will also help in adding medical value by providing help for unproductive medical decisions and structured and up to date medical policy evaluation etc. Additionally, it will also provide

Table 14.2 Stages of Healthcare Information

Situation	Process	Tools/Devices/Actions/Reports
Pre-Disease	Health Awareness	Smart sensor devices to provide health updates
	Regular health check-ups	Devices for health check-ups
	How to stay away from disease?	Training programs and devices for various exercises
In Disease	Diagnosis	Blood sample, X-Ray Image, Urine Sample, Biopsy, Devices for checking vital signs in the body (Oxygen, sugar, heartbeat, pulses, etc.)
	Treatment	Pre-surgery treatments, Minor surgery, Major surgery, Combined surgery, post-surgery treatments
	Medication	Drug dosage based on the nature of the body for a single disease, multiple diseases
Post Disease	Follow-ups	Prediction of the number of follow-ups or time period of follow-ups required
	Improvement comparison	Compare Pre, In and Post disease reports
	Future predictions	

support for gaining improvement in patient interactions with health professionals and the electronic health records, increasing health awareness in patients, improving qualitative care, and identifying patients who need critical health care. In healthcare, technologies of NLP and sequential DL has provided a boost to the health applications lies within domains like EHRs [43]. The various stages of Healthcare information are given in Table 14.2.

Figure 14.2 demonstrates various stages involved in processing of data.

A. **Unstructured EHR data**: Heterogeneity is often found in health records according to the storage policies, data structures and working mechanism of a particular healthcare facility. Therefore, it will vary from one healthcare facility to another.
B. **Data Standardization**: Data will be transformed into standard form into the similar format to associate data from various sources based on FHIR.
C. **Sequencing**: To sequence data into a patient timeline temporally, time-oriented DL techniques can be utilized to the EHR datasets entirely for delivering predictions about individual patients. NLP systems can prove very beneficial in the neurology domain too. The NLP system, "Edinburgh Information Extraction for Radiology reports (EdIE-R)", is a multiple staged pipelined process as demonstrated in Fig. 14.3, with XML rule-based text mining program at its internal level [47].

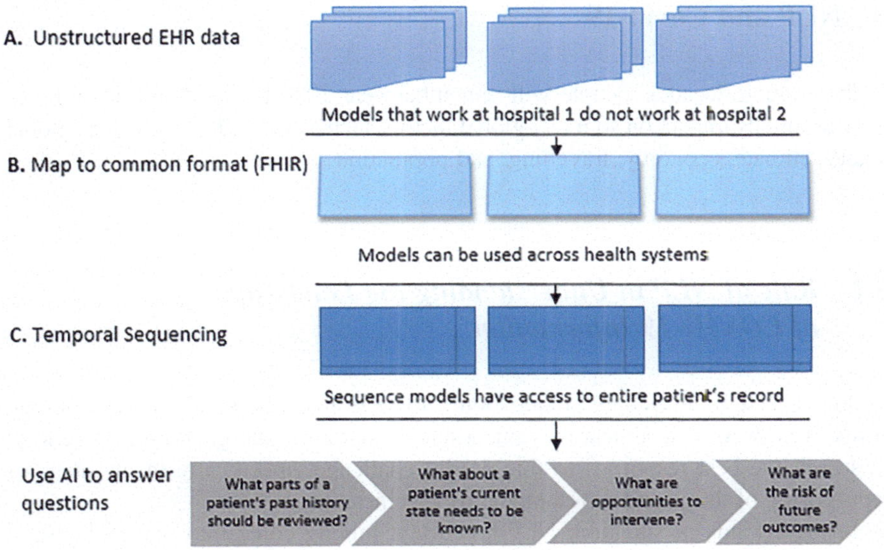

Fig. 14.2 Predicting using EHR'

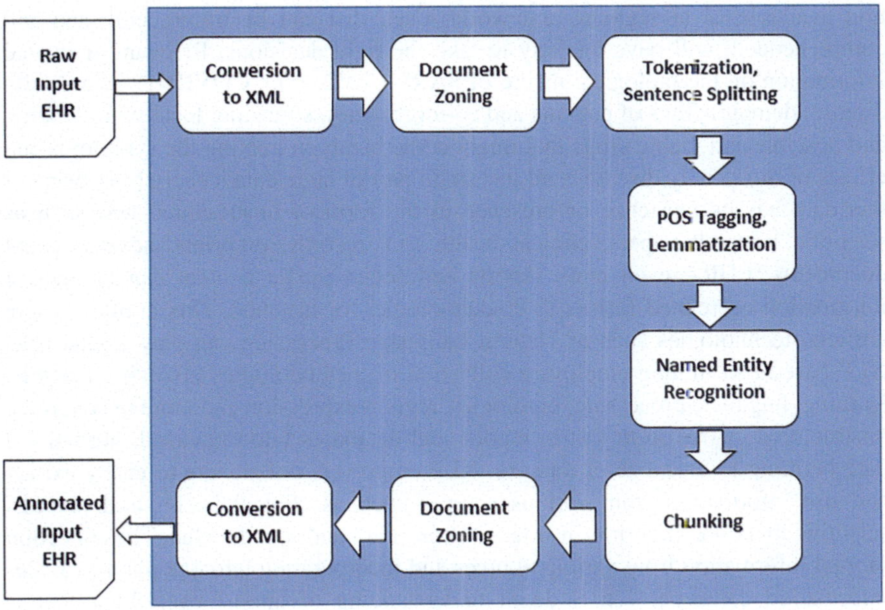

Fig. 14.3 Architecture of EdIE-R System

5 NLP and Covid-19

In the coming decades, people will remember year 2020 taking about novel coronavirus and its impact on so many global factors such as individual as well as global health, climate, economy, travelling, and population.

5.1 *Role of NLP in Understanding the Landscape of COVID-19 Information*

In this adverse time, as dark clouds looms, there is also a hope of coming from the collective efforts of healthcare organizations, institutions, and government agencies to search the best responses to this deadly challenge, specifically in the areas of repurposing of drugs and development of vaccines.

In these kinds of situation, NLP-based text mining come into scene playing a major role. Whenever researchers, scientists, healthcare professionals are met with such critical challenges, one crucial asset is to identify or stockpile as much informational data about the given problem as possible. Whatever kind of information available is, at regional and world level, that can be traced, collected and comprehended, will pave the way to take the right decisions. Relevant or related information on the biological nature of SARS-CoV2, from COVID-19 as a deadly disease, demographics of patients and co-morbidities, spreading locally or globally, and possible and viable drugs that might come handy in treating the symptoms and effects of this deadly disease is all just small part of huge data iceberg [48]. Most of this data has its existence or presence in the form of unstructured text such as scientific research papers, clinical health trial records, preprints, adverse event documents, EHRs, even news reports and social media content can all deliver information on related factors to epidemiologic, for instance. This is often where artificial technologies such as Natural Language Processing can play a vital role. NLP-based text mining employs a collection of methodologies involving machine learning, linguistic processing, ontologies, regular expression and more to covert the unstructured or free form text in reports and databases into organized, normalized data befitting to visualize or analyze. NLP empowers researchers to easily extract and use information from various sources such as clinical health trial records, scientific literature, preprints, insider sources, news and social media. The collection of vital information from various sources and incorporating into one place provides information consumers an in-depth understanding of almost everything that is happening all around. This approach can help in providing real time answers to main key questions to face the COVID-19 pandemic, such as:

- What are the best possible drugs for repurposing efforts?
- Where do I find the latest research, recent health trials, and the key health professionals and researchers in this field?

- Who are at more risk for deadly disease in the population?
- What are the main co-morbidities involved?
- What kind of additional health care activities are needed for patients post this deadly disease?

5.2 *Use of NLP for COVID-19 Understanding in Pharma and Healthcare Organizations*

An innovative approach, for example, for taking better care of patients arises from a large United States Healthcare System. Healthcare professionals in the system were perturbed about less reporting of COVID-19 cases, so they employed NLP techniques to extract incoming emails and chatting messages from their helpline for patient, for tracing symptoms related to COVID-19. They then performed analytical study for classification of these patients according to the possibility of possessing COVID-19. This automatic process helped in enabling healthcare professionals to manage the patient population in more effective manner. One more instance can be taken of a pharma company who ought to extract social media content to comprehend spreading and risk factors involved COVID-19. Again, a set of questionnaire were prepared for categorization of patient behaviors according to a variety of factors, e.g., mentioning of medical facilities being attended. They also performed a comparative analysis on the social media messages to comprehend COVID-19 status and risk across a spread of occupations and professions.

5.3 *Resources for NLP in Healthcare and COVID-19*

One of the ways in which NLP field can achieve more progress is sharing of different datasets, developed tools and resources used by various teams and groups of researchers. Shared databases provide assistance to various different teams of researchers in testing and comparing their systems analytically on the same datasets. Shared databases with appropriate annotations are very crucial, as they provide the provision for training of their NLP systems as well. As such, these NLP systems are very beneficial to the community. In last few years, there has been a relatively increase in the clinical and biological NLP communities to develop publicly available shared resources and tools, and in smooth conduction of challenges posed by community. Here we are presenting a few of publicly available datasets on COVID-19 data, but ever-evolving resources in the field, this list could prove to be obsolete. Therefore, we suggest the readers to explore the literature on COVID-19 and the WWW for the latest updates. Healthcare organizations are also utilizing NLP techniques to access the landscape of scientific research papers related to COVID-19 pandemic. Researchers working on developing COVID-19 cures employs NLP techniques to trace new and latest papers, specifically around safety of vaccine and drug. Many publishers have started offering free access to crucial scientific literature; for instance, "the CORD-19 Dataset compiled by Allen Institute for AI [48]; Coronavirus Dataset of Elsevier [49]; and Copyright Clearance Center COVID-19 resources [50]". These excellent resources can be harvested to identify efficacy of drug or safety related profiles, understanding co-morbidity profiles, the natural history of the severe virus and disease, and who are at more risk in the population for deadly disease. NLP can provide assistance in some way with enabling easy access to data, and hopefully therefore to dispel some of that uncertainty.

6 Conclusions and Future Directions

NLP in healthcare is giving birth to new and promising opportunities for delivery of healthcare facilities and patient experience. It will not be far away when these specialized NLP systems in healthcare will grant the opportunity to healthcare professionals to provide more quality care time with their patients, while providing assistance in deriving insightful outcomes based on precise data. In the decades to come, we will feel fortunate hearing the news, and witnessing the potential and functionalities of NLP technology, as it enables healthcare providers to contribute towards health conclusions positively. Technologies of NLP and Deep Learning will come into picture playing a significant role to accelerate the decision-making process in the healthcare sector. However, the actual rewards of designing efficient algorithms will rely largely on the data quality that they obtain and preserve. The rapid process of decision-making will empowers doctors and healthcare workers in focusing on the additional care of patients. Natural language processing with computer vision and deep learning can provide the greater help in processing a wide variety of data altogether to derive precise and accurate decisions. Collaborative research can provide the opportunity in achieving a higher level of medication and health treatment in healthcare sector. Keeping in mind, the impact of artificial technologies, systems using NLP require to be devised and developed using a cautionary approach in a larger socio-ecological view of healthcare facilities for provision of availing better care services in healthcare. Eventually, NLP tools may gain success in bridging the gap between the immeasurable amount of data accumulated on a daily basis and the limited coherent capability of the human mind. From the most arduous tasks to simpler tasks in healthcare, natural language processing has nearly never-ending possibilities to transform EHRs from burden to blessing. The success of NLP in healthcare will depend heavily on developing algorithms that are precise, intelligent, efficient, and healthcare-oriented and to design the user interfaces displaying healthcare decision support data effortlessly. If the healthcare organizations and industries succeed in meeting these dual goals of extracting and presenting information effectively, there will be no doubt about unbounded opportunities NLP in healthcare can bring in the future.

References

1. Sarosh P, Parah SA, Bhat GM, Muhammad K (2021) A security management framework for big data in smart healthcare. Big Data Res 25:100225
2. Ruder S. NLP-progress. Sebastian Ruder, London, UK. https://nlpprogress.com/. Accessed 18 Feb 2021
3. Topol EJ (2019) High-performance medicine: the convergence of human and artificial intelligence. Nat Med 25(1):44–56. https://doi.org/10.1038/s41591-018-0300-7
4. Jurafsky D, Martin JH (2019) Speech and language processing. Stanford University, Stanford, CA. https://web.stanford.edu/~jurafsky/slp3/. Accessed 18 Feb 2021
5. Nadkarni PM, Ohno-Machado L, Chapman WW (2011) Natural language processing: an introduction. J Am Med Inform Assoc 18(5):544–551. https://doi.org/10.1136/amiajnl-2011-000464
6. Gull S, Parah SA, Muhammad K (2020) Reversible data hiding exploiting Huffman encoding with dual images for IoMT based healthcare. Comput Commun 163:134–149
7. Tang B, Pan Z, Yin K, Khateeb A (2019) Recent advances of deep learning in bioinformatics and computational biology. Front Genet 10:214
8. Arcaya MC, Arcaya AL, Subramanian SV (2015) Inequalities in health: definitions, concepts, and theories. Glob Health Action 8:27106
9. Hirschberg J, Manning CD (2015) Advances in natural language processing. Science 349(6245):261–266
10. Kamili A, Fatima I, Hassan M, Parah SA, Vijaya Kumar V, Ambati LS (2020) Embedding information reversibly in medical images for e-health. J Intell Fuzzy Syst 39:8389–8398
11. Ghayvat H, Pandya SN, Bhattacharya P, Zuhair M, Rashid M, Hakak S, Dev K (2021) CP-BDHCA: blockchain-based confidentiality-privacy preserving Big Data scheme for healthcare clouds and applications. IEEE J Biomed Health Inform. https://doi.org/10.1109/JBHI.2021.3097237
12. Kumar I, Alshamrani SS, Kumar A, Rawat J, Singh KU, Rashid M, AlGhamdi AS (2021) Deep learning approach for analysis and characterization of COVID-19. Comput Mater Continua 70:451–468
13. Rashid M, Singh H, Goyal V, Parah S, Wani A (2020) Big data based hybrid machine learning model for improving performance of medical Internet of Things data in Healthcare systems. Healthc Paradig Internet Things Ecosyst. https://doi.org/10.1016/B978-0-12-819664-9.00003-X
14. Treasury Board Secretariat. Directive on automated decision-making. Government of Canada, Ottawa, ON. https://www.tbs-sct.gc.ca/pol/doc-eng.aspx?id=32592. Modified 5 Feb 2019; Accessed 27 Feb 2021
15. Jackson B, Huston P (2016) Advancing health equity to improve health: the time is now. Health Promot Chronic Dis Prev Can 36(2):17–20
16. Jiang F, Jiang Y, Zhi H, Dong Y, Li H, Ma S, Wang Y, Dong Q, Shen H, Wang Y (2017) Artificial intelligence in healthcare: past, present and future. Stroke Vasc Neurol 2(4):230–243. https://doi.org/10.1136/svn-2017-000101
17. Koleck TA, Dreisbach C, Bourne PE, Bakken S (2019) Natural language processing of symptoms documented in free-text narratives of electronic health records: a systematic review. J Am Med Inform Assoc 26(4):364–379
18. Carchiolo V, Longheu A, Reitano G, Zagarella L (2019) Medical prescription classification: a NLP-based approach. In: Proceedings of the 2019 federated conference on computer science and information systems, FedCSIS 2019, vol 18, pp 605–609. https://doi.org/10.15439/2019F197
19. Friedman C, Rindflesch TC, Corn M (2013) Natural language processing: state of the art and prospects for significant progress, a workshop sponsored by the National Library of Medicine. J Biomed Inform 46(5):765–773

20. Rashid M, Singh H, Goyal V (2020) The use of machine learning and deep learning algorithms in functional magnetic resonance imaging—a systematic review. https://doi.org/10.1111/exsy.12644
21. Harris JK, Mansour R, Choucair B, Olson J, Nissen C, Bhatt J (2014) Centers for Disease Control and Prevention. Health department use of social media to identify foodborne illness - Chicago, Illinois, 2013–2014. MMWR Morb Mortal Wkly Rep 63(32):681–685
22. Rashid M, Yousuf MM, Ram B, Goyal V (2019) Novel Big Data approach for drug prediction in health care systems. In: 2019 International conference on automation, computational and technology management (ICACTM), London, UK, pp 325–329. https://doi.org/10.1109/ICACTM.2019.8776823
23. Baclic O, Tunis M, Young K, Doan C, Swerdfeger H (2020) Challenges and opportunities for public health made possible by advances in natural language processing. Can Commun Dis Rep 46(6):161–168. https://doi.org/10.14745/ccdr.v46i06a02
24. Obermeyer Z, Powers B, Vogeli C, Mullainathan S (2019) Dissecting racial bias in an algorithm used to manage the health of populations. Science 366(6464):447–453
25. Penning de Vries BB, van Smeden M, Rosendaal FR, Groenwold RH (2020) Title, abstract, and keyword searching resulted in poor recovery of articles in systematic reviews of epidemiologic practice. J Clin Epidemiol 121:55–61
26. Rajkomar A, Hardt M, Howell MD, Corrado G, Chin MH (2018) Ensuring fairness in machine learning to advance health equity. Ann Intern Med 169(12):866–872
27. Jha N, Prashar D, Rashid M, Shafiq M, Khan R, Pruncu CI, Saravana Kumar M (2021) Deep learning approach for discovery of in silico drugs for combating COVID-19. J Healthc Eng 2021:6668985
28. Spasic I, Nenadic G (2020) Clinical text data in machine learning: systematic review. JMIR Med Inform 8(3):e17984
29. Holstein K, Vaughan JW, Daumé H, Dudík M, Wallach H (2019) Improving fairness in machine learning systems: what do industry practitioners need? In: CHI '19: Proceedings of the 2019 CHI conference on human factors in computing systems, vol 600, pp 1–16
30. Wiens J, Price WN, Sjoding MW (2020) Diagnosing bias in data-driven algorithms for healthcare. Nat Med 26(1):25–26
31. Montreal Declaration for a Responsible Development of Artificial Intelligence. Forum on the Socially Responsible Development of AI. 2–3 Nov 2017. Montréal, QC. Accessed 18 Feb 2021
32. Sheikhalishahi S, Miotto R, Dudley JT, Lavelli A, Rinaldi F, Osmani V (2019) Natural language processing of clinical notes on chronic diseases: systematic review. JMIR Med Inform 7(2):e12239
33. Ford E, Curlewis K, Wongkoblap A, Curcin V (2019) Public opinions on using social media content to identify users with depression and target mental health care advertising: mixed methods survey. JMIR Ment Health 6(11):e12942
34. Zhou M, Duan N, Liu S, Shum HY (2020) Progress in neural NLP: modeling, learning, and reasoning. Engineering 6(3):275–290. https://doi.org/10.1016/j.eng.2019.12.014
35. Radebaugh C, Erlingsson U (2021) Introducing tensorflow privacy: learning with differential privacy for training data. Medium.com. https://medium.com/tensorflow/introducing-tensorflowprivacy-learning-with-differential-privacy-for-trainingdata-b143c5e801b6. . Accessed 27 Feb 2021
36. Demner-Fushman D, Lin J (2007) Answering clinical questions with knowledge-based and statistical techniques. Comput Linguist 33(1):63–103. https://doi.org/10.1162/coli.2007.33.1.63
37. Kim ES, James P, Zevon ES, Trudel-Fitzgerald C, Kubzansky LD, Grodstein F (2020) Social media as an emerging data resource for epidemiologic research: characteristics of social media users and non-users in the Nurses' Health Study II. Am J Epidemiol 189(2):156–161
38. Chen IY, Joshi S, Ghassemi M (2020) Treating health disparities with artificial intelligence. Nat Med 26(1):16–17

39. Kreimeyer K, Foster M, Pandey A, Arya N, Halford G, Jones SF, Forshee R, Walderhaug M, Botsis T (2017) Natural language processing systems for capturing and standardizing unstructured clinical information: a systematic review. J Biomed Inform 73:14–29
40. Chapman D, Whitfield C, Felitti V, Dube S, Edwards V, Anda R (2004) Adverse childhood experiences and the risk of depressive disorders in adulthood. J Affect Disord 82:217–225. https://doi.org/10.1016/j.jad.2003.12.013
41. Hripcsak G, Elhadad N, Chen Y, Zhou L, Morrison F (2009) Using empiric semantic correlation to interpret temporal assertions in clinical texts. J Am Med Informatics Assoc 16:220–227. https://doi.org/10.1197/jamia.M3007
42. Conway M, Hu M, Chapman WW (2019) Recent advances in using natural language processing to address public health research questions using social media and consumer generated data. Yearb Med Inform 28(1):208–217
43. Esteva A, Robicquet A, Ramsundar B, Kuleshov V, DePristo M, Chou K, Cui C, Corrado G, Thrun S, Dean J (2019) A guide to deep learning in healthcare. Nat Med 25(1):24–29. https://doi.org/10.1038/s41591-018-0316-z
44. Xu C, Doshi T (2021) Fairness indicators: scalable infrastructure for fair ML system. Google, Mountain View, CA. Accessed 27 Feb 2021
45. Yin Z, Sulieman LM, Malin BA (2019) A systematic literature review of machine learning in online personal health data. J Am Med Inform Assoc 26(6):561–576
46. Juhn Y, Liu H (2020) Artificial intelligence approaches using natural language processing to advance EHR-based clinical research. J Allergy Clin Immunol 145(2):463–469. https://doi.org/10.1016/j.jaci.2019.12.897
47. Wheater E, Mair G, Sudlow C, Alex B, Grover C, Whiteley W (2019) A validated natural language processing algorithm for brain imaging phenotypes from radiology reports in UK electronic health records. BMC Med Inform Decis Mak 19(1):1–11. https://doi.org/10.1186/s12911-019-0908-7
48. The CORD-19 Dataset compiled by Allen Institute for AI. https://www.semanticscholar.org/cord19. Accessed 18 Feb 2021
49. Coronavirus Dataset of Elsevier. https://www.elsevier.com/clinical-solutions/coronavirus-research-hub/data-scientist. Accessed 18 Feb 2021
50. Copyright Clearance Center COVID-19 resources. https://www.copyright.com/covid19-resources/. Accessed 18 Feb 2021

Chapter 15
Prospects and Difficulties of Artificial Intelligence (AI) Implementations in Naturopathy

Akanksha Verma and Ishrat Naaz

Contents

1 Introduction

Innovative technologies like Artificial Intelligence are attaining a vital role in medicine as well for developing algorithms, which enables it to acquire information, and other datasets; and therefore, AI is primed and ready to play an extremely important role in healthcare treatment development [1–5]. Health care needs will increase by manifolds over the next 5 years.

Nowadays traditional medicine becomes the most important term in healthcare comparing western medicine because that is best treats and provides the best

A. Verma · I. Naaz (✉)
School of Education, Galgotias University, Greater Noida, Uttar Pradesh, India

S. A. Parah et al. (eds.), *Artificial Intelligence for Innovative Healthcare Informatics*,
https://doi.org/10.1007/978-3-030-96569-3_15

performance of modern medicine and also traditional medicine is more cost-effective. It is easier to obtain and it has several health benefits comparing modern medicine. (D.A.A.M. Dissanayake). The teaching model for Naturopathic medical school is similar to that of medical school in that it includes Biomedicine, Anatomy, Histology, Bacteriology, and Microbiology.

Naturopathy, on the other hand, emphasizes lifestyle-oriented self-care, preventive habits, diet, physical activity, and stress-management therapy before moving on to clinical nutrition (i.e., targeting pharmacologic activities by nutrients for specific diseases irrespective of nutrient status), herbal medicine, and homeopathy. Naturopathy emerged from nineteenth-century European "nature cure" and is based on nature to cure diseases. Naturopathy was developed in the United States and Canada in the early twentieth century, incorporating natural cure, homeopathy, spinal manipulation, and other therapies [6].

Naturopathy is a distinct form of treatment that has been recognized by the World Health Organization (WHO) and some countries are starting to follow this therapy model. In addressing the role of Naturopathy in the latest transformative trends like the introduction of Artificial Intelligence in the field of Alternative Medicine, this chapter will hopefully be a little more detailed.

There are many areas where artificial intelligence is applied Including healthcare and administrative decisions in hospitals, it is revolutionizing medical affairs, AI is being built to serve both purposes, symbolically and quantitatively (machine learning). Using symbolic data to work with computer vision and robotics is the main. An artificial neural network (ANN, which is also known as an intelligent data machine) uses neural network technology. In the healthcare industry, big data comes in several different shapes and forms, whether they are organized or semi-structured.

These types of data cannot be used on their own, but need to be integrated into algorithms so that other datasets and models can predict performance. Experts expect that the potential of artificial intelligence (AI) to affect the health care industry will be important, with areas like chronic disease treatment and clinical decision making [7].

2 Objective

To find out the prospects of AI in naturopathy.
To find out the difficulties in implementations of AI in naturopathy.

3 Methodology

An extensive review of the new literature on artificial intelligence research in the area of healthcare. A mix of databases, including artificial intelligence in healthcare, primary care naturopathy, machine learning, and deep learning, have been found in papers. A variety of search phrases, including Artificial Intelligence, implementation research, naturopathy, algorithmic bias, are the keywords used to classify documents. Often considered the reference lists of the relevant papers.

4 History of Naturopathy

For several decades, naturopathy has played a major role in Germany. Many of the theories and philosophies of naturopathy originated in Germany and Europe during the sixteenth and seventeenth centuries.

Before the 1900s, European doctors used hydrotherapy, herbal medicine, and other ancient healing practices to train the first naturopaths from all over the world. European countries now regard naturopathy as a healthcare system that has grown through the fusion of each country's traditional medicine with North American naturopathic beliefs, theories, modalities, and rituals.

However, European medical and naturing/naturopathic training and therapies are still dominant in traditional contexts. North America is regarded as the birthplace of naturopathic medicine, or naturopathic medicine, in modern times. The vast majority of schools in North America are government-accredited, and the majority of Canadian provinces, as well as all states and regions in the United States, are currently working toward oversight or licensure (with more than half of the provinces and 38% of all states and regions in the USA). They are using cutting-edge research methods and tools, such as artificial intelligence, to advance the field of naturopathy.

National and regional naturopathic associations, support groups, and prominent publications like the Journal of Natural life have numerous national and international links which provide the platform for several ongoing studies and researches to promote naturopathic medicine. North America is said to have codified naturopathic concepts and to have helped develop some of the known theories and methods that are still in use around the world.

It has been seen over some time, naturopathy has been developing together by qualified naturopaths and doctors, even in the case of North America and Europe the naturopath and mainstream doctors have come together and brought their expertise and skills for making naturopathy an effective healthcare system. In Europe and North America, educational techniques and conventional medical methods are combined as a part of their medical training.

4.1 Naturopathic Principles

There have been many disputes in the past regarding the concepts and practice of naturopathic medicine, but no single body was in charge of creating a standardized codification mechanism until 1986. That's why the American Association of Naturopathic Physicians (AANP) organized a committee that included Pamela Snider, Jared Zeff, and other naturopathic doctors.

These experts drew their conclusions after studying historical data and documents for over 3 years and interviewing over 1000 people. In 1989, the two North American National Naturopathic Associations (American Association of Naturopathic Physicians (AANP) and Canadian Association of Naturopathic Doctors (CAND) formally codified and accepted the definition of naturopathic medicine and the outline of the six naturopathic principles. These notions are based on the 2014/2015 global naturopathic workforce survey.

In most countries, the naturopathic principles that are taught include:

First, Do No Harm (*primum non nocere*)
Healing Power of Nature (*vis medicatrixnaturae*)
Treat the Cause (*tollecausam*)
Treat the Whole Person (*tolletotum*)
Doctor as Teacher (*docere*)
Disease Prevention and Health Promotion
Wellness

4.2 Modalities of Naturopathy

Many naturopathic modalities are used by people which differ from country to country. This includes some of the most common naturopathic treatments, like:

1. Clinical Nutrition
2. Botanical Medicine (Herbalism)
3. Homeopathic Medicine
4. Traditional Chinese Medicine/Acupuncture
5. Physical Medicine
6. Hydrotherapy—Water Cure
7. Prevention and Lifestyle Counselling
8. Hygiene Therapy
9. Nature Cure

4.3 Future of Naturopathy

The naturopathic medicine model is in the early stages of a systematic change in the world of medicine. There is now a range of analytical instruments that can be used to determine and understand natural medicines. For example, organizations such as the American Medical Association (AMA) that in the past have fiercely opposed naturopathic medicine have gradually come to accept lifestyle change, stress reduction, exercise, and toxin reduction as important naturopathic techniques.

The primary problem here is that patients expect a broader variety of health care services. The initial therapy for any disease has to be quick and short. Naturopathic doctors meet a void in the health care system, meeting a need and providing a bilingual health care provider with a sophisticated knowledge of both natural and allopathic medicine. Their expertise in holistic medicine empowers them to act as the leading authorities on integrative medicine, which is the health care system where healing comes from many sources (www.bharatvidya.org).

5 Correlation of AI with Naturopathy

The expert community is continuously developing ways to make precision naturopathy possible, which is why artificial intelligence (AI) and naturopathy would enable naturopaths to have more of an edge in their diagnostic capabilities and to be more effective and personalized in the treatment of patients. It can also be reviewed as Concerning clinical trials, concerning therapies, concerning diagnosis, Artificial intelligence and health systems given below:

5.1 Concerning Clinical Trials

Clinical trials are the part of research to evaluate the test and treatments along with their effects on patients' recovery. Technological advances such as Artificial Intelligence (AI) can effectively assist with the entire phase of clinical trials by analyzing data and extracting relevant patterns to discover similarities as well as correlations [8].

AI systems, in comparison to normal human systems, can collect and interpret mountains of data very quickly, and they can also conclude their study. This new technology will aid in predicting disease which is a difficult job in the best of situations for a human physician. Artificial Intelligence (AI) can assist naturopaths/doctors in determining an individual's risk of developing cancer, as well as heart attack, as opposed to a stroke [9].

5.2 Concerning Therapies

"AI is very effective in therapy management and lowering health costs," researchers confirmed. "It is expected that a patient should keep detailed records of the treatments they are taking, a record of other data points relating to their body functions, results of therapies, and adhere to guidelines on medication prescription usage and storage." researchers affirmed [10].

Traditional medicine, rather than modern medicine, is the most important idea of our modern culture because it is the most common therapy with the best outcomes than modern medicine. If you do get sick, traditional medicine is much easier to get, cheaper, and many times it's also more effective compared to modern medicine [11].

In ambulatory settings, NDs (Doctor of Naturopathy) are qualified as primary care physicians with a focus on natural medicine. Their scope of practice varies by state and territory but usually consists of the stimulation and encouragement of the natural healing processes of the body to diagnose, prevent, and treat illness.

Normal procedures used for diagnosis and prevention include physical examination, laboratory testing, and diagnostic imaging. Additional laboratory tests and evaluation techniques can be used by NDs to further determine nutritional status, metabolic function, and toxicity. Diet and clinical nutrition, behavioral modification, hydrotherapy, homeopathy, botanical medicine, and physical medicine are the treatment modalities used by NDs (Doctor of Naturopathy) and AI can contribute a revolutionary enhancement of more precise treatment modalities.

NDs may also be approved to carry out minor office procedures and surgery, administer vaccines, and prescribe certain prescription medications, depending on the state.

5.3 Concerning Diagnosis

By manipulating mass electronic health records, Artificial Intelligence has been able to greatly assist doctors in patient diagnosis (EHRs) [12]. Medical problems have become more complex, and with a vast history of building electronic medical records, the risk of replication of cases is high. While anyone with a rare condition today is less likely to be the only person with any given disease, the failure to access cases of similarly symptomatic origins is a significant roadblock for doctors [12].

Implementing AI not only helps find similar cases and treatments but also to factor in the main symptoms and to help doctors ask the most suitable questions helps the patient to receive the most precise diagnosis and treatment possible [13].

5.4 Artificial Intelligence and Health Systems

On a theoretical level, if one could reliably forecast likely primary outcomes, the utilization of hospital palliative care services may be more effective and precise. This term is used as an example of an algorithm that may use current clinical criteria to forecast the probability of a patient's impending hospital readmission, even if the conventional clinical criteria would not reflect it. This approach might be useful if steps could be done to prevent discharge and better align resources with the underlying issues [14–17].

Our diagnostic capabilities can benefit from integrating AI, which will allow us to identify those patients who need palliative care and also for them to identify those

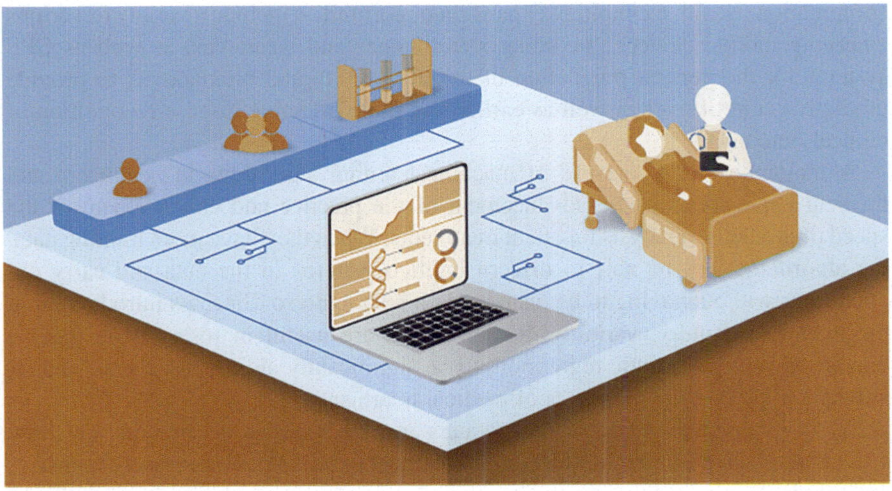

Fig. 15.1 GAO-21-7SP—Artificial intelligence in health care: benefits and challenges of technologies to augment patient care (Published: Nov 30, 2020)

who may go on to septic shock. With the help of electronic health record data, a machine-learning algorithm and a deep learning model were able to predict several important clinical parameters, including Alzheimer's disease [18–20].

In recent research, reinforcement learning was used to evaluate the effectiveness of vasopressors, intravenous fluids, and/or drugs, as well as the dosage of the preferred treatment for patients with sepsis, using two large datasets. On average, the care prescribed by the 'AI Clinician' was more successful than that recommended by humans [21].

There has been a fair amount of variability when it comes to both the size of the study cohorts and the level of AUC accuracy, as well as all of these studies being retrospective and still being evaluated in the real-world clinical setting. But as the days have gone on, several others have emerged to sell algorithms of this kind, including Care's kore, which offers electronic health records with a predicted risk of readmission and mortality calculated from EHR data. These individuals are aggressively selling these algorithms [22]. AI increases the capacity of healthcare providers to help the patients they serve, both by gathering information about their condition and enhancing their efficiency as shown in Fig. 15.1.

These rapid increases in AI in healthcare implementation of diagnosis and therapy advances have taken place with the introduction of disease identification and treatment capabilities for individual patients in mind. As a large number of cancer patients are diagnosed every year and vast quantities of medical data are produced in the course of cancer care, the use of AI is warranted.

AI refers to a machine's ability to do tasks that are commonly associated with intelligent human activity. It was first characterized in the 1950s. A subset of this description is Mandelbrot sets or folds, which are a collection of iterative, "self-learning" systems that can employ stored connections to unfold a dataset for computation. Health technology expansion opportunities include a variety of various emerging mobile devices, including smartphones and wearables, as well as GPS systems for the general population that could use "digital biomarkers" to provide predictive control over as well as earlier and more effective disease recognition of clinical outcomes.

A major benefit of the use of machine learning algorithms in healthcare and medical applications is the advancement of the practice and enhancement of the speed of predictive analysis inpatient treatments. When they have more training data, the algorithms will be able to discern implicit patterns in the data and carry out operations without having to be instructed on how to do so. Since its introduction in the twentieth century, various ML algorithms are useful in research on disease diagnosis, such as logistic regression, to be significantly aiding physicians in their attempts to predict the outcomes of medical treatments [23].

AI is required to modify how patients get medications, treatments and how specialists reach their clinical decisions. Diagnostics will be quicker, less expensive, and relatively precise than at any time ever. In any case, to lead the advent of the AI period, one must be aware of the attributes and the restrictions of this innovation as well. AI strategies require a lot of data for their training and approval, which additionally beg the inquiries of computerized trust, information sharing, and privacy concerns. With the outburst of electronic data; improvement in the technological foundation and noteworthy research in DL (deep learning) neural systems, AI is all set to impact practice in the clinical field and healthcare.

6 Prospects of AI in Healthcare with Naturopathy

Future technologies like AI are notoriously difficult to reliably forecast, but it can certainly be confirmed that they will play a role in medicine in aiding clinical research and care. The features of AI-based systems have been evaluated with the use of the methods used to this end. Thanks to synthesized and processed and combined information such as the product of which far exceeds the human capacity, such as that found in Watson, a digital device such as this has the ability to combinatoriality and resources to comb through thousands of reference articles and discover facts that no doctor possesses in the scale of depth or breadth of knowledge [9].

Although there are undoubtedly many questions about the creation of artificial intelligence, we still believe that artificial intelligence as an assistance tool for doctors and naturopaths makes very good clinical decisions and even can substitute human judgment in some areas of treatment (Fig. 15.2).

This ML/or other AI solutions could help solve some of these problems, namely better healthcare coverage, especially in rural and low-income settings, disadvantaged regions, as well as personalized training for physicians/naturopaths and nurses [24]. Additionally, they could aid in fixing the problem of having not enough qualified candidates to perform complicated medical procedures by growing the

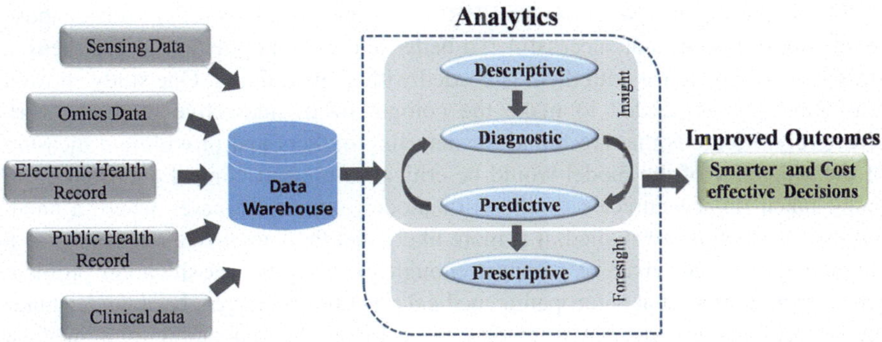

Fig. 15.2 Big data in healthcare: management, analysis, and prospects [24]

population and facilitating personalized healthcare delivery on a large scale in naturopathy treatments.

7 Adopting and Adapting the Digital World

Currently, naturopathy is being used in combination with artificial intelligence and used to promote modern living. The perceived change to the online world has already begun to destabilize the conventional naturopathy market. AI in the naturopathy sector could theoretically make a considerable profit, given the shift. A research study from Accenture says, "By the year 2035, AI is expected to add an average of 55% to healthcare industry profitability" [25].

For a long time, the beauty and wellness industry has been alongside us, starting with the history of naturopathic inheritance. Despite the rapid shift to the digital era, in which personal beauty and wellness products manufacturers utilize AI to produce highly customized products, naturopathic beauty, and wellness products manufacturers are also opting for customization. While AI has facilitated the production of customized beauty products, it has also allowed for a rapid rise in its prevalence [26].

There is a significant amount of excitement about digital health care due in part to the expectation that by digitizing health records, we will be able to better use computer information systems and better understand with enhancing medical care. That said, a vast amount of patient health data is accumulating that approaches the size of whole-genome sequencing in complexity and volume.

However, it is important to note that much of this knowledge has not yet been applied in the types of predictive statistical models that clinicians could use to improve the delivery of treatment. There is good reason to suggest that the widespread use of these practices, if effective, may have huge monetary and medical benefits beyond improving patient safety and quality and reducing healthcare costs [27].

Simply putting inexperience with EHRs (electronic health records) override those trends doesn't seem that successful. To better allow the population to use them, a strong early experience with them is needed with some training. One study showed that training was needed to make the computerized, interactive methods work effectively. Methods that are found for detecting outliers and providing a measure of the reliability of the model would be critical to prevent clinical decisions from being taken on inaccuracies (outliers) of model outputs. In cases where a small number of patients are studied, it is more likely that the knowledge resides inside a singular dataset that may be compact enough to solve the classification problem [28]. It is important that naturopathic medical practitioners have a basic understanding of artificial intelligence principles to maintain the reputation of a medical professional and can participate "in both effectively and critically" (in a way that amplifies or enhances) AI systems in naturopathy treatments [29].

8 What Is Artificial Intelligence (AI) and How It Is Useful in Healthcare?

AI is a field of study that explores and develops a technical system capable of dealing with complex tasks in a manner that is comparable to human intelligence [30]. With the interaction of engineering, computer science, and other applied sciences, progress in robotics, machine learning (ML), computer vision, and other fields of applied research is augmenting the fundamental fields of applied research.

Artificial intelligence will act on the concept of self-improvement by gaining new functionality from the digital sector, and information and communication technology will result in a major mechanical and social shift in economic frameworks [31]. The use of artificial intelligence (AI) in healthcare is to enhance disease detection and treatment, as well as the development of persuasive therapies, has exploded.

There is a lot of interest in using AI to enhance oncologic care because there are a lot of patients diagnosed with different diseases every year and a lot of data produced during treatment. AI, which was first described in the 1950s, refers to a machine's ability to perform tasks that are generally associated with intelligent human activity [32]. AI can be thought of as a collection of iterative, "self-learning" systems, similar to Mandelbrot sets, which recognize connections within data that can be unraveled and performed more efficiently [as in the addition,] where the use of artificial intelligence can also be coupled to many rising mobile health interfaces such as cell phones and wearables, the introduction of digital biomarkers can enhance, educate, and predict the effects of clinical outcomes.

A great majority of DL (or deep learning) strategies use neural architectures, explaining why DL models are often defined as deep neural networks. Although it usually refers to the majority of neural circuits, the term "deep" is used to speak about how many layers there are in the neural system. This is shown in Fig. 15.3. Deep neural systems can have up to 150 hidden layers, whereas traditional neural

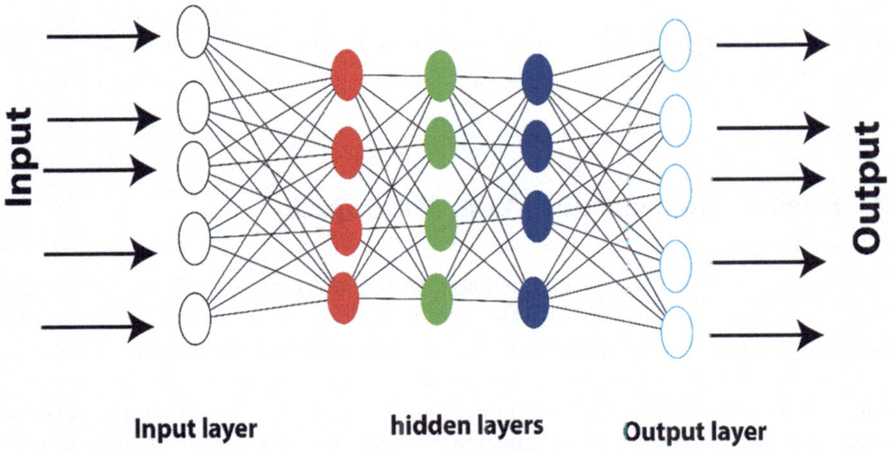

Fig. 15.3 Neural networks are organized in layers consisting of a set of interconnected nodes. Networks can have tens or hundreds of hidden layers

systems only have 2–3. Researchers are developing increasingly larger neural networks and non-manual networked learning models by employing massive amounts of labeled data and continuous data sets and training them with real data in long-based iterations [33, 34].

In the spring of 1956, computer scientist and AI pioneer John McCarthy made new use of the word, "artificial intelligence," and defined it as "the science and engineering of creating intelligent machines" [35].

Artificial intelligence (AI) is a branch of computer science that seeks to build complex machines that imitate human intelligence. This term can be summed up as "General AI," which refers to computers that can think, interpret, and even see and hear in the same way as humans can [36, 37].

In short, it is an IT industry that produces "smart" machines for functioning and responding to something other than the human brain. Examples include computer programs (e.g. web platforms) and machines (e.g., robots). These machines are capable of processing data, patterns, and models to interpret, reason, prepare, solve problems, predict, and manipulate objects. One of the key benefits is that AI spends time automating complex and time-consuming tasks.

Another concept of Artificial Intelligence is the ability of a computer or other engine to perform activities in which [human] intelligence is normally considered to be essential. Modified from [38]. The rise of AI which has access to big data will assist physicians to increase the quality of patient care by making diagnoses simpler than ever. With AI, medical imaging procedures can be improved by automating them, thus making the process quicker and more efficient at the same time.

AI is well-suited to manage repetitive work processes, handling vast volumes of data, and can provide another layer of decision support to minimize errors. Most businesses and analysts believe that this technology can boost patient outcomes by 30–40% at a cost savings of up to 50% and the company has already made loans to AI companies [38].

9 Scope of Implementing AI in Naturopathy

The problem with statistical methods for extracting meaningful predictions from the training data is the amount of uninterpretable data. If these objectives can be achieved, they can lead to profound changes in the standard of naturopathy care.

Cancer, Diabetes, Arthritis, and Asthma are some of the few chronic diseases that naturopathy can handle. With AI, the complete integration of technology enables computers and machines to work intelligently and upgrade this ancient and valuable system of medicine.

We all know that technology has enormous potential for reducing human workloads, increasing storage capacity, lowering costs, and much more. However, some people can find its use in naturopathy difficult to absorb. That's because naturopathy is seen as outdated and obsolete in comparison to AI (Artificial Intelligence), which has only been around for a few years and is seen as revolutionary and futuristic. Artificial intelligence is making a revolutionary shift in the field of naturopathy by embracing and adapting to this combination.

The purpose of the ND (naturopathy doctor) is to restore health by recognizing and mitigating these disturbances in naturopathic theory. To have a healthy body, the ND first considers what factors decide health. When a body part is affected in some way, it may become a part of the disease. His care aims to restore a stable life and he follows a strict, but adaptable, treatment regimen that starts with minimal interventions and progresses to higher-level interventions as appropriate [39]. Skin lesions and rashes, ear infections, migraine headaches, and retinal diseases like diabetic retinopathy and age-related macular degeneration are among the medical conditions for which smartphone exams with AI are being pursued.

It is heavily supported by Artificial Intelligence (AI) and the development of a public system that gives patients access to their medical data and makes this easy for the general public to follow, as well (Fig. 15.4).

Some mobile applications, such as Ai Cure (NCT02243670), use AI to monitor medical adherence by making patients take a selfie video while swallowing their prescribed pill. Some other apps use image recognition of food content, such as the food and nutrition information [40]. There are now attempts to use the same approach for matching patients with primary care physicians to engender higher levels of confidence, which could be seen as an outgrowth of dating apps that use AI nearest-neighbor analysis to find matches [41].

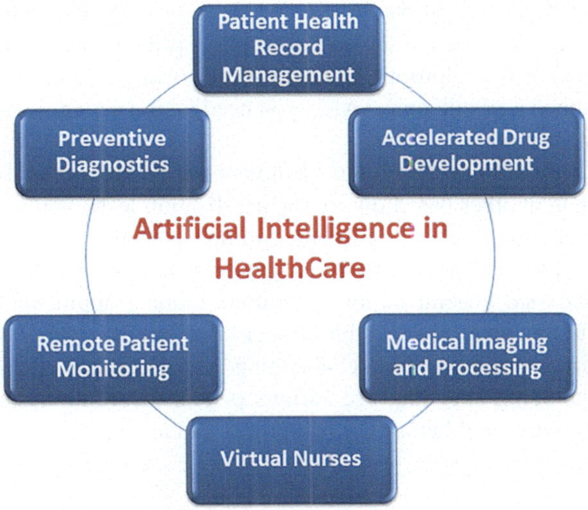

Fig. 15.4 AI in the healthcare world

10 Difficulties in Implementations of AI in Naturopathy

Although saying what lies ahead for medicine's future about AI is extremely uncertain, there is a strong reason to suggest that AI would be useful in assisting naturopaths. This evaluation is focused on certain AI-based device characteristics. Watson, for example, can browse through millions of pages of data and read countless medical papers, far beyond the depth and scope of expertise of any human physician [9].

An overworked doctor can overlook a patient's vulnerability to a drug's side effects, but an AI-based system would not. In conjunction with virtual reality programs, AI can also aid with surgery. We know that one of AI's greatest strengths is its ability to collect and analyze vast quantities of data and draw conclusions from it. This will assist in disease detection, which is a daunting job for human naturopaths in the best of circumstances.

AI will help doctors calculate the risk of cancer or compare the risk factors of heart attacks and strokes [9]. Patients could be spared from these diseases shortly, thanks to the availability of future doctors who could have a strategy for coping with them [9]. To increase the performance of medicine's future standards of excellence, all these innovations are on the verge of introduction.

The next advancement in medicine will be in discovering illnesses and protecting patients from harm through the expansion of accuracy and efficiency, and precision, and the decrease in side effects that is due to tests and diagnoses dependent on complexity. Thus, it is of significant benefit to all parties involved, including patients, their relatives, and the medical community.

AIs (artificial intelligence applications) can fail at being implemented without any preparation history, show bias and become compromised due to unexplained causes, and have the line of defects of ignorance and blindness [42].

As described above, data needs to be collected carefully because it may change over time. Also, if the data you collect is the focus of clinical practice you need to be sure it is foolproof. Also, you need to improve the precision of your algorithm's analysis of outcomes. Also, you need to find a more accurate measure of your trust in your model.

Finally, because your method could be more effective for one group of patients than another based on your generalization tests, you need to be confident that your technique is effective in other groups as well.

For most forms of medical data, the majority of AI systems are far from achieving accurate generalizability, let alone clinical applicability. In trying to predict the future, there are still blind spots that people cannot see. Analyzing data can be time-consuming and challenging because there is a range of variance in sites, including sites that use various patient recording systems, coding concepts, EHR systems, and laboratory equipment and assays.

11 Algorithmic Bias

Researchers also found evidence that the performance of computers can be substantially impacted by the geographical, socio-economic, and educational context of the consumer. This has created a pet issue for individuals who are discriminated against because of their ethnicity, gender, and socio-economic background [43].

According to the medical literature, the algorithm, it was widely believed that medical problems varied in their likelihood of success depending on ethnicity. There are three forms of algorithmic unfairness, (1) a model bias, Minorities, and vulnerable groups are underrepresented in the model collection, (2) an algorithm variance, there is a lack of adequate data about minorities, and (3) outcome noise the influence of a collection of unobserved variables that potentially interfere with the model's predictions to assess the model, a larger group of observations must be quantified [44]. As we see it, we need to properly face up the issues of prejudice in healthcare.

We think we should be more aware of these issues, and assist healthcare providers in identifying and eradicating the biases. Algorithms should be designed with the global community in mind, and clinical validation should be done on a representative sample of the projected deployment population. Population subgroups should conduct a thorough performance analysis, taking into account age, race, gender, socioeconomic status, and location. The research is especially important to understand the effects of a new algorithm, i.e., if the spectrum of illnesses observed using the AI system differs from current clinical practice, then the benefits of this different spectrum must be calculated.

12 Key Challenges in the Implementation of Artificial Intelligence in Naturopathy

Metrics also do not show clinical significance or validity: To reflect the fact that accuracy does not inherently signify clinical effectiveness, the word 'AI chasm' has been introduced [45]. The region under the curve (or RUC) is a widely used machine learning technique and is commonly used in research studies. However, it should not be assumed that RUC is appropriate for any clinical use since the applicability is individual [46]. Clinicians with many specialties find it challenging to understand. For the general public (who are not medical professionals), AI-related practices, such as creating an AI-related awareness, are useful. They will become conscious of new things by reading, listening, and watching.

For public use, medical procedures that include AI are not as complex as the implementation of AI-related technology, so the general public, who are not medical practitioners, can use these techniques without apprehension.

Challenges concerning the science of machine learning. A machine learning algorithm can be defeated and it does not have broad applicability outside of training, it is very susceptible to being fooled [42]. It would be important to consider several different variables to obtain proper treatment. This includes the many possible data adjustments, the possibility that rare confounders will be identified during research, the incorporation of bias in the clinical process, a lack of information about the drugs because of how they are being programmed, and the potential for generalization errors.

Difficult to compare various algorithms. There are some complex and difficult issues involved in comparing algorithms; each analysis is conducted using a different approach by different people using different trials of the algorithm, with different populations and different distributions of the population. Algorithms must be subject to comparison on the same independent test set that is representative of the target population, using the same output metrics, to allow fair comparisons.

In healthcare, human obstacles to AI adoption Human barriers to adoption are important, even with a highly successful algorithm that overcomes all of the above challenges. It will be important to retain a focus on clinical applicability and patient outcomes, advance methods for algorithmic interpretability, and develop a deeper understanding of human-computer interactions to ensure that this technology will reach and support patients.

Susceptibility to coercion or adversarial attack It has been shown that algorithms are vulnerable to the possibility of adversarial attacks. An adversarial attack describes an otherwise successful model, albeit somewhat theoretical at present. That is susceptible to manipulation by inputs intentionally designed to fool them. In one research, for example, by incorporating adversarial noise or even only rotation, photographs of benign moles were misdiagnosed as malignant.

Developing a deeper understanding of human-algorithm interactions: We have a very limited understanding of how algorithms in clinical practice affect humans, but our understanding is growing. Our work should be conducted in the clinical setting so that we can gain an even deeper understanding of the dynamic and evolving relationship between clinicians and human-centered AI instruments.

Dataset movement: When a new predictive algorithm is implemented, the algorithm's usage patterns which shift, which could lead to an entirely new distribution as opposed to the one used to train the algorithm. In summary, there are methods to detect drift and/or upgrade models as part of an effort to preserve current levels of efficiency. These mitigations to manage this issue involve diligent quantification of output over time so that issues can be identified before they occur and ultimately resolved before they cause substantial damage.

Data-driven testing procedures have been proposed to choose the most suitable form of software-hardware upgrades, such as a simple recalibration, to maintenance-only mode, or complete model retraining, to obtain consistent results over time [47]. Very crucial for EHR (electronic health record) algorithms, the fact that all input data are generated in a non-stationary setting with changing patient populations must be understood. Because clinical and organizational procedures change over time, EHR algorithms must be able to process and manage these constantly shifting realities [48].

Achieving good supervision and strict monitoring of quality: For successful and secure deployment of AI algorithms, a foundational prerequisite is the creation of the appropriate regulatory frameworks. Machine learning poses an important challenge considering the current speed of progress, as well as major risks and the probability of machine learning models being unreliable over time.

Proactive legislation would improve the trust of healthcare professionals and the healthcare systems. Latest U.S. activities Food and Drug Administration (FDA) guidance has started the process of creating a new regulatory system to help ensure that successful and healthy artificial intelligence devices can effectively advance to patients (Food and Drug Administration 2019).

13 Conclusion

Throughout this chapter, we study the current literature to find out what skills and expertise traditional medicine practitioners would have in an age of increasing AIs precision and personalized medicine become more common, the avalanche of medical data in the form of clinical, genomic, and imaging data can only grow. Consequently, to be anticipated, with this nexus between naturopathy and AI more prominent, more of an overall picture of patient well-being would be determined by the application of knowledge derived from science. More and more medical schools are recognizing the fact that new technologies are important in the education they provide. Medical schools are adding technology, data analysis, and data processing classes to their curriculum as well as a result of industry demand for both in the area and growth in the sector, as well as the need for these specializations [49]. New models of nutrition analysis and administration will help naturopathic treatment in the years to come by keeping track of the detailed data generated by patients and healthcare facilities and by both gatherings and by discovering ways to exploit it. AI would most certainly help and augment naturopaths by removing the mundane aspects of their practice, allowing them to spend more time with their patients, and strengthening the human touch. Although AI is unlikely to completely replace physicians shortly, medical practitioners must learn both the basics of AI technology and how AI-based technologies will assist them in delivering better care at work [50].

More research is required in this area to (1) identify algorithmic bias and unfairness themes and develop mitigations to address them, (2) reduce brittleness and improve generalizability, and (3) develop methods for improving the interpretability of machine learning predictions. If these goals are met, the benefits to patients will almost certainly be transformative.

Acknowledgments The authors are grateful to Dr. Md. Zubbair Malik, Young Scientist at the Department of Health & Research, MoHFW, School of Computational and Integrative Sciences, Jawaharlal Nehru University, and School of Education, Galgotias University for their valuable suggestions and timely support and providing the research infrastructure.

References

1. Gull S, Mansour RF, Aljehane NO, Parah SA (2021) A self-embedding technique for tamper detection and localization of medical images for smart-health. Multimed Tools Appl 80(19): 29939–29964
2. Kaw JA, Loan NA, Parah SA, Muhammad K, Sheikh JA, Bhat GM (2019) A reversible and secure patient information hiding system for IoT driven e-health. Int J Inf Manag 45:262–275
3. Gull S, Parah SA, Khan M (2020) Reversible data hiding exploiting Huffman encoding with dual images for IoMT based healthcare. Comput Commun 163:134–149
4. Loan NA, Parah SA, Sheikh JA, Akhoon JA, Bhat GM (2017) Hiding electronic patient record (EPR) in medical images: a high capacity and computationally efficient technique for e-healthcare applications. J Biomed Inform 73:125–136. https://doi.org/10.1016/j.jbi.2017.08.002
5. Gull S, Loan NA, Parah SA, Sheikh JA, Bhat GM (2020) An efficient watermarking technique for tamper detection and localization of medical images. J Ambient Intell Humaniz Comput 11(5):1799–1808
6. Fleming SA, Gutknecht NC (2010) Naturopathy and the primary care practice. Prim Care 37(1): 119–136. https://doi.org/10.1016/j.pop.2009.09.002
7. Bresnick J (2018) Machine learning, imaging analytics predict kidney function. https://healthitanalytics.com/news/machine-learning-imaging-analytics-predict-kidney-function
8. Singh KU, Abu-Hamatta HS, Kumar A, Singhal A, Rashid M, Bashir AK (2021) Secure watermarking scheme for color DICOM images in telemedicine applications. Comput Mater Continua 70(2):2525–2542
9. Sappin E (2018) 4 ways AI could help shape the future of medicine. https://venturebeat.com/2018/02/20/4-ways-ai-could-help-shape-the-future-of-medicine/

10. Kent J (2019) Artificial intelligence could increase clinical trial success rates. Trends Pharmacol Sci. HealthITAnalytics.com
11. Dissanayake A, Gunathilaka G, Dias M, Jayasinghe G, Kasthurirathna D (2018) "Niwarana"-an artificial intelligence-based system for traditional medicine. https://doi.org/10.13140/RG.2.2.19949.23522
12. Liang H, Tsui BY, Ni H, Valentim CC, Baxter SL, Liu G, Cai W, Kermany DS, Sun X, Chen J, He L, Zhu J, Tian P, Shao H, Zheng L, Hou R, Hewett S, Li G, Liang P, et al. (2019). Evaluation and accurate diagnoses of pediatric diseases using artificial intelligence. Nat Med 25(3): 433–438. https://doi.org/10.1038/s41591-018-0335-9
13. Hussan M, Parah SA, Gull S et al (2021) Tamper detection and self-recovery of medical imagery for smart health. Arab J Sci Eng 46:3465–3481
14. Mansour RF, Parah SA (2021) Reversible data hiding for electronic patient information security for telemedicine applications. Arab J Sci Eng 46:9129–9144
15. Sarosh P, Parah SA, Bhat GM, Muhammad K (2021) A security management framework for big data in smart healthcare. Big Data Res 25:100225
16. Hussan M, Parah SA, Gull S, Qureshi GJ (2021) Tamper detection and self-recovery of medical imagery for smart health. Arab J Sci Eng 46(4):3465–3481
17. Showkat S, Parah SA, Gull S (2021) Embedding in medical images with contrast enhancement and tamper detection capability. Multimed Tools Appl 80:2009–2030
18. Walsh CG, Ribeiro JD, Franklin JC (2017) Predicting risk of suicide attempts over time through machine learning. Clin Psychol Sci 5(3):457–469. https://doi.org/10.1177/2167702617691560
19. Yang Z, Huang Y, Jiang Y, Sun Y, Zhang Y, Luo P (2018) Undefined. Sci Rep 8(1). https://doi.org/10.1038/s41598-018-24389-w
20. Bhagwat N, Viviano JD, Voineskos AN, Chakravarty MM (2018) Modeling and prediction of clinical symptom trajectories in Alzheimer's disease using longitudinal data. PLoS Comput Biol 14(9):e1006376. https://doi.org/10.1371/journal.pcbi.1006376
21. Komorowski M, Celi LA, Badawi O, Gordon AC, Faisal AA (2018) The artificial intelligence clinician learns optimal treatment strategies for sepsis in intensive care. Nat Med 24(11): 1716–1720. https://doi.org/10.1038/s41591-018-0213-5
22. Zaidi D (2017) AI is transforming medical diagnosis, prosthetics, and vision aids. https://venturebeat.com/2017/10/30/ai-is-transforming-medical-diagnosis-prosthetics-and-vision-aids/
23. Kourou K, Exarchos TP, Exarchos KP, Karamouzis MV, Fotiadis DI (2015) Machine learning applications in cancer prognosis and prediction. Comput Struct Biotechnol J 13:8–17. https://doi.org/10.1016/j.csbj.2014.11.005
24. Rashid M, Yousuf MM, Ram B, Goyal V (2019) Novel big data approach for drug prediction in health care systems. In: 2019 International conference on automation, computational and technology management (ICACTM). IEEE, New York, pp 325–329
25. Purdy M, Daugherty P (2017) How AI industry profits and innovation. Accenture. https://www.accenture.com/fr-fr/_acnmedia/36dc7f76eab444cab6a7f44017cc3997.pdf
26. Kamili A, Hurrah NN, Parah SA, Bhat GM, Muhammad K (2020) DWFCAT: dual watermarking framework for industrial image authentication and tamper localization. IEEE Trans Ind Informatics 17(7):5108–5117
27. Rajkomar A, Oren E, Chen K, Dai AM, Hajaj N, Hardt M, Liu PJ, Liu X, Marcus J, Sun M, Sundberg P, Yee H, Zhang K, Zhang Y, Flores G, Duggan GE, Irvine J, Le Q, Litsch K, Dean J (2018) Scalable and accurate deep learning with electronic health records. NPJ Dig Med 1(1). https://doi.org/10.1038/s41746-018-0029-1
28. Chilamkurthy S, Ghosh R, Tanamala S, Biviji M, Campeau NG, Venugopal VK, Mahajan V, Rao P, Warier P (2018) Deep learning algorithms for detection of critical findings in head CT scans: a retrospective study. Lancet 392(10162):2388–2396. https://doi.org/10.1016/s0140-6736(18)31645-3
29. Organization for Economic Co-operation and Development (OECD) (2018) Education and AI: preparing for the future & AI, attitudes and values. EDU/EDPC(2018)45/ANN2. https://doi.org/10.7717/peerj.7702

30. Iafrate F (2018) Artificial intelligence and big data. ISTE Ltd and John Wiley & Sons, New York. https://doi.org/10.1002/9781119426653
31. Geuna A, Guerzoni M, Nuccio M, Pammolli F, Rungi A (2017) Digital disruption and the transformation of Italian manufacturing. People + AI Research. https://pair.withgoogle.com/
32. Russell S, Norvig P (2016) Artificial intelligence: a modern approach, 3rd edn. Createspace Independent Publishing Platform, Scotts Valley, CA
33. Rathour N, Alshamrani SS, Singh R, Gehlot A, Rashid M, Akram SV, AlGhamdi AS (2021) IoMT based facial emotion recognition system using deep convolution neural networks. Electronics 10(11):1289
34. Mondal S, Agarwal K, Rashid M (2019) Deep learning approach for automatic classification of x-ray images using convolutional neural network. In: 2019 Fifth International conference on image information processing (ICIIP). IEEE, New York, pp 326–331
35. The Society for the Study of Artificial Intelligence and Simulation of Behaviour–AISB (2018) What is AI? https://aisb.org.uk/new_site/?p=73. Accessed 4 Dec 2019
36. Copeland M (2016) What's the difference between artificial intelligence, machine learning, and deep learning? The Official NVIDIA Blog. https://blogs.nvidia.com/blog/2016/07/29/
37. Jha N, Prashar D, Rashid M, Shafiq M, Khan R, Pruncu CI, Kumar SM (2021) Deep learning approach for discovery of in silico drugs for combating COVID-19. J Healthc Eng 2021: 6668985
38. Hsieh P (2017) AI in medicine: the rise of the machines. https://www.forbes.com/sites/paulhsieh/2017/04/30/ai-in-medicine-rise-of-the-machines
39. Washington Association of Naturopathic Physicians (2009) http://www.wanp.org/mc/page.do?sitePageId=58070&orgId=wanp
40. Levine B, Brown A (2018) On duo delivers diabetes clinic and coaching to your smartphone. Diatribe. https://diatribe.org/onduo-delivers-diabetes-clinic-and-coaching-your-smartphone
41. Han Q, Ji M, de Rituerto M, de Troya I, Gaur M, Zejnilovic L (2018) A hybrid recommender system for patient-doctor matchmaking in primary care. In: 2018 IEEE 5th international conference on data science and advanced analytics (DSAA). https://doi.org/10.1109/dsaa.2018.00062
42. Marcus G (2019) Deep learning: a critical appraisal. https://arxiv.org/abs/1801.00631
43. Barocas S, Selbst AD (2016) Big data's disparate impact. SSRN Electron J. https://doi.org/10.2139/ssrn.2477899
44. Chen IY, Johansson FD, Sontag D (2018) Why is my classifier discriminatory? [Paper presentation]. Conference on neural information processing systems (NeurIPS)
45. Keane PA, Topol EJ (2018) With an eye to AI and autonomous diagnosis. NPJ Dig Med 1(1). https://doi.org/10.1038/s41746-018-0048-y
46. Saito T, Rehmsmeier M (2015) The precision-recall plot is more informative than the ROC plot when evaluating binary classifiers on imbalanced datasets. PLoS One 10(3):e0118432. https://doi.org/10.1371/journal.pone.0118432
47. Davis SE, Greevy RA, Fonnesbeck C, Lasko TA, Walsh CG, Matheny ME (2019) A nonparametric updating method to correct clinical prediction model drift. J Am Med Inform Assoc 26(12):1448–1457. https://doi.org/10.1093/jamia/ocz127
48. Nestor B, McDermott M, Chauhan G, Naumann T, Hughes MC, Goldenberg A (2018) Rethinking clinical prediction: why machine learning must consider the year of care and feature aggregation [Paper presentation]. In: Machine learning for health (ML4H) NeurIPS. https://arxiv.org/abs/1811.12583
49. Dyche J (2018) The promise of artificial intelligence in diagnosing illness
50. Ahuja AS (2019) The impact of artificial intelligence in medicine on the future role of the physician. PeerJ 7:e7702. https://doi.org/10.7717/peerj.7702

The manufacturer's authorised representative in the EU is Springer Nature Customer Service Centre GmbH, Europaplatz 3, 69115 Heidelberg, Germany. If you have any concerns regarding our products, please contact ProductSafety@springernature.com

Printed and bound by CPI Group (UK) Ltd, Croydon, CR0 4YY
22/09/2026
02221055-0014